# Delmar's
# Fundamentals of Anatomy & Physiology

## Volume 1

## Donald C. Rizzo, PH.D.

Biology Department Head
Professor of Biology
Marygrove College
Detroit, Michigan

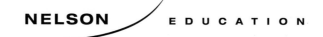

NELSON EDUCATION

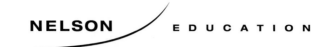

ISBN-13: 978-0-17-649161-1
ISBN-10: 0-17-649161-9

Consists of:

*Delmar's Fundamentals of
Anatomy and Physiology*
Donald C. Rizzo
ISBN-10: 0-7668-0498-4, © 2001

# Contents

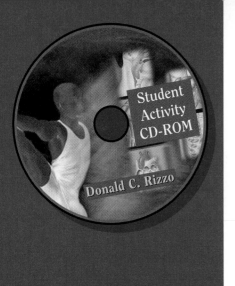

# How to Use The Student Activity CD-ROM

The Student Activity CD-ROM was designed as an exciting enhancement to *Delmar's Fundamentals of Anatomy and Physiology* to help you learn about the structure and function of the body. As you study each chapter in the text, be sure to explore the corresponding unit on the CD-ROM.

Each chapter is divided into two major sections: exercises and activities. Exercises can be used for additional practice, review, or self-testing. Activities provide an opportunity to play and practice.

Getting started is easy. Follow the simple directions on the CD label to install the program on your computer. Then take advantage of the following features:

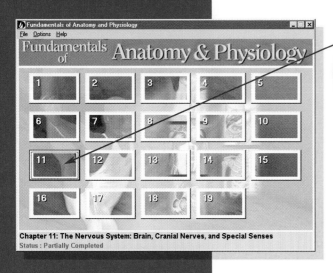

## Main Menu

**1** The main menu follows the chapter organization of the text exactly—which makes it easy for you to find your way around. Just click on the button for the chapter you want, and you'll come to the chapter opening screen.

## Toolbar

The Back button at the top left of every screen allows you to retrace your steps, while the Exit button gets you out of the program quickly and easily. As you navigate through the software, check the toolbar for other features that help you use individual exercises or games.

## On-Line Help

If you get stuck, just press F1 to get help. The on-line help includes instructions for all parts of the Student Activity CD-ROM.

## The Chapter Screen

Here you have the opportunity to choose how you want to learn. Select one of the exercises for additional practice, review, or self-testing. Or click on an activity to practice the terms for that chapter in a fun format.

**2**

# Exercises

**3** The Student Activity CD-ROM acts as your own private tutor. For each exercise, it chooses from a bank of over 900 questions covering all 19 chapters. Putting these exercises to work for you is simple:

- Choose a multiple choice, fill-in-the-blank, or matching exercise, whichever one appeals to you.

- You'll encounter a series of 10 questions for each exercise format; each question gives you two chances to answer correctly.

- Instant feedback tells you whether you're right or wrong—and helps you learn more quickly by explaining why an answer was correct or incorrect.

- The Student Activity CD-ROM displays the percentage of correct answers on the chapter screen. An on-screen score sheet (which you can print) lets you track correct and incorrect answers.

- Review your previous questions and answers in an exercise for more in-depth understanding. Or start an exercise over with a new, random set of questions that gives you a realistic study environment.

- When you're ready for an additional challenge, try the timed Speed Test. Once you've finished, it displays your score and the time you took to complete the test, so you can see how much you've learned.

# Activities

**4**

To have fun while reinforcing your knowledge, enjoy each of the five simple activities on this disk. You can play alone, with a partner, or on teams.

- **Concentration:** Match terms to their corresponding definitions under the cards as the seconds tick by.

- **Hangman:** Review your spelling and vocabulary by choosing the correct letters to spell anatomy and physiology terms before you're "hanged."

- **Tic-Tac-Toe:** You or your team must correctly answer a anatomy or physiology question before placing an X or an O.

- **Anatomy and Physiology Championship Game:** Challenge your classmates and increase your knowledge by playing this Jeopardy style question-and-answer game.

- **Drag & Drop:** Art labeling exercises are included to help you learn in an interactive environment.

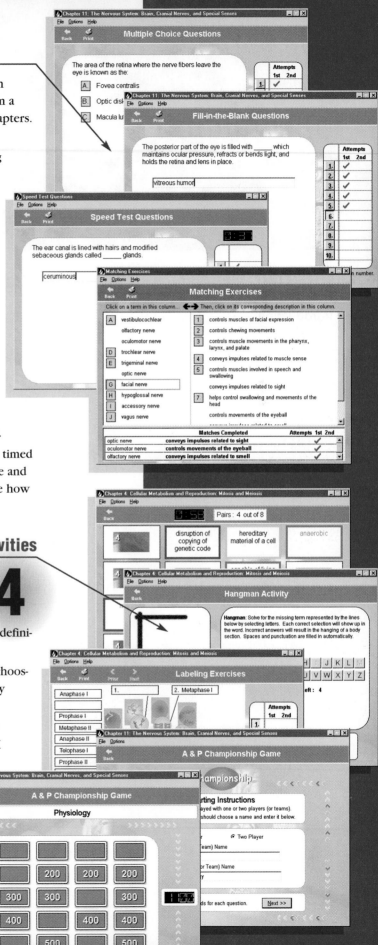

# 1

# The Human Body

## CHAPTER OBJECTIVES

After studying this chapter, you should be able to:

1. Define the anatomic terms used to refer to the body in terms of directions and geometric planes.

2. Describe the major cavities of the body and the organs they contain.

3. Explain what a cell is.

4. Describe the major functions of the four types of human tissue.

5. List the major systems of the body, the organs they contain, and the functions of those systems.

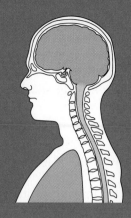

# KEY TERMS

# INTRODUCTION

Interest in the human body and how it functioned probably developed when our ancestors began to think about the reasons people became ill and died. All earlier cultures had someone designated as a healer who was responsible for finding plants and herbs that cured body disorders. This healer also was responsible for praying/or invoking the assistance of past ancestors to help in the healing process.

As cultures developed and science began to evolve, interest in and knowledge about the human body advanced. Leonardo da Vinci, an Italian (1452–1519) was the first to correctly illustrate the human skeleton with all of its bones. Andreas Vesalius, Flemish (1514–1564), wrote a book on the human body, and the English anatomist William Harvey (1578–1657) discovered how blood circulates through the body. These were just a few of the many contributors who added to our understanding of the human body and how it functions.

**Anatomy** is the study of the structure or morphology of the body and how the body parts are organized. **Physiology** is the study of the functions of body parts, what they do, and how they do it. These two areas of the organization of the body are so closely associated that it is difficult to separate them. For example, our mouth has teeth to break down food mechanically, a tongue that tastes the food and manipulates it, and salivary glands that produce saliva containing enzymes that break down complex carbohydrates into simple sugars, thus beginning the process of digestion. **Pathology** is the study of the diseases of the body.

We still do not know everything about how the human body functions. Research is still going on today to discover the mysteries of this complex unit we call ourselves.

To facilitate uniformity of terms, scientists have adopted four basic reference systems of bodily organization. These systems are directions, planes, cavities, and structural units. When referring to terms of direction, planes, and cavities, the human body is erect and facing forward. The arms are at the sides and the palms of the hand and feet are positioned toward the front (Figure 1-1). All descriptions of location or position assume the body to be in this posture.

# TERMS OF DIRECTION

When an anatomist (one who studies the human body's structures) is describing parts of the body, it is necessary to make reference to their positions in regard to the body as a whole. The following directional terms have been established to facilitate these references. Use Figure 1-2 as your guide as these terms are defined.

**Superior** means uppermost or above. Example: the head is superior to the neck, the thoracic cavity is superior to the abdominal cavity. **Inferior** means lowermost or below. Example: the foot is inferior to the ankle, the ankle is inferior to the knee. **Anterior** means toward the front. Example: the mammary glands are on the anterior chest wall. The term **ventral** can also be used for anterior. Ventral means the belly side. **Posterior** means toward the back. Example: the vertebral column is posterior to the digestive tract, the esophagus is posterior to the trachea. The term **dorsal** can also be used for posterior. Dorsal means the back side.

**Cephalad** (**SEF**-ah-lad) or **cranial** means toward the head. It is synonymous with superior. Example: the thoracic cavity lies cephalad (or superior) to the abdominopelvic cavity. Occasionally **caudal** (**KAWD**-al) is synonymous with inferior. However, caudal specifically means toward the tail and, as we know, humans do not have tails.

**Medial** means nearest the midline of the body. Example: the nose is in a medial position on the face, the ulna is on the medial side of the forearm. **Lateral** means toward the side or away from the midline of the body. Example: the ears are in a lateral position on the face, the radius is lateral to the ulna. **Proximal** means nearest the point of attachment or origin. Example: the elbow is proximal to the wrist, the knee is proximal to the ankle. **Distal** means away from the point of attachment or origin. Example: the wrist is distal to the elbow. The ankle is distal to the knee.

# PLANES

Occasionally it is useful to describe the body as having imaginary flat geometric surfaces passing through it called planes (Figure 1-1). These terms are most useful when describing dissections to

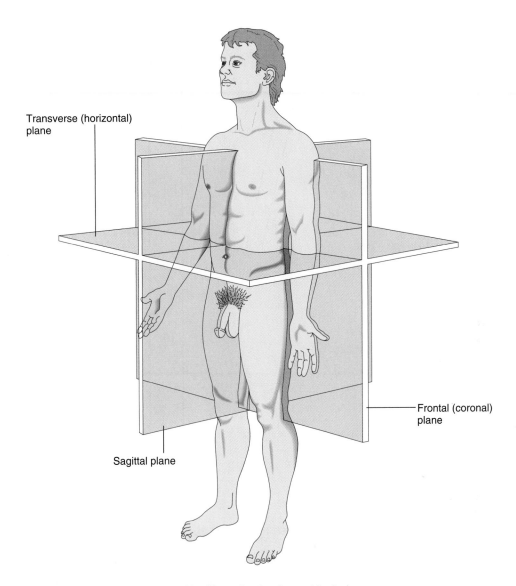

Transverse (horizontal)
plane

Frontal (coronal)
plane

Sagittal plane

**FIGURE 1-1.** The human body in correct anatomic position illustrating the planes of the body.

look inside an organ or the body as a whole. A **midsagittal** (mid-**SAJ**-ih-tal) plane vertically divides the body through the midline into two equal left and right portions or halves. This is also referred to as a median plane. A **sagittal** plane is any plane parallel to the midsagittal or median plane vertically dividing the body into unequal right and left portions.

A **horizontal** or **transverse** plane is any plane dividing the body into superior and inferior portions. A **frontal** or **coronal** plane is one that divides the anterior (or ventral) and posterior (or dorsal) portions of the body at right angles to the sagittal plane. When organs are sectioned to reveal

internal structures, two other terms are often used. A cut through the long axis of an organ is called a longitudinal section, and a cut at right angles to the long axis is referred to as a transverse or cross section.

## CAVITIES

The body has two major cavities, the dorsal cavity and the ventral cavity (Figure 1-3). Each of these is further subdivided into lesser cavities. The organs of any cavity are referred to as the **viscera** (**VISS**-er-ah).

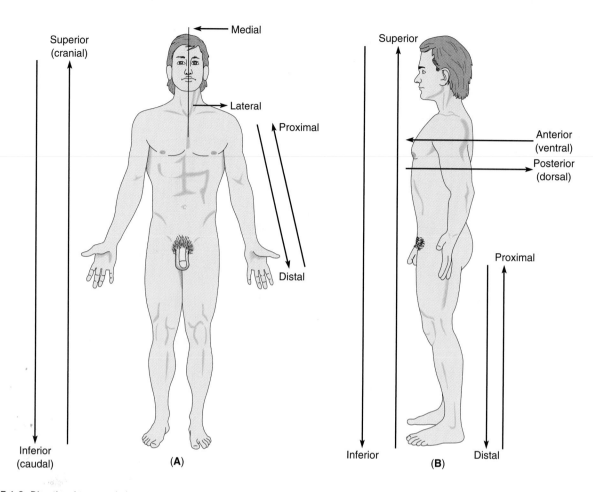

**FIGURE 1-2.** Directional terms relating to anatomic position.

The dorsal cavity contains organs of the nervous system that coordinate the body's functions. It is divided into the **cranial cavity**, which contains the brain, and the **spinal cavity**, which contains the spinal cord.

The ventral cavity contains organs that are involved in maintaining homeostasis or a constant internal environment within small ranges of deviation (Figure 1-4). The first subdivision of the ventral cavity is the **thoracic** (tho-**RASS**-ik) **cavity**. It is surrounded by the rib cage. The thoracic cavity contains the heart in a pericardial sac referred to as the **pericardial cavity**, and the two lungs each covered by the pleural membrane referred to as the **pleural cavities**. A space called the **mediastinum** (**mee**-dee-ass-**TYE**-NUM) is found between the two pleural cavities. It contains the heart, thymus gland, lymph and blood vessels, trachea, esophagus, and nerves. The diaphragm muscle separates the thoracic cavity from the abdominopelvic cavity.

The **abdominopelvic cavity** is the second subdivision of the ventral cavity. It contains the kidneys, stomach, liver and gallbladder, small and large intestines, spleen, pancreas, and the ovaries and uterus in women.

Two other terms are used when discussing the cavities of the body. The term **parietal** (pah-**RYE**-eh-tal) refers to the walls of a cavity. Example: the parietal peritoneum lines the abdominal wall. The term **visceral** refers to the covering on an organ. Example: the visceral peritoneum covers abdominal organs.

## STRUCTURAL UNITS

All living material is composed of cells, the smallest units of life. Cells are organized into tissues. Tissues are organized into organs, and organs are part of the major systems of the body (Figure 1-5). The cell is the basic unit of biologic organization. The liquid

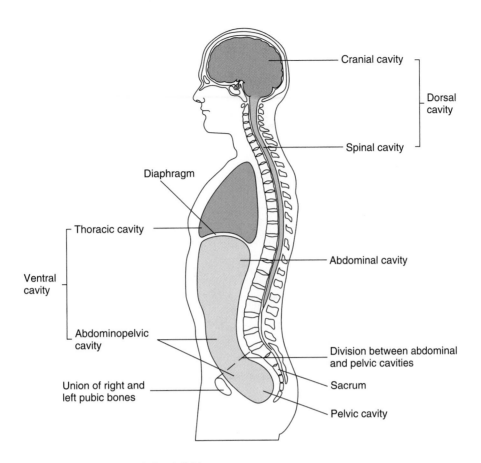

**FIGURE 1-3.** The major cavities of the body and their subdivisions.

part of a cell is called **protoplasm** (**PRO**-toh-plazm). This protoplasm is surrounded by a limiting membrane, the cell membrane also called the plasma membrane, which selectively determines what may enter or exit the cell. This protoplasm is an aqueous (watery), colloidal (grouping of large molecules) solution of various proteins, lipids, carbohydrates, and inorganic salts that are organized into cellular structures referred to as organelles. These organelles, such as the mitochondria, ribosomes, lysosomes, among others will be discussed in further detail in Chapter 3.

A cell performs all the activities necessary to maintain life including metabolism, assimilation, digestion, excretion, and reproduction. Different kinds of cells make up a tissue (muscle or bone). Different types of tissues make up an organ (stomach or heart). Finally organs are grouped into organ systems (digestive system or nervous system). Each system of the body serves some general function to maintain the body as a whole. All of the diverse tissues of the body can be placed into one of four cat-

egories: **epithelial (ep**-ih-**THEE**-lee-al), **connective**, **muscle**, or **nervous**. We will study these tissues in greater detail in Chapter 5.

Epithelial tissue covers surfaces and protects (both the outer surface like the skin and inner surfaces of organs like the intestine), forms glands, and lines cavities of the body. It is made up of one or more layers of cells with very little, if any, intercellular material. Connective tissue binds together and supports other tissues and organs. In many instances it is highly specialized (blood, bone, lymphatic tissue). It is made up of different kinds of cells that produce various fibers (elastin and collagen) embedded in a matrix (substance) of nonliving intercellular material. Muscle tissue is characterized by elongated cells (so long in fact they are often referred to as muscle fibers) that generate movement by shortening or contracting in a forcible manner. There are three types of muscle tissue. Skeletal or voluntary muscle pulls on bones and causes body movements. Smooth or involuntary muscle is found in the intestines where it pushes food along the

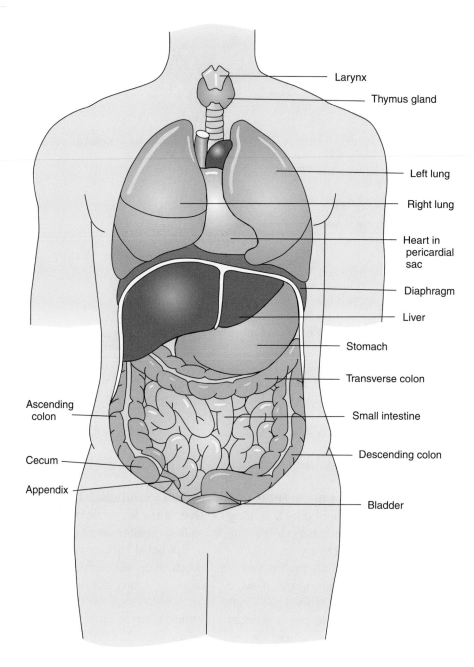

**FIGURE 1-4.** The thoracic and abdominopelvic cavities of the body and some of the organs they contain.

digestive tract. It is also found in arteries and veins where it pushes blood forward. Cardiac muscle is found only in the heart. It is also involuntary and causes contractions of the heart; these contractions pump the blood through thousands of miles of blood vessels. Finally nervous tissue is composed of nerve cells forming a coordinating system of fibers connecting the numerous sensory (touch, sight) and motor (muscular) structures of the body.

Organs are composed of cells integrated into tissues serving a common function (skin, liver, stomach, heart, lungs). A system is a group of organs. The **integumentary system** is made up of two layers: the epidermis and the dermis. It includes the skin, hair, nails, sebaceous glands, and sweat glands (Figure 1-6). Its functions include insulation of the body, protection from environmental hazards such as the ultraviolet radiation of the sun and certain

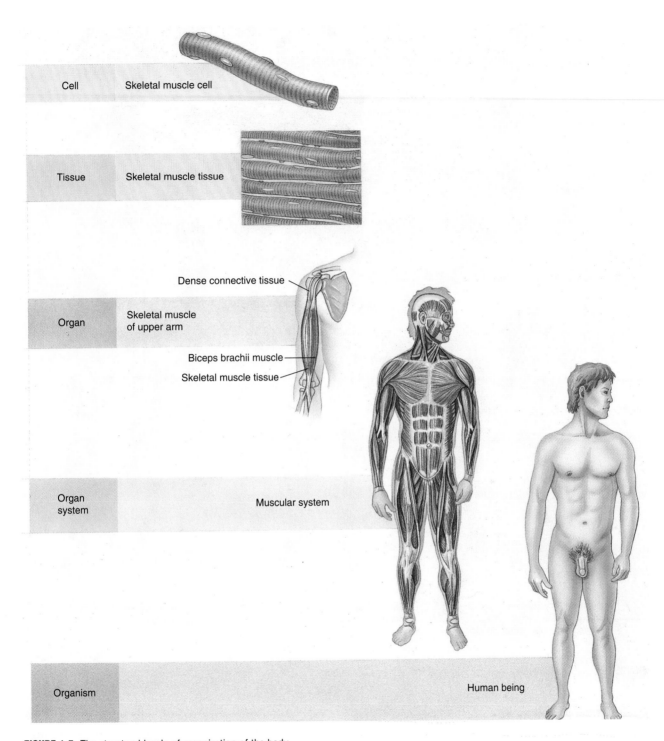

**FIGURE 1-5.** The structural levels of organization of the body.

chemicals; and temperature and water regulation. It also has receptor sites to detect changes in temperature and pressure.

The **skeletal system** is composed of bones, cartilage, and the membranous structures associated with bones (Figure 1-6). It protects the soft and vital parts of the body and provides support for body tissues. Its bones act as levers for movement. This system also manufactures blood cells in red bone marrow and stores fat in yellow bone marrow.

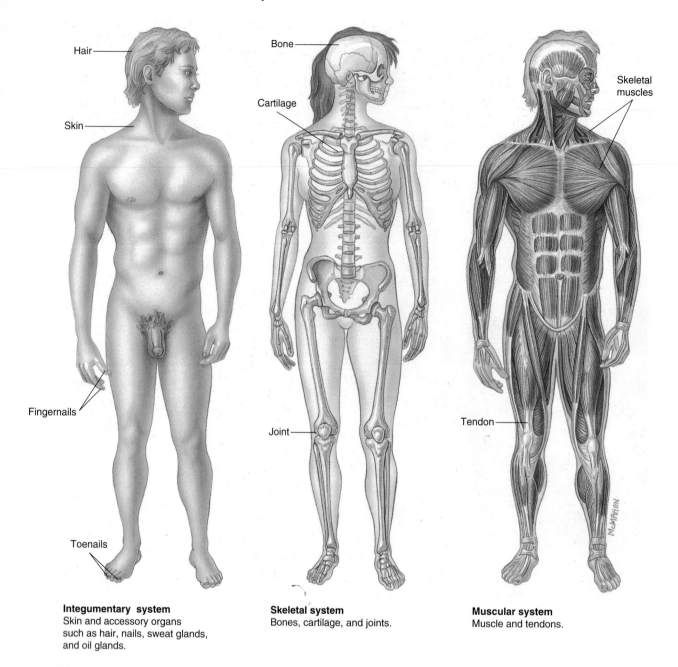

**Integumentary system**
Skin and accessory organs
such as hair, nails, sweat glands,
and oil glands.

**Skeletal system**
Bones, cartilage, and joints.

**Muscular system**
Muscle and tendons.

**FIGURE 1-6.** The integumentary, skeletal, and muscular systems of the body.

The **muscular system** consists of muscles, fasciae (fibrous connective tissues), tendon sheaths, and bursae (fibrous sacs) (see Figure 1-6). Skeletal muscles pull on bones to allow movement; smooth muscle pushes food through the digestive tract and blood through the circulatory system; and cardiac muscle causes contraction of the heart.

The **nervous system** consists of the brain, the spinal cord, the cranial nerves, the peripheral nerves, and the sensory and motor structures of the body (Figure 1-7). Its functions include controlling, correlating, and regulating the other systems of the body; interpreting stimuli from the outside world; and controlling the special senses of sight, hearing, taste, and smell.

The **endocrine system** consists of the endocrine (ductless) glands (Figure 1-7). The master gland or pituitary controls the other glands—thyroid, renal

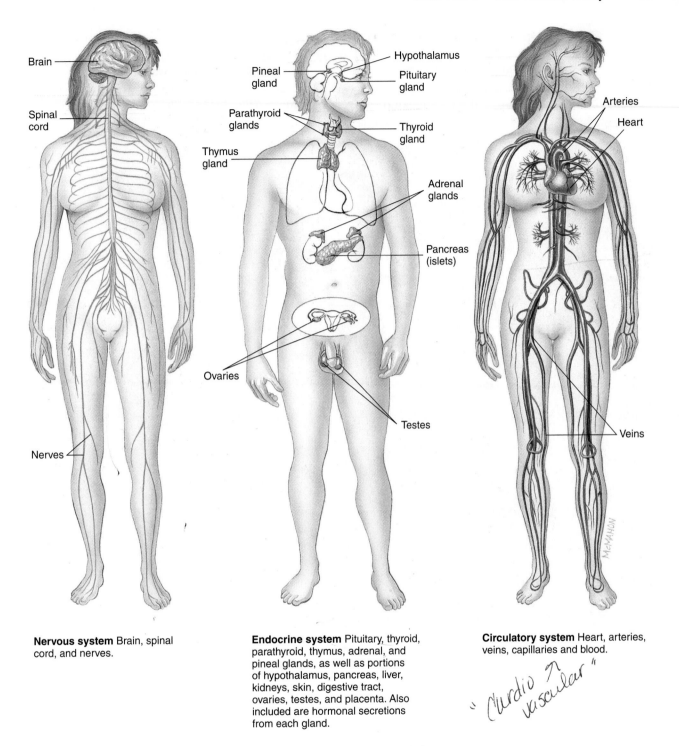

**Nervous system** Brain, spinal cord, and nerves.

**Endocrine system** Pituitary, thyroid, parathyroid, thymus, adrenal, and pineal glands, as well as portions of hypothalamus, pancreas, liver, kidneys, skin, digestive tract, ovaries, testes, and placenta. Also included are hormonal secretions from each gland.

**Circulatory system** Heart, arteries, veins, capillaries and blood.

**FIGURE 1-7.** The nervous, endocrine, and cardiovascular or circulatory systems of the body.

glands, ovaries, and testes. These glands produce hormones that chemically regulate the body's functions. This system works with the nervous system through the hypothalamus of the brain, which controls the pituitary gland.

The **cardiovascular** or blood circulatory system consists of the heart, arteries, veins, and capillaries (Figure 1-7). Its function is to pump and distribute the blood that carries oxygen, nutrients, and wastes to and from the cells of the body.

The **lymphatic system** or immune system is made up of the lymph nodes, the thymus gland, the spleen, and the lymphatic vessels (Figure 1-8). Its function is to drain tissue spaces of excess interstitial fluids and to absorb fats from the intestine and carry them to the blood. It also protects the body from disease by developing immunities and destroying most invading disease-causing microorganisms.

The **respiratory system** is composed of the nasal cavities, pharynx, larynx, trachea, bronchi, and lungs (Figure 1-8). It brings oxygen to and eliminates carbon dioxide from the blood.

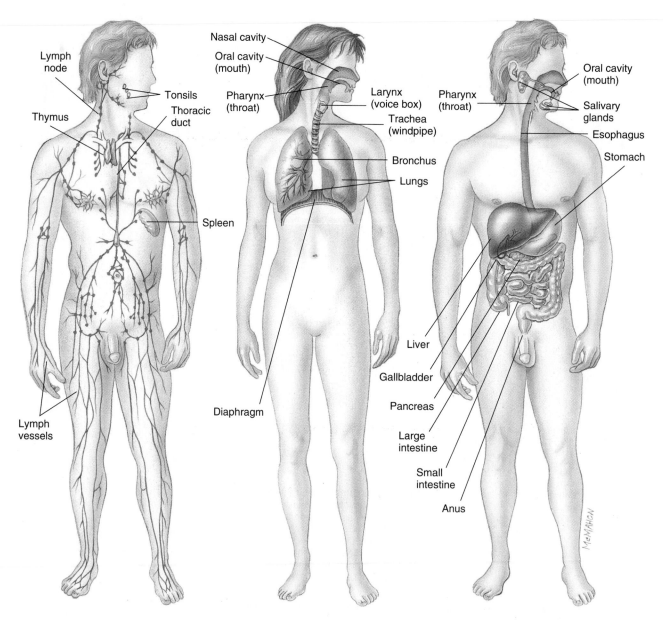

**Lymphatic and immune systems**
Thymus, bone marrow, spleen, tonsils, lymph nodes, lymph capillaries, lymph vessels, lymphocytes, and lymph.

**Respiratory system** Lungs, nasal cavity, pharynx, larynx, trachea, bronchi, and bronchioles.

**Digestive system** Mouth, pharynx, esophagus, stomach, small intestine, large intestine, salivary glands, pancreas, gallbladder, and liver.

**FIGURE 1-8.** The lymphatic or immune, respiratory, and digestive systems of the body.

The **digestive system** includes the alimentary canal (mouth, esophagus, stomach, small and large intestine, rectum, and anus) with its associated glands (salivary, liver, and pancreas) (Figure 1-8). Its function is to convert food into simpler substances that can be absorbed along with other nutrients by the cells of the body and to eliminate indigestible wastes.

The **urinary system** is made up of two kidneys, two ureters, the bladder, and the urethra (Figure 1-9). Its functions include the chemical regulation of the blood, the formation and

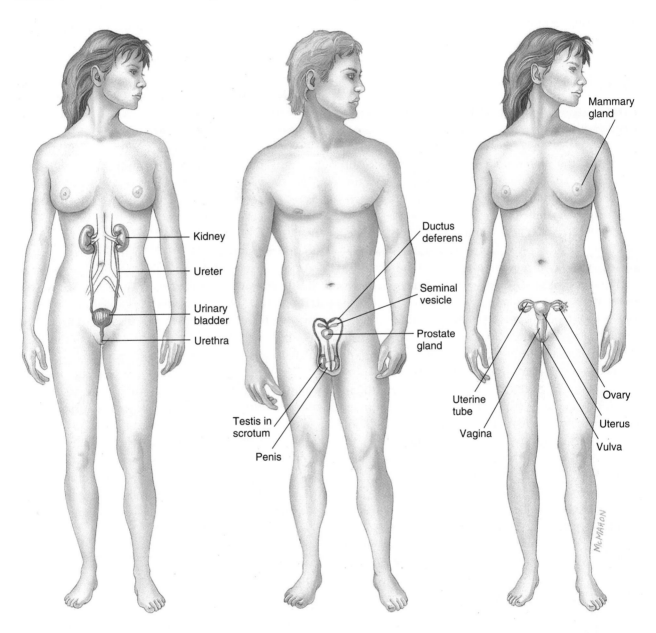

Kidney

Ureter

Urinary bladder

Urethra

Ductus deferens

Seminal vesicle

Prostate gland

Testis in scrotum

Penis

Mammary gland

Uterine tube

Vagina

Ovary

Uterus

Vulva

**Urinary system** Kidneys, ureters, urinary bladder, urethra.

**Reproductive systems** Male: testes, epididymides, vas deferens, ejaculatory ducts, penis, seminal vesicles, prostate gland, and bulbourethral glands.

**Reproductive systems** Female: ovaries, uterine tubes, uterus, vagina, external genitalia, and mammary glands.

**FIGURE 1-9.** The urinary and reproductive systems of the body.

elimination of urine, and the maintenance of homeostasis.

The **reproductive system** consists of the ovaries, uterine tubes, uterus, and vagina in the female and the testes, vas deferens, seminal vesicles, prostate gland, penis, and the urethra in the male (see Figure 1-9). Its functions include maintenance of sexual characteristics and the perpetuation of our species.

# HOMEOSTASIS

**Homeostasis** (hom-ee-oh-**STAY**-sis) is the maintenance (within varying narrow limits) of the internal environment of the body. One of the first scientists to discuss the significance of homeostasis to the survival of an organism was a French scientist, Claude Bernard (1813–1878). Homeostasis is essential to survival; hence, many of the body's systems are concerned with maintaining this internal environment. Some examples of homeostasis are blood sugar levels, body temperature, heart rate, and the fluid environment of cells. When homeostasis is maintained, the body is healthy. This is the reason your doctor takes your temperature and blood pressure as part of a routine examination.

We shall examine two examples of maintaining homeostasis. After ingesting a meal, which is predominately carbohydrates (salad, vegetables, bread, and perhaps fruit), the blood glucose level increases dramatically due to the breakdown of the complex carbohydrates by the digestive system into sugars such as glucose. Cells take in the glucose they need carried by the blood, but so much glucose is in the blood that now the pancreas secretes insulin, which moves the excess blood glucose into the liver where it is stored as glycogen or animal starch. Between meals when the blood glucose level drops below normal, the pancreas secretes glucagon that breaks down the glycogen into glucose and returns it to the blood circulatory system for distribution to body cells. Thus, the glucose level in the blood plasma remains at a nearly constant level so that it does not remain elevated after a meal nor does it drop too low between meals.

Body temperature regulation is another important example of homeostasis. When we go out on a hot summer day and our body temperature rises above 98.6°F, the hypothalamus of the brain detects this change and sends signals to various organs so that we sweat (sweating is a cooling process). As water is excreted by the sweat glands onto the skin, it evaporates in the air (evaporation is a cooling mechanism). In addition our blood vessels dilate to bring the blood near the skin's surface to dissipate body heat. When our body temperature falls below 98.6°F, as when we go out on a cold winter day, the hypothalamus sends signals to muscles causing us to shiver to raise our body temperature; it also causes our blood vessels to constrict to conserve body heat.

Our body must constantly monitor itself to correct any major deviations in homeostasis. It does this by using what is referred to as a *negative feedback loop*. Feedback responses that revise disturbances to our body's condition are examples of negative feedback. A good example of a negative feedback loop is the relationship between your home thermostat and your furnace. You set the thermostat at a temperature of 72°F. When the temperature in your home drops below 72°F, the furnace turns on to raise the house temperature. When the temperature goes above 72°F, the thermostat causes the furnace to turn off.

Our organ systems help control the internal environment of the body and cells so that it remains fairly constant. Our digestive, urinary, circulatory, and respiratory systems work together so that every cell receives the right amount of oxygen and nutrients and that waste products are eliminated fairly quickly and do not accumulate to toxic levels. If homeostasis is not maintained, the body experiences disease and eventually death.

## Summary Outline

### INTRODUCTION

1. The four basic reference systems of body organization are directions, planes, cavities, and structural units.

### TERMS OF DIRECTION

1. Superior means uppermost or above; inferior means lowermost or below.

2. Anterior means toward the front, ventral is synonymous with anterior. Posterior means toward the back; dorsal is synonymous with posterior.
3. Cephalad or cranial means toward the head; it is synonymous with superior.
4. Medial means nearest the midline; lateral means toward the side.
5. Proximal means nearest the point of attachment; distal means away from the point of attachment.

## PLANES

1. A midsagittal or median plane vertically divides the body into equal halves. A sagittal plane is parallel to a median or midsagittal plane.
2. A horizontal or transverse plane divides the body into superior and inferior portions.
3. A frontal or coronal plane divides the anterior or ventral and the posterior or dorsal portions of the body at right angles to the sagittal planes.

## CAVITIES

1. The body has two major cavities: the dorsal cavity and the ventral cavity.
2. The dorsal cavity is subdivided into the cranial cavity, which contains the brain, and the spinal cavity, which contains the spinal cord.
3. The ventral cavity is divided into two lesser cavities. The first is the thoracic cavity, which contains the heart in the pericardial cavity and the two lungs each in a pleural cavity. The second is the abdominopelvic cavity, which contains many of the digestive organs and some urinary and reproductive organs.
4. The term parietal refers to the walls of a cavity.
5. The term visceral refers to the covering of an organ.

## STRUCTURAL UNITS

1. The cell is the basic unit of the body's organization.
2. Different types of cells make up the four tissues of the body: epithelial, connective, muscle, and nervous.
3. Organs are composed of cells integrated into tissues serving a common function.

4. A system is a group of organs that perform a common function.
5. The integumentary system includes skin, hair, nails, and sweat and sebaceous glands. It protects, insulates, and regulates water and temperature.
6. The skeletal system includes bones and cartilage. It allows movement, makes blood cells, stores fat, protects, and supports.
7. The muscular system is made of skeletal, smooth, and cardiac muscle. It causes movement.
8. The nervous system includes the brain, spinal cord, and cranial and spinal nerves. It is the controlling, regulatory, and correlating system of the body.
9. The endocrine system consists of the endocrine glands and their hormones. In conjunction with the nervous system it regulates chemical aspects of the body.
10. The cardiovascular or blood circulatory system consists of the heart, arteries, veins, and capillaries. It distributes blood, carrying oxygen, nutrients, and wastes to and from body cells.
11. The lymphatic or immune system is made up of the lymph nodes, lymphatic vessels, the thymus gland, and the spleen. It drains tissues of excess fluids, transports fats, and develops immunities.
12. The respiratory system includes the nose, pharynx, larynx, trachea, bronchi, and lungs. It brings oxygen to and eliminates carbon dioxide from the blood.
13. The digestive system is composed of the organs of the alimentary tract from the lips to the anus and its associated glands. It converts food into simpler substances that can be absorbed along with other nutrients by the body's cells.
14. The urinary system includes the kidneys, ureters, bladder, and urethra. It functions in the chemical regulation of the blood.
15. The reproductive system includes the ovaries, uterine tubes, uterus, and vagina in women and the testes, seminal vesicles, prostate gland, penis, and urethra in men. It maintains sexual characteristics and perpetuates the species.

## HOMEOSTASIS

1. Homeostasis is the maintenance of the internal environment of the body within certain narrow ranges.
2. Some examples of homeostasis are blood sugar levels, body temperature, heart rate, and the fluid environment of the cell.

## REVIEW QUESTIONS

1. Name the systems of the body and their functions. Indicate what major organs each system contains.

2. The body has two major cavities, each divided into two lesser cavities. List them and explain what each cavity contains.
*3. Discuss how the body maintains homeostasis in terms of the blood glucose level.
*4. Discuss how the body maintains homeostasis in regards to maintaining normal body temperature.
5. Explain what a cell is.

*Critical Thinking Questions

## Matching

Place the most appropriate number in the box provided.

2 Superior
7 Anterior
11 Inferior
1 Posterior
10 Medial
3 Lateral
4 Proximal
6 Distal
5 Horizontal
8 Midsagittal

1. Toward the back, dorsal
2. Uppermost or above
3. Toward the side
4. Nearest the point of attachment or origin
5. Any plane dividing the body into superior and inferior
6. Away from the point of attachment
7. Toward the front, ventral
8. The plane vertically dividing the body into equal right and left halves
9. Toward the heart
10. Nearest the midline of the body
11. Lowermost or below
12. Frontal

# 2

# The Chemistry of Life

## CHAPTER OUTLINE

■ **Introduction**

■ **Atomic structure**

■ **Elements, isotopes, compounds**

■ **Bonds and energy**

■ **Common substances in living systems:**
*Water, Carbon dioxide, Molecular oxygen,
Ammonia, Mineral salts, Carbohydrates, Lipids,
Proteins, Nucleic acids, Adenosine triphosphate*

■ **Movement of materials into and out of cells:**
*Diffusion, Osmosis*

■ **pH**

## CHAPTER OBJECTIVES

After studying this chapter, you should be able to:

1. Define the structure of an atom and its component subatomic particles.

2. List the major chemical elements found in living systems.

3. Compare the differences between ionic and covalent bonding and how molecules formed by either ionic or covalent bonds react in water.

4. Understand the basic chemical structure of water, carbon dioxide and oxygen gas, ammonia, the mineral salts, carbohydrates, lipids, proteins, the nucleic acids DNA and RNA, ATP, and their role in living systems.

5. Explain the difference between diffusion, osmosis, and active transport and their role in maintaining cellular structure and function.

6. Define pH and its significance in the human body.

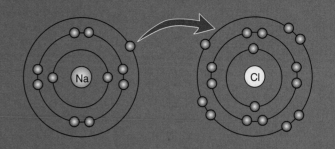

# KEY TERMS

# INTRODUCTION

Because all of the structures of the body (cells, tissues, and organs) are composed of chemicals, it is necessary to have a basic understanding of the science of chemistry. In addition, the body functions through chemical reactions. For example, in the digestive process complex foods are broken down through chemical reactions into simpler substances such as sugars that can be absorbed and used by the body's cells. Later these simple substances are converted into another kind of chemical fuel, **adenosine triphosphate (ATP)** (ah-**DEN**-oh-seen try-**FOS**-fate), which allows the body cells to do work and to function. Chemistry is the science that deals with the elements, their compounds, the chemical reactions that occur between elements and compounds, and the molecular structure of all matter. Students of anatomy need to have some basic knowledge of this field of study.

This chapter will introduce you to some basic principles of chemistry that will assist in your comprehension of human anatomy and physiology. To understand the human body, it is necessary to understand the chemical basis of life. We will look at the structure of the atom, how atoms interact with one another to form compounds, and how those compounds form the building blocks of life. All nonliving and living things are made of matter. Matter is composed of elements, which are primary substances from which all other things are constructed. Elements cannot be broken down into simpler substances. There are 92 elements that occur naturally. Other elements have been created artificially in the laboratory.

# ATOMIC STRUCTURE

**Atoms** are the smallest particles of an element that maintain all the characteristics of that element and enter into chemical reactions. Each atom consists of a relatively heavy, compact central nucleus composed of **protons** and **neutrons**. Lighter particles called **electrons** orbit the nucleus at some distance from its center.

Electrons are practically weightless and each one carries a negative electrical charge ($^-$). Atomic nuclei are composed of protons and neutrons, except for the hydrogen nucleus, which contains only one proton (Figure 2-1). Each proton and neutron has one unit of atomic weight and is about 1800 times heavier than an electron. Thus an atom's weight results almost entirely from its protons and neutrons. A proton carries a positive charge ($^+$), whereas a neutron is neutral and has no charge. Like charges repel—they push away from each other. Thus when you brush your hair on a dry day, like electrical charges build up on the brush and your hair so your hair flies away from the brush. Unlike charges attract. The clinging of clothes taken out of a dryer is due to the attraction of unlike electrical charges.

# ELEMENTS, ISOTOPES, COMPOUNDS

Each element has a distinctive number of protons. An **element** is a substance whose atoms all contain the same number of protons and the same number of electrons. Because the number of protons equals the number of electrons, an atom is electrically neutral. The theory that suggested that all matter consists of atoms was proposed in 1808 by John Dalton (1766–1844). He stated that atoms were responsible for the combinations of elements found in compounds. The atomic theory developed from his proposal. The atomic theory proposed that:

- All matter is made up of tiny particles called atoms.
- All atoms of a given element are similar to one another but different from the atoms of other elements.

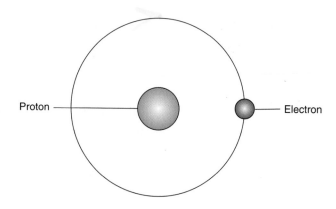

**FIGURE 2-1.** The hydrogen atom is unique because its nucleus contains only one proton.

- Atoms of two or more elements combine to form compounds.
- A chemical reaction involves the rearrangement, separation, or combination of atoms.
- Atoms are never created or destroyed during a chemical reaction.

In the atoms of some elements, the number of neutrons varies. Carbon is the element found in all living matter. Life on earth is based on the carbon atom. In fact, a whole branch of chemistry called organic chemistry studies the nature of the carbon atom and its chemical reactions. Different atoms of carbon may have different numbers of neutrons. Atoms of carbon may have one of three different atomic weights—12, 13, or 14—depending on the number of neutrons. These different kinds of atoms of the same element are called **isotopes** and are designated as $C^{12}$, $C^{13}$, and $C^{14}$. Each of these isotopes contains six protons and six electrons but $C^{12}$ has six neutrons, $C^{13}$ has seven neutrons, and $C^{14}$ has eight neutrons. $C^{14}$ is mildly radioactive and is used to estimate the age of fossilized human remains. A radioactive isotope of iodine is used to treat disorders of the thyroid gland. The **atomic number** is the number of protons or the number of electrons. By the late 1800s, scientists discovered similarities in the behavior of the known elements. It was a Russian chemist, Dimitri Mendeleev (1834–1907) who suggested that the elements could be arranged in groups that showed similar physical and chemical properties. From his work we have the modern **periodic table** of the elements, which arranges the elements by increasing atomic number in such a way that similar properties repeat at periodic intervals (Figure 2-2).

In summary, protons and neutrons make up the nucleus of an atom. Electrons orbit the nucleus. It is impossible to know exactly where any given electron is located at any given moment but the area where it is found can be referred to as the electron's orbital. **Orbitals** are grouped together to form **electron shells**. Shells can contain more than one electron. Thus, atoms are represented as a round nucleus (containing protons and neutrons) surrounded by concentric circles representing the electron shells. Carbon has two electrons in the first shell and four electrons in the second shell.

Hydrogen has a single electron in its first shell and no other shells. Oxygen has two electrons in the first shell and six electrons in the second shell.

## BONDS AND ENERGY

Atoms combine chemically with one another in one of two ways, that is, they form **bonds**. Chemical bonds are formed when the outermost electrons are transferred (gained or lost) or shared between atoms. When the atoms of two or more different elements combine in this way, a **compound** (such as water, $H_2O$) is created. This symbol $H_2O$ also represents a **molecule**. A molecule or compound is the smallest combination or particle retaining all the properties of the compound itself.

One type of bond is called an **ionic bond**. This kind of bond is formed when one atom gains electrons while the other atom loses electrons from its outermost shell or orbit. Atoms that gain electrons become negatively charged, whereas those that lose electrons become positively charged each having originally been electrically neutral. The new charged atoms are called **ions**. Negatively charged ions ($Cl^-$, for example) are attracted to positively charged ions ($Na^+$). The resulting force that binds these ions together is an ionic bond. Referring to Figure 2-3, notice that the sodium atom has a completely filled innermost shell with two electrons, a completely filled second shell with eight electrons, but only one electron in its third shell. The chlorine atom has a completely filled innermost shell with two electrons, a completely filled second shell with eight electrons, but only seven in its third shell. Because eight electrons would fill the outermost shell, in forming the ionic bond sodium loses its one electron to the chlorine atom's outermost shell thus filling chlorine's outermost shell with new eight electrons. The resulting compound, sodium chloride ($Na^+ Cl^-$), is common table salt formed an ionic bond, held together by the attraction of opposite electric charges of the ions. When immersed in water, compounds held together ionic bonds tend to separate or dissociate into constituent ions because of the attraction of the water molecule (which we shall discuss later this chapter). Many of the substances required by

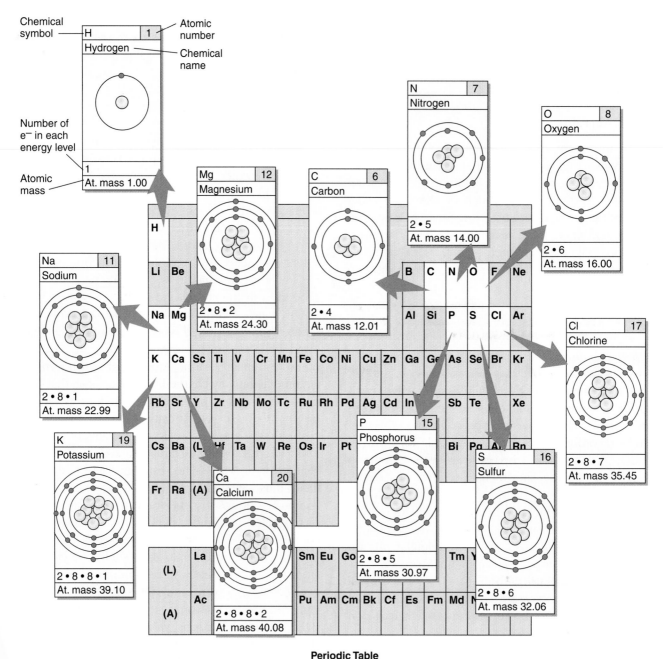

**Periodic Table**

**FIGURE 2-2.** The periodic table of the elements.

human cells exist in nature in ionic form. Some examples are the mineral salts; such as sodium, chloride, potassium, calcium, and phosphate.

A second type of bond found in many molecules the **covalent bond**. In this type of bond, the atoms share electrons to fill their outermost shells. Molecules containing covalent bonds do not dissociate when immersed in water. Four of the most important elements found in cells form this type of bond. They are carbon (C), oxyen (O), hydrogen (H), and nitrogen (N). They constitute about 95% of the materials found in cells. All of the cell's larger molecules and many of its smaller ones contain such bonds. The formation of the covalent bond between two hydrogen atoms forms the compound hydrogen gas ($H_2$) (Figure 2-4).

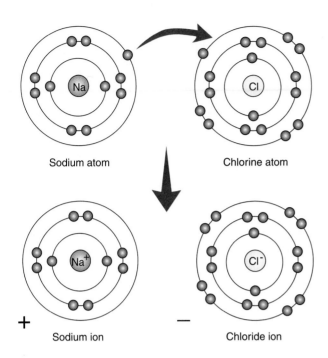

**FIGURE 2-3.** The formation of an ionic bond between sodium and chloride forms Na⁺Cl⁻ (sodium chloride or table salt).

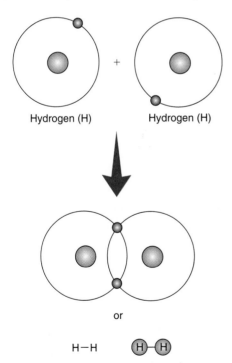

**FIGURE 2-4.** The formation of compounds through covalent bonding.

Another type of bond is the **hydrogen bond**. Hydrogen bonds are very weak bonds and help hold water molecules together by forming a bridge between the negative oxygen atom of one water molecule and the positive hydrogen atoms of another water molecule. Hydrogen bonds also help to bind various parts of one molecule into a three-dimensional shape such as a protein molecule like an enzyme.

Molecules furnishing electrons during a reaction are called **electron donors** (e.g., sodium); those that gain electrons during the process are called **electron acceptors** (e.g., chlorine when salt was formed). Some very special molecules will gain electrons only to lose them to some other molecule in a very short time; these are designated as **electron carriers**. These molecules will be discussed in Chapter 4 and are very important in making the cellular energy molecule ATP.

Bonds contain **energy**, the ability to do work. This results from the interaction of the electrons and the nuclei of the bonded atoms. If we measure the amount of energy present between two atoms, we discover that the amount varies as the distance between the atoms changes. When atoms are close to one another, the paths of their electrons overlap. The natural repulsion of these negatively charged electrons tends to drive the two atoms apart. Thus, the amount of energy necessary to keep them together is quite high. This type of bond contains a high degree of energy. If we break these bonds, as in the breakdown of a glucose ($C_6H_{12}O_6$) molecule inside a cell, electron carriers in the cell will use the energy of the released electrons to put together an ATP molecule. ATP is the high-energy fuel molecule that the cell needs to function. This high-energy molecule that is used in the cell is called adenosine triphosphate. This molecule is constantly being created and broken down to release its energy to do the cell's work. It is abbreviated as ATP. It is created by adding a phosphate to adenosine diphosphate. When it is broken down (ATP → ADP + $PO_4$) it releases the energy contained in the phosphate bond. We shall discuss this in further detail in Chapter 4.

# COMMON SUBSTANCES IN LIVING SYSTEMS

There are ten common substances found in living systems. They are water, carbon dioxide gas, molecular oxygen, ammonia, mineral salts, carbohydrates, lipids, proteins, nucleic acids, and adenosine triphosphate.

## Water

**Water** is the most abundant substance in living cells, approximately 60% to 80%; plasma, which is the liquid portion of blood, is 92% water. Water is a small, simple molecule composed of two hydrogen atoms covalently bonded to one oxygen atom. Because the oxygen atom attracts electrons more strongly than do the hydrogen atoms, water molecules are polar with a partial positive charge by the hydrogen atoms and a partial negative charge by the oxygen atom (Figure 2-5). This unique feature of the water molecule determines why ionic bonded molecules dissociate in water. Negatively charged ions (e.g., chloride) are attracted to the positively charged hydrogen atoms and positively charged ions (e.g., sodium) are attracted to the negatively charged oxygen atoms. Thus, the ionic bonded molecule salt dissociates in water.

Water has a number of roles in cells. It takes part in some reactions, such as photosynthesis in plant cells, which supplies our earth with molecular oxygen, and respiration in both plant and animal cells, which produces energy.

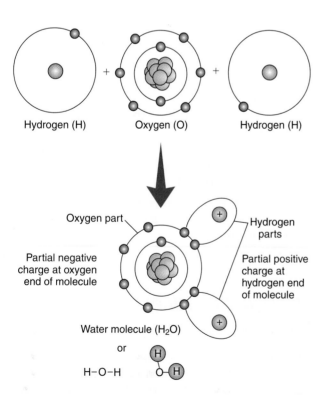

**FIGURE 2-5.** The uniqueness of the water molecule.

Photosynthesis:
$$6CO_2 + 12H_2O \rightarrow C_6H_{12}O_6 + 6\ O_2 + 6H_2O;$$

Respiration: $C_6H_{12}O_6 + 6O_2 \rightarrow 6CO_2 + 6H_2O$ + energy in the form of ATP

Digestion of food requires water to break down larger molecules. This is called hydrolysis. Water serves as a medium or **solvent** for other reactions, and water is referred to as the universal solvent. The chemistry of life is dominated by the chemistry of water. Chemical reactions occur in cells between individual atoms, ions, or molecules not between large aggregations of these particles. It is as these particles move about in the water that they come in contact with other particles and chemical reactions occur. In addition, water is a basis for the transport of materials such as hormones and enzymes in the plasma of blood.

Water also absorbs and releases high levels of heat before its temperature changes, thus helping control normal body temperature. Vigorous exercise liberates heat from contracting muscle cells. This excess heat is absorbed by the water in the cells and then released. Water is part of amniotic fluid and protects the developing fetus. It is also part of the cerebrospinal fluid and protects the brain and spinal cord by functioning as a shock absorber. Finally water is the base for all body lubricants such as mucus in the digestive tract and synovial fluid in joints.

## Carbon Dioxide

The small **carbon dioxide** molecule ($CO_2$) contains one carbon atom covalently bonded to two oxygen atoms. It is produced as a waste product of cellular respiration and must be eliminated quickly from the body through expiration via the respiratory system and the cardiovascular system. It is also necessary for photosynthesis in plant cells to convert the radiant energy of the sun into usuable chemical energy such as glucose for both plant and animal cells. It is also a source of the element carbon, found in all organic compounds of living systems. If carbon dioxide is allowed to accumulate within cells, it becomes toxic by forming carbonic acid as it reacts with water. Hence, we exhale it quickly from the lungs.

## Molecular Oxygen

**Molecular oxygen** ($O_2$), formed when two oxygen atoms are covalently bonded together, is required by all organisms that breathe air. It is necessary to convert chemical energy (food), such as the energy found in a glucose ($C_6H_{12}O_6$) molecule, into another form of chemical energy ATP that can be used by cells to do work. Because $O_2$ is a product of photosynthesis, it becomes obvious how dependent we animals are on plants for our survival. Without plants there would be no molecular oxygen in our atmosphere and without $O_2$ there would be no life on our planet as we know it. The level of $O_2$ in our atomosphere is maintained at a nearly constant level (about 21% of the gas in the atomosphere is oxygen) by the many different kinds of plants found on our earth.

## Ammonia

The **ammonia** molecule ($NH_3$) comes from the decomposition of proteins via the digestive process and the conversion of amino acids in cellular respiration to ATP molecules. Note that an important element in ammonia is nitrogen. Nitrogen is an essential element in amino acids, which are the building blocks of proteins. Because even a small amount of ammonia is injurious to cells, the human body must quickly dispose of this material. Through enzymes, the liver converts the toxic ammonia to a harmless substance called urea. Because urea is soluble in water, the blood then carries the urea to the kidneys to be filtered and eliminated from the body as urine. Because many plants are able to use $NH_3$ or the products of bacterial action on $NH_3$ as a nitrogen source for protein synthesis, ammonia is a common constituent of fertilizers.

## Mineral Salts

**Mineral salts** are composed of small ions. They are essential for the survival and functioning of the body's cells. They function in numerous ways as parts of enzymes or as portions of the cellular environment necessary for enzyme or protein action.

Calcium ($Ca^+$) is necessary for muscle contraction and nervous transmission as well as being necessary to build strong bones. Phosphate ($PO_4^-$) is necessary to produce the high energy molecule ATP. Chloride ($Cl^-$) is necessary for nervous transmission. Sodium ($Na^+$) and potassium ($K^+$) are also necessary for muscle cell contraction and nervous transmission.

## Carbohydrates

**Carbohydrates** (kar-boh-**HIGH**-draytz) are made of the atoms of carbon, hydrogen, and oxygen in a 1:2:1 ratio (e.g., glucose or $C_6H_{12}O_6$). The smallest carbohydrates are the simple sugars that cannot be made to react with water to produce a simpler form. Sugars are generally chains of either five or six carbon atoms. Important five-carbon sugars are **ribose** and **deoxyribose** which are parts of the RNA and DNA **nucleic acid** molecules. Important six-carbon sugars are **glucose** and **fructose** (the suffix ose denotes a sugar) (Figure 2-6). Note the repetition of the H-C-OH unit in the molecule. This is typical of sugars. Starch, **glycogen** (animal starch), cellulose (the material of plant cell walls that forms fiber in our diets), chitin (**KYE**-tin) (the exoskeleton of arthropods such as insects and lobsters), as well as many other complex carbohydrates, are formed by bonding together a number of glucose molecules. Besides glucose there are other six-carbon sugars. Combinations of these with glucose results in another series of sugars such as common table sugar or sucrose, a disaccharide.

Carbohydrates have two important functions: energy storage (sugars, starch, glycogen) and cell strengthening (cellulose of plant cell walls and chitin in the external skeleton of arthropod animals). Energy storage is the more common function of carbohydrates.

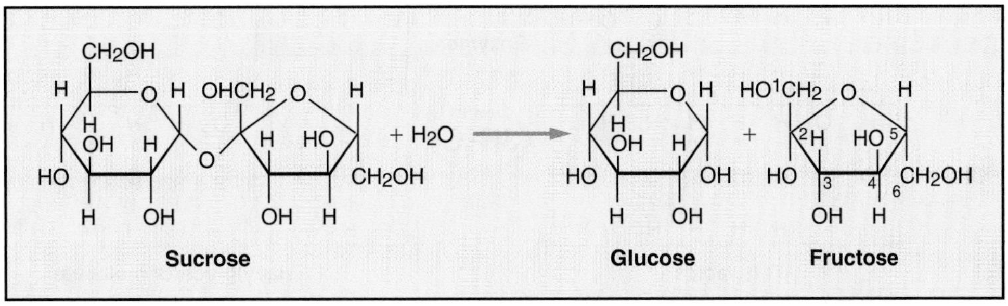

**FIGURE 2-6.** The chemical structure of the six-carbon sugars, glucose and fructose. When combined they produce the disaccharide sucrose.

## Lipids

There are a number of different kinds of **lipids**. Lipids are substances that are insoluble in water. Fats, phospholipids, steroids, and prostaglandins are examples of these different kinds of molecules. We will concentrate on fats, which are a major kind of lipid. Of the fats in the human body, 95% are triglycerides, now called **triacylglycerols** (try-**ass**-il **GLISS**-er-allz). They consist of two types of building blocks: **glycerol** and **fatty acids**. Glycerol is a simple molecule similar to a sugar except that it has only a three-carbon chain. Each carbon of the chain is bonded to a hydrogen and a **hydroxyl** (-OH) **group** as well as to the carbons of the chain (Figure 2-7). Fatty acids are composed of long chains of carbon atoms of different lengths. All the carbon atoms are bonded to  hydrogen atoms except the carbon at one end of the chain. This carbon atom is bonded to the **carboxyl** (-COOH) **group**, which makes these molecules slightly acidic. Most naturally occurring fatty acids contain an even number of carbon atoms, 14 to 18. A fatty acid is **saturated** if it contains only single covalent bonds as those found in whole milk, butter, eggs, beef, pork, and coconut and palm oils. Too much of these fatty acids contributes to cardiovascular disease. However, if the carbon chain has one or more double covalent bonds between the carbon atoms, it is an **unsaturated** fatty acid. These fatty acids are good for you and are found in sunflower, corn, and fish oils. Fats have a number of major roles in the body. Like car-bohydrates they contain stored chemical energy. Fat found under the skin acts as an insulator to prevent heat loss. Any animal that lives in the Arctic or Antarctic region (polar bears, seals, whales, or penguins) has a thick layer of insulatory fat. The camel's hump is a thick deposit of fat to protect its internal organs from excessive rises in temperature in the hot desert. Fat also protects organs as a surrounding layer such as the layer around our kidneys to protect the kidney from severe jolts.

## Proteins

**Proteins** are composed of carbon, hydrogen, oxygen, and nitrogen covalently bonded. Most proteins also contain some sulfur. The basic building blocks of proteins are the 20 amino acids. They vary in both the length of their carbon chain backbones and the atoms connected to that backbone. However, each amino acid has a carboxyl group (-COOH), an **amine group** (-NH$_2$), a hydrogen atom, and the R group. The R group refers to the different types of atoms and length of the chain (Figure 2-8). Covalent bonds form between different amino acids to form proteins. These are referred to as **peptide bonds** (Figure 2-9).

Proteins function in a number of very important ways in the human body. Many are structural proteins. Proteins are part of a cell's membranous structures: plasma membrane, nuclear membrane, endoplasmic reticulum, mitochondria. In addition, actin and myosin are structural proteins found in a muscle

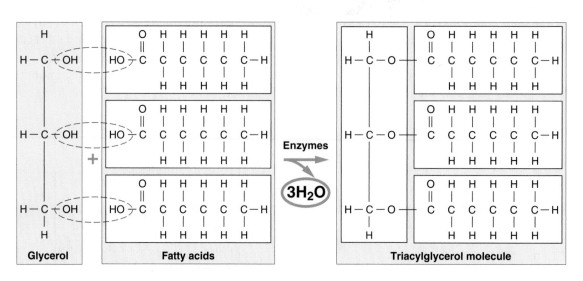

**FIGURE 2-7.** The structure of a fat like triacylglycerol is composed of a glycerol molecule and fatty acids.

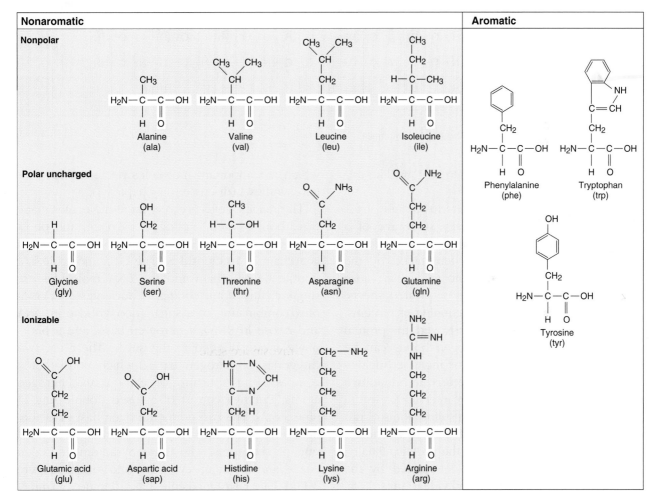

**FIGURE 2-8.** The general structure of an amino acid and the list of the 20 amino acids found in the human body.

cell. We could not move, talk, digest, or circulate blood without the proteins actin and myosin. Inside a cell it is chemical reactions that allow a cell to function properly. These chemical reactions would not occur in cells without the assistance of **enzymes**. Enzymes are protein **catalysts,** which increase the rate of a chemical reaction without being affected by the reaction. In addition, our immune system functions because antibodies, which are proteins of a high molecular weight, are formed to combat foreign proteins called antigens that get into our body. Some examples of foreign proteins would be bacterial cell membranes, virus protein coats, or bacterial flagella. Finally proteins are also a source of energy and can

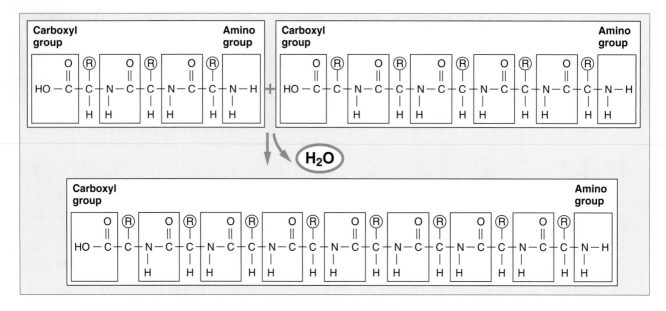

**FIGURE 2-9.** The formation of a dipeptide bond to form a protein.

be broken down and converted to ATP just like carbohydrates and fats.

Proteins are also discussed in terms of their structure (Figure 2-10). The **primary structure** of a protein is determined by its amino acid sequence. The **secondary structure** is determined by the hydrogen bonds between amino acids that cause the protein to coil into helices or pleated sheets. This shape is crucial to the functioning of proteins. If those hydrogen bonds are destroyed, the protein becomes nonfunctional. Hydrogen bonds can be broken by high temperatures or increased acidity resulting in changes in pH. The **tertiary structure** is a secondary folding caused by interactions within the peptide bonds and between sulfur atoms of different amino acids. Changes affecting this structure can also affect the function of the protein. Finally, the **quaternary structure** is determined by the spatial relationships between individual units.

## Nucleic Acids

Two very important nucleic acids  are found in cells. **Deoxyribonucleic** (dee-ock-see-rye-boh-noo-**KLEE**-ik) **acid** (**DNA**) is the genetic material of cells located in the nucleus of the cell. It determines all of the functions and characteristics of the cell. **Ribonucleic** (rye-boh-noo-**KLEE**-ik) **acid** (**RNA**) is structurally related to DNA. Two important types of RNA are **messenger RNA** and **transfer RNA**,

which are important molecules necessary for protein synthesis (discussed in Chapter 3).

The nucleic acids are very large molecules made of carbon, oxygen, hydrogen, nitrogen, and phosphorous atoms. The basic structure of a nucleic acid is a chain of **nucleotides**. The DNA molecule is a double helical chain and the RNA molecules are single chains of nucleotides. A nucleotide is a complex combination of a sugar (deoxyribose in DNA and ribose in RNA), a nitrogren base, and a phosphate group bonded to the sugar. There are two categories of nitrogen bases, which consist of a complex ring structure of carbon and nitrogen atoms. **Purines** consist of a fused double ring of nine atoms. The two purine nitrogen bases are adenine and guanine. **Pyrimidines** consist of a single ring of six atoms. The three pyrimidine nitrogen bases are thymine, cytosine, and uracil (Figure 2-11). The DNA molecule has adenine, thymine, guanine, and cytosine. The RNA molecule substitutes uracil for thymine and also has adenine, cytosine, and guanine. In the DNA molecule adenine joins thymine while cytosine always joins guanine in forming the double helical chain. We will discuss this structure in detail in Chapter 4.

## Adenosine Triphosphate

Adenosine triphosphate (ATP) is the high energy molecule or fuel that runs the cell's machinery. All

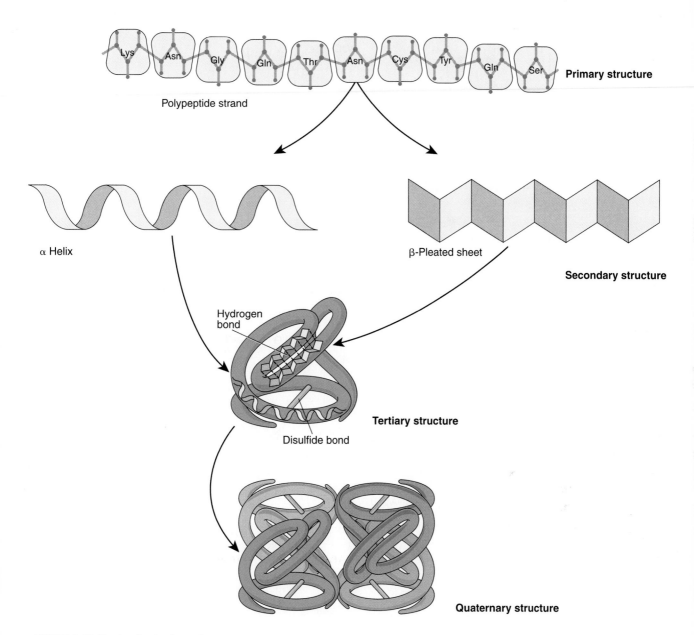

**FIGURE 2-10.** The four levels of protein structure.

the food that we eat (which is a form of chemical energy) must be transformed into another form of chemical energy (ATP) that allows our cells to maintain, repair, and reproduce themselves. The ATP molecule consists of a ribose sugar, the purine adenine, and three phosphate groups (Figure 2-12). The energy of the molecule is stored in the second and third phosphate groups.

The breakdown of the glucose molecule and other nutrients provides the energy to make ATP molecules (discussed in greater detail in Chapter

4). An ATP molecule is made by putting together an adenosine diphosphate (ADP) with a phosphate group ($PO_4$): ADP + $PO_4$ + energy $\rightarrow$ ATP. The energy stored in the ATP molecule is then used to run the cell and to perform activities such as structural repair, reproduction, assimilation, and transport of materials across cell membranes. This occurs when we break down an ATP molecule by releasing the energy in the phosphate bonds: ATP $\rightarrow$ ADP + $PO_4$ + energy (to do cell processes).

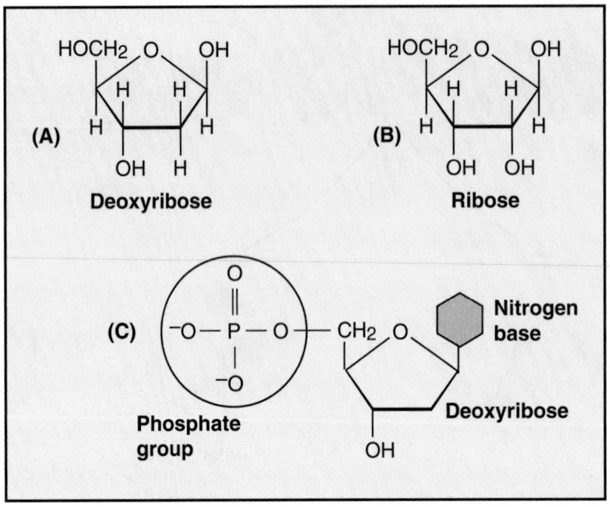

**(A)**

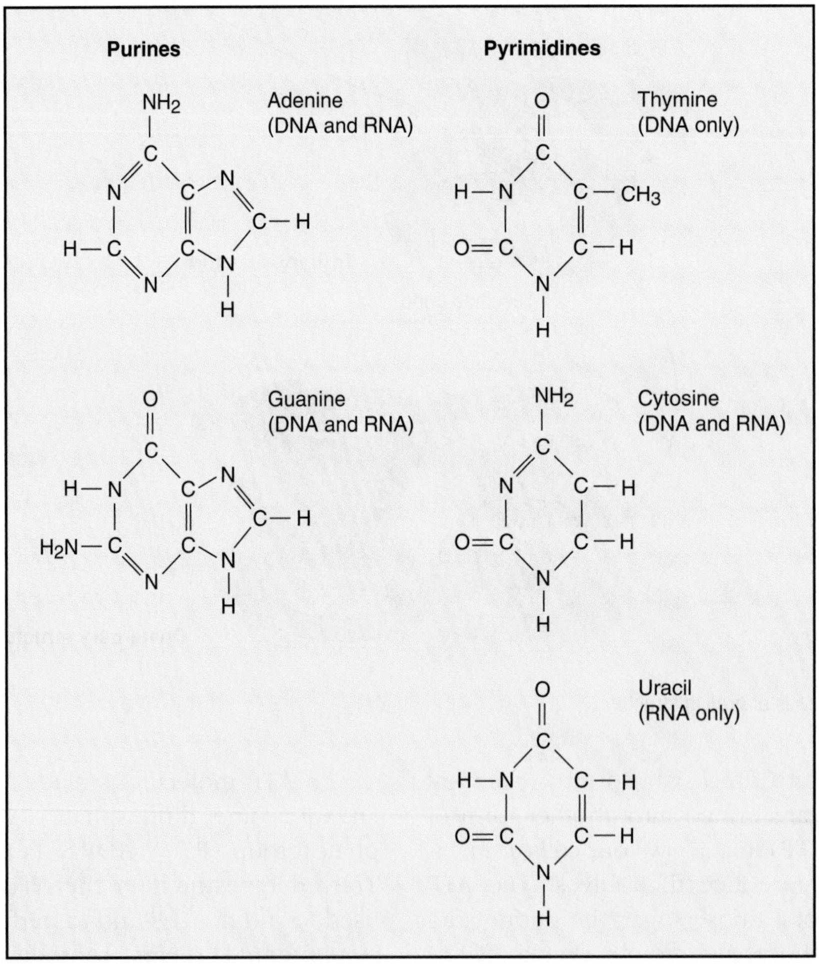

**(B)**

**FIGURE 2-11.** (A) The structure of a nucleotide and (B) their nitrogen bases.

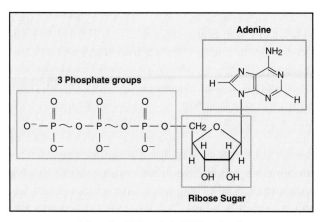

Adenosine triphosphate (ATP) molecule

**FIGURE 2-12.** The structure of the adenosine triphosphate (ATP) molecule.

# MOVEMENT OF MATERIALS INTO AND OUT OF CELLS

The plasma membrane of cells is a **semipermeable membrane**. This means that only selected materials are capable of getting into and out of cells. The chemical structure of the cell membrane is responsible for this quality. The cell membrane is composed of an outer and inner layer of protein with a double phospholipid layer in between. This chemical arrangement allows water to pass into and out of the cell with ease. However, water is not the only material needed for the cell's survival. Cells need food like sugars, amino acids to make proteins, and nutrients like the mineral salts, to mention just a few. Materials pass through the cell's membrane in three different ways: diffusion, osmosis, and active transport.

## Diffusion

**Diffusion** is the movement of molecules through a medium from an area of high concentration of those molecules to an area of low concentration of those molecules. As an example of diffusion think of a closed perfume bottle in a room. Within the stoppered bottle perfume molecules are in constant motion; they are in the liquid and the gaseous state. Those in the gaseous state are in faster motion than those in the liquid state. In the air of the room, there are also molecules in motion—water vapor, oxygen, nitrogen, and carbon dioxide gas to name a few.

When the perfume bottle is opened, perfume molecules randomly move out of the bottle and randomly bump or collide with those other molecules in the air. The collisions are like bumping billiard balls on a pool table. The random collisions eventually bump the perfume molecules toward the walls of the room and eventually throughout the room. If the perfume bottle is opened at one end of the room and you are standing at the opposite end of the room, you would eventually smell the perfume once the molecules reached your end of the room. A person standing near the perfume bottle when it was opened would smell the perfume molecules before you did. The random collisions of diffusing molecules are referred to as **brownian movement** after Sir Robert Brown an English scientist who discussed this kind of movement in 1827.

Despite the randomness of these collisions, over time there is a net displacement of perfume molecules from areas of high concentration (on and near the perfume bottle) to areas of low concentration (at the other end of the room). This is diffusion. Eventually the proportion of perfume molecules being bumped back to the perfume bottle will equal the proportion of perfume molecules being bumped away from the bottle and the molecules will be evenly spread throughout the room.

Temperature has an effect on diffusion. The higher the temperature the faster the movement. Think of a chunk of ice; low temperature keeps the molecules moving very slowly, so the water is in a solid state. As temperature increases, molecular motion increases and the water moves to a liquid state; the ice melts. Continued heating, such as putting a pot of water on a stove, increases molecular motion even further so that the water becomes water vapor and moves into the gaseous state.

An example of an important diffusion in the human body is the uptake of oxygen by the blood in the lungs and the release of carbon dioxide gas to the lungs from the blood. Blood returning to the lungs is low in oxygen but high in carbon dioxide gas as a result of cellular respiration. When we breathe in air, we take in oxygen gas, so the lungs have lots of oxygen but little carbon dioxide gas. The oxygen moves from an area of high concentration (the lungs) to an area of low concentration (the blood) by diffusion. Similarly the carbon dioxide gas moves from an area of higher concentration (the blood) to an area of low concentration (the lungs) by diffusion and we exhale to get rid of the carbon dioxide gas now in the lungs.

## Osmosis

**Osmosis** (oz-**MOH**-sis) is a special kind of diffusion. Osmosis pertains only to the movement of water molecules through a semipermeable membrane (e.g., a plasma membrane) from an area of high concentration of water molecules (e.g., pure water) to an area of low concentration of water molecules (e.g., water to which a **solute** such as salt or sugar has been added).

Osmosis can be demonstrated fairly simply by separating pure distilled water with a semipermeable membrane (a barrier that will allow only water to pass through it, but not solutes such as salt) and

adding a 3% salt solution to the water on the other side of the membrane (Figure 2-13). The water level on the solute side will rise, and the water on the pure water side will drop. The rise in water on the open-ended flask tube opposes atmosphere pressure and gravity and will eventually stop rising. At this equilibrium level, the number of water molecules entering the solute area equals the number of water molecules leaving the solute area. The amount of pressure required to stop osmosis is a measure of osmotic pressure. The solution stops rising when the weight of the column equals the osmotic pressure.

The mechanism of osmosis is simple. The salt in the column of water in solution cannot pass through the semipermeable membrane. Salt is in higher concentration in the solution. Water is in lower concentration in the column because salt has

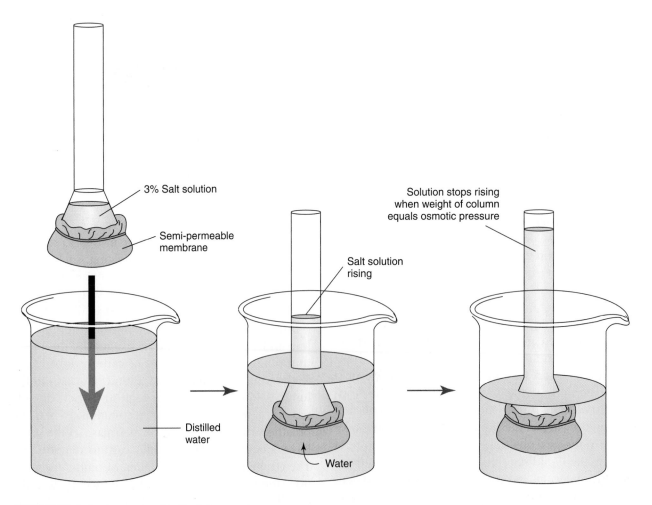

**FIGURE 2-13.** A simple experiment to illustrate osmosis.

been added to the water. However, the water in the beaker is pure distilled water; there are no solutes in it. The water, which can move through the semipermeable membrane, causes the observed increased height of the water column in the flask. The water "tries" to equalize its concentration in both the beaker and the flask. Thus, the water moves from an area of high concentration in the beaker through the semipermeable membrane to an area of low concentration (the salt solution in the flask).

Many biologic membranes are semipermeable, such as the membranes of cells. The effects of osmosis on red blood cells can easily be demonstrated (Figure 2-14). If a red blood cell is placed in a normal saline solution (an **isotonic solution**) where the salt concentration outside the red blood cell equals the salt concentration inside the red blood cell, water molecules will pass into and out of the red blood cell at an equal rate and there will be no observed change in the shape of the red blood cell (Figure 2-14A). If, however, the red blood cell is placed in pure distilled water (a **hypotonic solution**) where the water molecules are in a higher concentration outside the red blood cell, water will move into the red blood cell causing it to swell and eventually rupture (Figure 2-14B). If the red blood cell is placed in a 5% salt solution (a **hypertonic solution**) where there is more water inside the red blood cell than in the solution, the red blood cell will lose water to the solution and will shrivel up or crenulate (Figure 2-14C).

Because blood in the circulatory system is under pressure due to the beating of the heart, much blood plasma (the fluid part of blood, which is predominantly water with dissolved and colloidal suspended materials in it) is lost into surrounding tissues in the highly permeable one-cell thick capillaries. Colloidally suspended proteins in the blood cannot pass through the capillary cell membranes; thus, they cause an osmotic pressure large enough to reabsorb most of the fluid that escapes from the capillaries.

Although water and a few other substances with small molecular weights can osmose into the cells that need them, osmotic transportation is insufficient for most of the cell's needs. Sugars, amino acids, larger proteins, and fats are needed by the cell to produce ATP and to maintain and create structure. Cells obtain these nonosmotic or nondiffusable materials by a special mechanism called **active transport**. This mechanism, however, needs energy in the form of ATP to overcome the osmotic/diffusional barriers—another major reason that ATP is so important to a cell's survival. Active transport is the transportation of materials against a concentration gradient or in opposition to other factors that would normally keep the material from entering the cell.

## pH

**pH** is defined as the negative logarithm of the hydrogen ion concentration in a solution: $pH = -\log(H^+)$. Pure water has a pH of 7. Remember that when distilled water ($H_2O$) dissociates, for every $H^+$ ion formed an $OH^-$ ion is also formed. Or in other words, the dissociation of water produces $H^+$ and

---

### Health Alert

#### ■ ACID RAIN

We are all aware of the term **acid rain**. Excess industrial pollutants emitted into the air from coal-fired power plants and automobiles can change the pH of our environment. These pollutants fall back to the earth as acid precipitation (rain, snow, or fog). This *acid rain* can cause respiratory problems when breathed in or gastric problems when reaching the stomach and digestive systems. We are aware of how serious this problem can be when we see lakes whose fish have all been killed or whole forests destroyed near industrial plants with high pollution rates. Acid precipitation is of global concern.

Buildings and monuments made of limestone (calcium carbonate) are easily eroded by even weak acids. The United States passed and implemented the Clean Air Act of 1990 to help lower the levels of acid precipitation to protect our health and our environment.

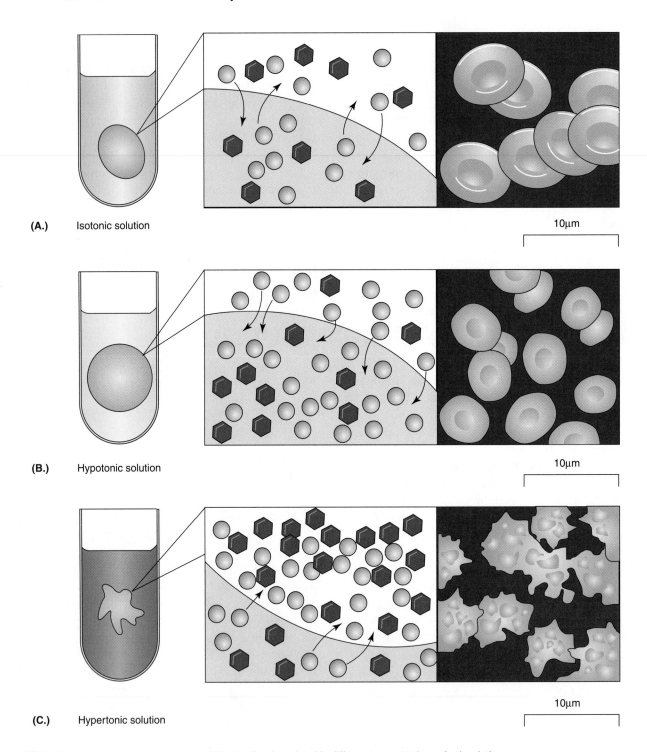

**(A.)**      Isotonic solution

10μm

**(B.)**      Hypotonic solution

10μm

**(C.)**      Hypertonic solution

10μm

**FIGURE 2-14.** The effects of osmosis on red blood cells when placed in different concentrations of salt solutions.

OH⁻ in equal amounts. Therefore, a pH of 7 indicates neutrality on the pH scale. Figure 2-15 shows the pH of various solutions.

If a substance dissociates and forms an excess of H⁺ ions when dissolved in water, it is referred to as an **acid.** All acidic solutions have pH values below 7. The stronger an acid is, the more H⁺ ions it produces and the lower its pH value. Because the pH scale is logarithmic, a pH change of 1 means a tenfold change in the concentration of hydrogen ions.

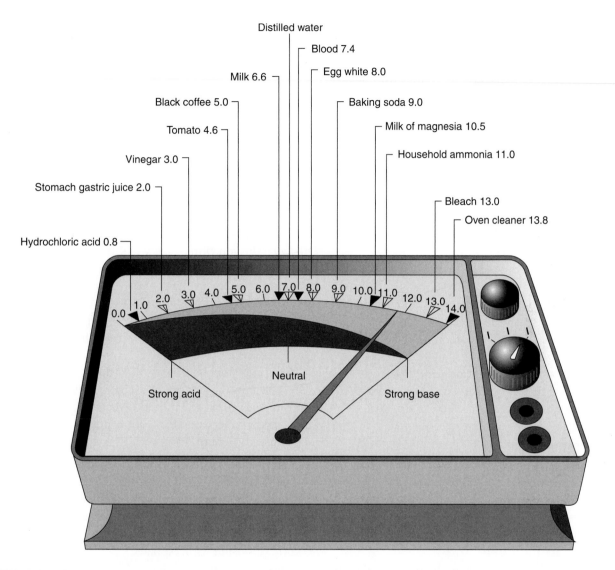

**FIGURE 2-15.** The pH of various solutions. A pH above 7 indicates a base; a value below 7 indicates an acid.

So lemon juice with a pH value of 2 is 100 times more acidic than tomato juice with a pH of 4.

A substance that combines with $H^+$ ions when dissolved in water is called a **base**. By combining with $H^+$ ions, a base therefore lowers the $H^+$ ion concentration in that solution. Basic, also called alkaline, solutions have pH values above 7. Seawater with a pH of 8 is 10 times more basic than pure distilled water with a pH of 7. In our bodies, saliva in our mouths has a pH value slightly lower than 7 so it is just slightly acidic, whereas the stomach with its gastric juice and hydrochloric acid is very acidic with a pH value near 1. Our blood on the other hand has a pH value of 7.4 making it just slightly basic. Urine has

a pH of 6 thus although acidic it is not as acidic as tomato juice with a pH of 4.

The pH inside most cells and in the fluid surrounding cells is fairly close to 7. Because enzymes are extremely sensitive to pH, even a small change can render them nonfunctional; thus, our bodies have **buffers**. A buffer is a substance that acts as a reservoir for hydrogen ions, donating them to a solution when their concentration falls and taking the hydrogen ions from a solution when their concentration rises. Buffers are necessary because the chemical reactions in cells constantly are producing acids and bases. Buffers help maintain homeostasis within cells in regard to pH levels. Most buffers consist of pairs of substances, one an acid and the other a base. For example, the key buffer in human blood is the acid–base pair bicarbonate (a base) and carbonic acid (an acid). Carbon dioxide and water combine chemically to form carbonic acid ($H_2CO_3$). The carbonic acid then can dissociate in water freeing $H^+$ ions and bicarbonate ions $HCO_3^-$. The blood's pH can be stabilized by the equilibrium between these forward and reverse reactions that interconvert the $H_2CO_3$ carbonic acid and the $HCO_3^-$ bicarbonate ion (base).

## Summary Outline

### INTRODUCTION

1. Because the body's cells, tissues, and organs are all composed of chemicals and function through chemical reactions, it is necessary to understand some basic chemistry.
2. Chemistry is the science that studies the elements, their compounds, the chemical reactions that occur between elements and compounds, and the molecular structure of all matter.

### ATOMIC STRUCTURE

1. Atoms are the smallest particles of elements that maintain all the characteristics of that element and enter into chemical reactions.
2. An atom consists of a nucleus containing positively charged protons and neutral neutrons.
3. Electrons have a negative charge and orbit the nucleus of an atom in shells at some distance from the compact heavy nucleus.

### ELEMENTS, ISOTOPES, COMPOUNDS

1. An element is a substance whose atoms all contain the same number of protons and the same number of electrons. Atoms are electrically neutral.
2. A compound is a combination of the atoms of two or more elements.
3. An isotope is a different kind of atom of the same element where the number of neutrons in the nucleus varies.
4. Carbon is the element found in all living matter.
5. The periodic table of the elements arranges elements in categories with similar properties.

### BONDS AND ENERGY

1. Atoms combine chemically with one another to form bonds by gaining, losing, or sharing electrons.
2. An ionic bond is formed when one atom gains electrons while the other atom in the bond loses electrons. Ionically bonded molecules disassociate when immersed in water. The mineral salts form ionic bonds.
3. A covalent bond is formed when atoms share electrons. Carbon, oxygen, hydrogen, and nitrogen form covalent bonds. These bonds do not dissociate when placed in water.
4. Hydrogen bonds are weak bonds. They help hold water molecules together and bind other molecules into three-dimensional shapes.
5. Molecules furnishing electrons during a chemical reaction are called electron donors; those that gain electrons are called electron acceptors.
6. Bonds contain energy. It is the electrons that contain the energy of a chemical bond.
7. Special molecules called electron carriers accept electrons for a short period of time and use the energy of the electrons to make ATP molecules.

### COMMON SUBSTANCES IN LIVING SYSTEMS

The common substances found in living systems are water, carbon dioxide, oxygen, ammonia, mineral salts, carbohydrates, lipids, proteins, nucleic acids, and adenosine triphosphate.

#### Water

1. Sixty to 80% of a cell is water ($H_2O$). Water is a slightly polar molecule: the two hydrogen atoms have a partial positive charge and the oxygen atom a partial negative charge. This explains why ionically bonded molecules dissociate when placed in water.
2. Water has many important roles in cells: it takes part in some reactions; it serves as a medium or solvent for other reactions to occur in; it serves as a basis for the transportation of materials; it absorbs and releases heat maintaining body temperature; it protects; and it is the base for all body lubricants.

#### Carbon Dioxide

1. Carbon dioxide gas ($CO_2$) is produced as a waste product of cellular respiration.

**2.** It is necessary for plants to produce oxygen gas in the photosynthetic reaction, which converts the sun's radiant energy into usable chemical energy like glucose for plant and animal survival.

**3.** All of the carbon in the carbon-containing molecules of life comes either directly or indirectly from carbon dioxide gas.

## Oxygen

**1.** Molecular oxygen ($O_2$) is required by all organisms that breathe air.

**2.** It is necessary for cellular respiration to occur, converting glucose into ATP molecules $C_6H_{12}O_6$ + $6O_2 \rightarrow$ ATP (energy) + $6CO_2$ + $6H_2O$.

**3.** Oxygen comes from plants in the photosynthesis process $6CO_2$ + $12H_2O \rightarrow$ $C_6H_{12}O_6$ (glucose) + $6O_2$ + $6H_2O$.

## Ammonia

**1.** Ammonia ($NH_3$) is produced as a by-product of the break down of amino acids.

**2.** Amino acids contain nitrogen and amino acids are the building blocks of proteins.

**3.** Ammonia, which is toxic, is converted to harmless urea by enzymes in our liver.

## Mineral Salts

**1.** The mineral salts are calcium ($Ca^+$), phosphate ($PO_4^-$), chloride ($Cl^-$), sodium ($Na^+$), and potassium ($K^+$).

**2.** Calcium is needed for muscle contraction and strong bones.

**3.** Phosphate is needed to make ATP.

**4.** Sodium, potassium, and chloride are necessary for muscle contraction and nervous transmission.

## Carbohydrates

**1.** Carbohydrates are composed of carbon, hydrogen, and oxygen in a 1:2:1 ratio. The simplest carbohydrates are five- and six-carbon sugars.

**2.** Important five-carbon sugars are deoxyribose and ribose; important six-carbon sugars are glucose and fructose.

**3.** Carbohydrates have two important functions: energy storage and structural strengthening of the cell.

## Lipids

**1.** Fat is a major type of lipid; 95% of fats in the human body are triacylglycerols, which are composed of glycerol and fatty acids.

**2.** A fat is called saturated if the fatty acids contain single covalent bonds. These can contribute to cardiovascular disease. A fat is called unsaturated if the fatty acids have one or more double covalent bonds. These are good for you.

**3.** Fats are a source of energy, act as insulators for the body, and protect organs.

## Proteins

**1.** Proteins contain carbon, oxygen, hydrogen, nitrogen, and sulfur.

**2.** Amino acids are the building blocks of protein.

**3.** Proteins are a source of energy. There are structural proteins like actin and myosin in muscle cells and proteins are an essential part of a cell's membranous structures.

**4.** Enzymes are protein catalysts that make chemical reactions occur in cells. The functioning of our immune system is based on proteins.

**5.** Proteins have four types of structure based on bonding: primary (amino acid sequences), secondary (based on hydrogen bonds between amino acids, causing coiling), tertiary (secondary folding based on sulfur atoms), and quaternary (based on spatial relationships between units).

## Nucleic Acids

**1.** Deoxyribonucleic acid (DNA) is the genetic material of the cell found in the nucleus that determines all of the characteristics and functions of the cell.

**2.** Ribonucleic acid (RNA) exists in two forms necessary for protein synthesis: messenger RNA and transfer RNA.

**3.** Nucleic acids are composed of chains of nucleotides.

**4.** A nucleotide is a complex combination of a nitrogen base (purine or pyrimidine), a sugar (deoxyribose), and a phosphate group.

**5.** The two purine bases are adenine and guanine. The three pyrimidine bases are thymine, cytosine, and uracil (uracil is found in RNA only and is substituted for thymine).

## Adenosine Triphosphate

**1.** ATP is a high-energy molecule that is the fuel that allows cells to function and to maintain themselves.

2. The ATP molecule consists of a ribose sugar, adenine, and three phosphate groups. The energy of the molecule is stored in the second and third phosphate groups.
3. The breakdown of the glucose molecule and other nutrients provides the energy to make ATP molecules.

### MOVEMENT OF MATERIALS INTO AND OUT OF CELLS

Materials move through plasma membranes in three different ways: diffusion, osmosis, and active transport.

### Diffusion

1. Diffusion is the movement of molecules through a medium from an area of high concentration of those molecules to an area of low concentration of those molecules.
2. The random collision of diffusing molecules is called brownian movement.
3. Increased temperature accelerates the rate of diffusing molecules.
4. An example of diffusion in the human body is the uptake of oxygen by the blood in the lungs and the release of carbon dioxide gas to the lungs from the blood.

### Osmosis

1. Osmosis is a special kind of diffusion.
2. Osmosis is the movement of water molecules through a semipermeable membrane, such as a plasma membrane, from an area of higher concentration of water molecules (e.g., pure water) to an area of low concentration of water molecules (e.g., water to which a solute like salt or sugar has been added).
3. An isotonic solution (e.g., normal saline) is a solution in which the salt concentration outside a cell is the same as that inside a cell. The cell would neither gain nor lose appreciable amounts of water.
4. A hypotonic solution (e.g., pure distilled water) is a solution in which the salt concentration inside the cell is higher than outside the cell. The cell would absorb water in such a solution.
5. A hypertonic solution (e.g., a 5% salt solution) is one in which the salt concentration is greater outside the cell than inside the cell. The cell would lose water in such a solution.

6. Active transport is the transportation of materials against a concentration gradient in opposition to other factors that would normally keep the material from entering the cell. This mechanism requires energy in the form of ATP and is the main mechanism by which most cells obtain the materials they need for normal functioning.

### pH

1. pH is the negative logarithm of the hydrogen ion concentration in a solution: $pH = -\log(H^+)$.
2. If a substance dissociates and forms an excess of $H^+$ ions when dissolved in water, it is referred to as an acid. Acids have pH values below 7.
3. A substance that combines with $H^+$ ions when dissolved in water is called a base. Basic solutions have a pH value above 7.
4. Distilled pure water has a pH value of 7 and is neutral.
5. Buffers are special substances that act as reservoirs for hydrogen ions, donating them to a solution when their concentration falls and taking them from a solution when their concentration rises. Buffers help maintain homeostasis within cells in regard to pH levels, keeping them fairly close to 7.

### REVIEW QUESTIONS

1. Describe the nature and structure of an atom.
2. List the major chemical elements found in living systems.
*3. Compare ionic and covalent bonding and indicate which major four elements found in cells bond covalently.
*4. Why is it necessary for a cell to have nucleic acids in its nucleus?
5. Explain the roles that water plays in living systems.
6. What two major roles do carbohydrates play in living cells?
7. List three functions of fats in the human body.
*8. List four functions of proteins necessary for the function and survival of the human body.
*9. Compare the differences and similarities between osmosis and diffusion and how they function in the body.

*10. What is the significance of active transport to the survival of a cell?

*11. Why is pH important to the maintenance of homeostasis in the body?

*Critical Thinking Questions

## Fill in the Blank

Fill in the blank with the most appropriate term.

1. Molecules that contain carbon, hydrogen, and oxygen are known as _Covalent Bond_. Glucose (a sugar) is one of these molecules.

2. Molecules known as _____ are the building blocks of protein.

3. All the carbon in the larger organic compounds found in living systems comes directly or indirectly from _____.

4. The smallest particles of elements that enter into chemical reactions are _____.

5. An _____ is a substance whose atoms all contain the same number of protons and the same number of electrons.

6. In the atoms of some elements, the number of neutrons varies. These different kinds of atoms are called _____.

7. Two kinds of chemical bonds found in living matter are _____ and _____ bonds.

8. The most abundant molecule found in living cells is _____.

9. Carbohydrates have two basic functions: _____ and _____.

10. Nucleotides bonded together between the phosphate group of one and the sugar of another form long chain molecules called _____.

## Matching

Place the most appropriate number in the blank provided.

____ $NH_3$

____ $C_6H_{12}O_6$

____ Glycogen

____ Starch

____ $CO_2$

____ OH

____ COOH

____ $NH_2$

____ $PO_4^-$

____ $C_5$

1. Plant carbohydrate
2. Hydroxyl group
3. Amino group
4. Ammonia
5. Glycerol
6. Carboxyl group
7. Inorganic phosphate group
8. Animal carbohydrate
9. Fatty acid
10. Ribose
11. Glucose
12. Carbon dioxide

_Laboratory Exercise: The Chemistry_

## LABORATORY EXERCISE: THE CHEMISTRY OF LIFE

Materials needed: A pH meter, osmosis kit, models of chemical molecules.

1. pH measurements: With the assistance of a pH meter provided by your instructor, measure the pH of tap water, distilled water, tomato juice, orange juice, apple juice, your saliva, a baking soda solution, ammonia, and household bleach. Prepare a chart to place these items under the basic or acidic category.

2. Demonstration of osmosis: Your instructor will demonstrate the effects of osmosis with the assistance of an osmosis kit from a biologic supply company. The experiment shown in Figure 2-13 will be demonstrated using first a 3% salt solution and then a 3% sugar solution.

3. Examine the chemical models, provided by your instructor, illustrating the molecular structures and bonding of some common substances found in living systems.

# 3

# Cell Structure

## CHAPTER OUTLINE

- **Introduction**

- **History of the cell theory**

- **Anatomy of a typical cell:** *Cell membrane; Cytoplasm of the cell; Nucleus:* Nuclear membrane, Nucleoplasm, Chromatin, Nucleolus; *Mitochondria; Lysosomes; Endoplasmic reticulum:* Rough or granular ER, Agranular or smooth ER; *Golgi apparatus; Ribosomes:* Protein synthesis; *Centrioles; Cilia and flagella; Plastids of plant cells:* The cell wall of plant cells

## CHAPTER OBJECTIVES

After studying this chapter, you should be able to:

1. Name the major contributors to the cell theory.

2. Explain the molecular structure of a cell membrane.

3. Describe the structure and function of cellular organelles.

4. Explain the significance and process of protein synthesis.

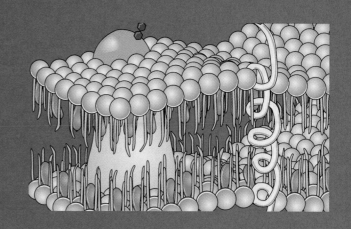

# KEY TERMS

## INTRODUCTION

The cell is the basic unit of biological organization of the human body. Our bodies are made up of trillions of cells. Although cells have different functions in the body, they all have certain common structural properties. All cells are composed of **protoplasm**, which is an aqueous colloidal solution of carbohydrates, proteins, lipids, nucleic acids, and inorganic salts surrounded by a limiting cell membrane. This protoplasm (proto meaning first and plasm meaning formed) is predominantly water with organic compounds in a colloidal suspension and inorganic compounds in solution. These compounds are the building blocks of structures within the protoplasm called **organelles**. Some organelles are common to most cells. Higher cells like those of the human body are called **eukaryotic** cells (eu = true); cells that do not have membrane-bound organelles (e.g., bacteria) are called **prokaryotic** cells.

Organelles that are common to all eukaryotic cells are the nucleus, the mitochondria, the endoplasmic reticulum, ribosomes, the Golgi apparatus, and lysosomes. If a cell has a specialized function that other cells do not have, for example, movement, the cell will have specialized organelles. Cells in our bodies that move materials across their exposed or free surface will be covered with row on row of hundreds of cilia. (For instance, cells in our respiratory tract produce mucus to trap dust and microorganisms that get past the hairs in our nose then move the material to our throat to be swallowed and passed out through the digestive system.) The human sperm cell, which must travel up the uterus of the female to the upper one-third of the fallopian or uterine tube to fertilize an egg, has a flagellum to propel it along its journey. Plant cells that do photosynthesis (the conversion of light energy into chemical energy, i.e., foods like sugars) have special organelles called chloroplasts.

When one observes a cell under the microscope in a laboratory, the most prominent structure in the cell is the nucleus, which is the control center of the cell. For this reason, the protoplasm of the cell is subdivided into two sections: the protoplasm inside the nucleus is called **nucleoplasm** and the protoplasm outside the nucleus is called the **cytoplasm**. Cells vary in size and most cells are too small to be seen with an unaided eye. Cells are measured in terms of **microns** (**MY**-kronz) more commonly called **micrometers** (my-**KROM**-ee-terz). One micrometer ($\mu$/m) equals one thousandth ($10^{-3}$) of a millimeter. Most eukaryotic cells range in size from 10 to 100 micrometers in diameter (10 to 100 millionths of a meter). Light microscopes allows us to see general features of cells with magnifications from 10× to 1000×. These are the microscopes we use in the laboratory. However to "see" or study the details of cells, an electron microscope must be used. These microscopes use a beam of electrons to visualize structures and are quite complex. A person must be specially trained to use one of these sophisticated instruments. Our current knowledge of cellular structure comes from research done on cell structure using electron microscopes. The diagrams of a typical animal cell (Figure 3-1) and a typical plant cell (Figure 3-2) illustrate a three-dimensional view of ultrastructure.

## HISTORY OF THE CELL THEORY

Because cells are too small to be seen with the naked eye, cells were not observed until the invention of the first microscope in the mid-17th century. Robert Hooke was an English scientist who first described cells in 1665. He built one of the first primitive microscopes to look at a thin slice of cork. Cork is nonliving plant tissue that comes from the bark of trees. Because this was dead plant tissue, he observed the cell walls of dead cells. They resembled tiny rooms so he called them cellulae (small rooms) from the Latin. Thus, the term cells has been used ever since.

Living cells were observed a few years later by the Dutch naturalist Anton von Leeuvenhoek. He observed pond water under his microscope and was amazed at what he saw in what he believed was pure water. He called the tiny organisms in the water animalcules (meaning little animals). It took, however, almost another 150 years before the significance of cells as the building blocks of biologic organization was to take hold.

It was two German scientists who laid the foundation of what we call today the cell theory. In 1838, Matthias Schleiden, a botanist, after careful study of plant tissues, stated that all plants are composed of individual units called cells. In 1839, Theodor Schwann, a zoologist, stated that all ani-

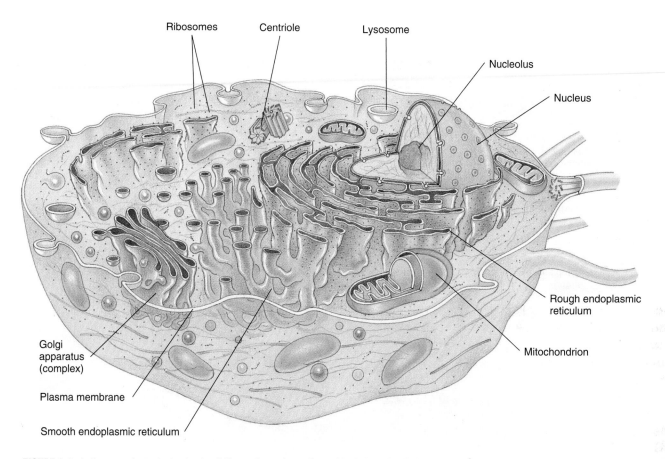

**FIGURE 3-1.** A diagram of a typical animal cell illustrating a three-dimensional view of cell ultrastructure.

Ribosomes  Centriole  Lysosome  Nucleolus  Nucleus  Rough endoplasmic reticulum  Mitochondrion  Golgi apparatus (complex)  Plasma membrane  Smooth endoplasmic reticulum

mals are also composed of individual units called cells. Thus the foundation of our modern cell theory was formed.

The modern cell theory consists of the following principles:

1. Cells are the smallest complete living things—they are the basic units of organization of all organisms.
2. All organisms are composed of one or more cells in which all life processes occur.
3. Cells arise only from preexisting cells through the process of cell division.
4. All of today's existing cells are descendants of the first cells formed early in the evolutionary history of life on earth.

## ANATOMY OF A TYPICAL CELL

The following structures of a cell will be discussed: cell membrane, cytoplasm, nucleus, nuclear membrane, nucleoplasm, chromatin, nucleolus, mito-chondria, lysosomes, endoplasmic reticulum (both rough and smooth), Golgi apparatus, and ribosomes.

### The Cell Membrane

All cells are surrounded by a cell membrane. This membrane is often called the **plasma membrane** or the **plasmalemma**. (Figure 3-3). Under the high magnification of an electron microscope, this membrane is composed of a double phospholipid layer with proteins embedded in the phospholipid layer. The phospholipids look like balloons with tails. The round balloon-like part is hydrophilic (attracts water) and the double tails are hydrophobic (repels water). This arrangement allows for the easy passage of water molecules through the cell membrane via osmosis (discussed in Chapter 2). The proteins embedded in the double phospholipid layer allow for the passage of molecules and ions across the cell membrane (Figure 3-4). Some proteins make transport channels for small dissolved ions, others act as enzymes for the active transport of materials into the cell against a concentration gradient and

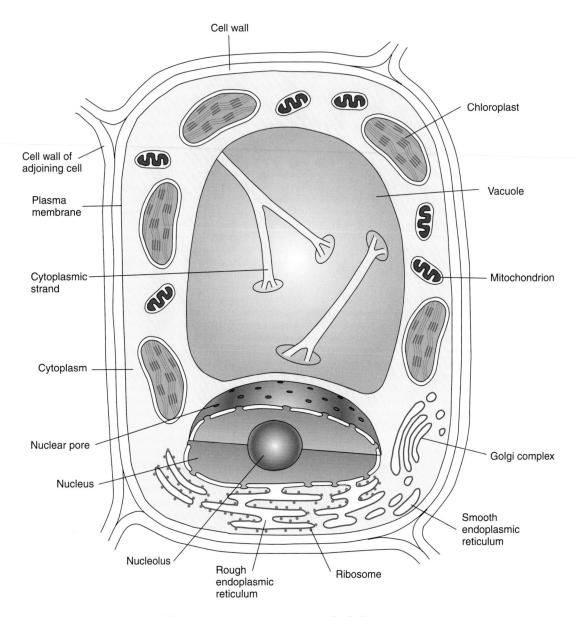

**FIGURE 3-2.** A diagram of a typical plant cell illustrating a three-dimensional view of cell ultrastructure.

need adenosine triphosphate (ATP) to function, other proteins act as receptor sites for hormones to gain entrance into the cell, and still other proteins act as cell identity markers. In addition, some proteins in the phospholipid layer act as cementing materials for cell adhesion on the outside of cells to hold cells together; others act as structural supports inside the cell attaching to cytoskeleton structures, which hold organelles in place in the cytoplasm. Proteins also make up the structure of the sodium–potassium pump, a unique feature of certain cell membranes like muscle cell membranes and nerve cell membranes (Figure 3-5).

These molecules of proteins and phospholipids are currently referred to in their arrangement as a **fluid mosaic pattern**. The molecules are like the tiles of a mosaic but rather than being embedded in a solid cement-like material, they are embedded in a fluid and can move slightly to allow the passage of materials across the cell membrane and thus into the cytoplasm of the cell. This basic molecular structure of the cell membrane is the

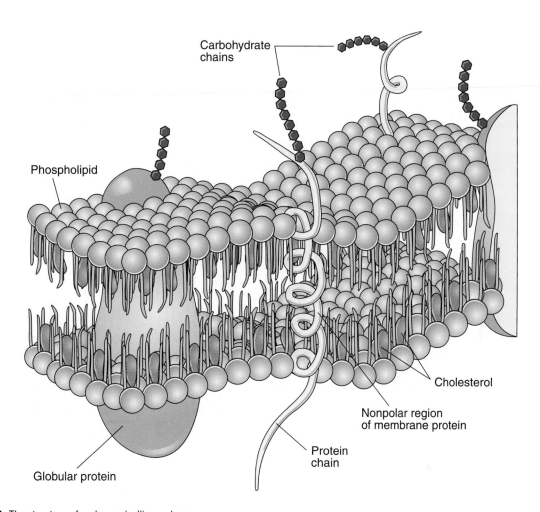

**FIGURE 3-3.** The structure of a plasma (cell) membrane.

same for all other membrane-bound organelles of the cell.

## Cytoplasm of the Cell

The liquid portion of a cell is called protoplasm. The protoplasm outside the nucleus is called cytoplasm; the protoplasm inside the nucleus is called nucleoplasm. The main constituent of cytoplasm is water. This water, however, has many different kinds of chemical compounds distributed among the water molecules. Some of these compounds are nucleic acids like transfer ribonucleic acid (RNA) and messsenger RNA, enzymes, hormones, and various other chemicals involved in the functioning of the cell. Some of these compounds are in solution in the water, whereas others are in a colloidal suspension. In both solutions and colloids, substances are uniformly distributed throughout the water medium. In a solution, however, *individual* atoms or ions are distributed throughout the medium. In a colloid, *clumps* of atoms rather than individual atoms are distributed throughout the medium.

The factor that determines whether a substance will go into solution or a colloidal suspension in water is the electronic interaction between the molecules of the substance and the molecules of water. Because the oxygen atom in $H_2O$ has a stronger attraction for the electrons in the H-O bond than the hydrogen atom does (it shares the electrons unequally), the oxygen atom is *slightly* negative and the two hydrogen atoms are *slightly* positive. Refer to Figure 2-5 in Chapter 2. A molecule with such an unequal electron distribution of bonding electrons is said to be **polar.** Because of this polarity of the water molecule, other polar compounds, like ionically bonded compounds such as salt (sodium

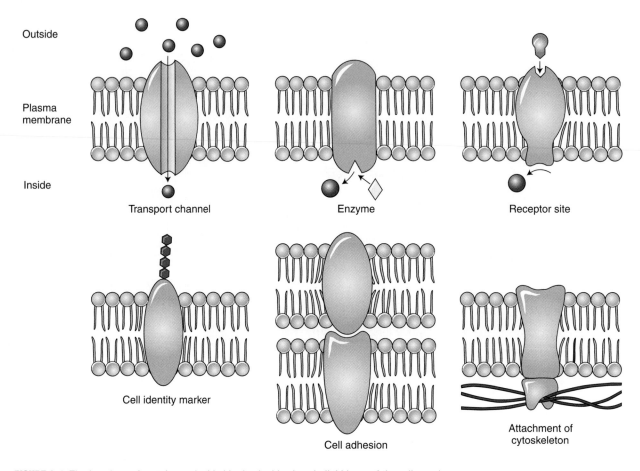

Outside

Plasma
membrane

Inside

Transport channel

Enzyme

Receptor site

Cell identity marker

Cell adhesion

Attachment of
cytoskeleton

**FIGURE 3-4**. The functions of proteins embedded in the double phospholipid layer of the cell membrane.

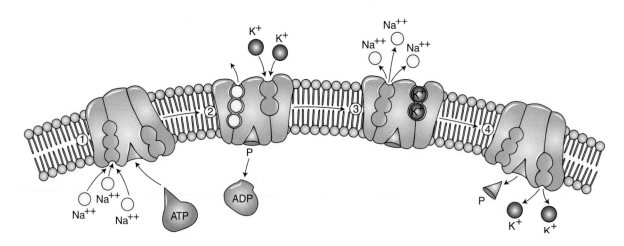

**FIGURE 3-5.** The protein nature of the sodium–potassium pump of the cell membrane of muscle and nerve cells.

chloride: $Na^+Cl^-$) are readily *soluble* in water and go into solution. The polarity of the water molecules lessens the electrostatic forces holding ionically bonded molecules together so that they dissociate into individual ions and dissolve in the water.

Other compounds such as covalently bonded molecules are made up of atoms that have equal attraction for the bonding electrons that hold them together. Thus, the bonding electrons are not attracted to one atom of the bond more than the other. Compounds with such unpolarized bonds are called **nonpolar** and do not dissolve readily in water. The organic compounds with the C-H bonds are nonpolar and thus they go into a colloidal suspension in the watery medium of the cytoplasm. Proteins, carbohydrates, fats, and nucleic acids are colloidally suspended in the cytoplasm while the mineral salts like sodium, potassium, calcium, chlorine, and phosphorous are in solution.

Some cellular components, such as storage granules and fat droplets, are neither dissolved nor suspended in the cytoplasm. These compounds are products of cellular functions that have collected at certain specific sites within the cytoplasm. The cytoplasm will also contain structures called **vacuoles**. A vacuole is an area within the cytoplasm that is surrounded by a vacuolar membrane. This membrane has the same structure as the cell membrane. A vacuole is generally filled with a watery mixture but can also contain stored food (food vacuole) or waste products of the cell.

## The Nucleus

The **nucleus** is the most prominent structure in the cell. It is clearly visible with a light compound microscope. It is a fluid-containing structure that is separated from the cytoplasm by the **nuclear membrane**, sometimes referred to as the nuclear envelope. The nucleus is the control center of the cell. Cells whose nuclei have been removed lose their functions and eventually die. Cells with a nucleus transplanted from a different cell take on the characteristics of the cell from which the nucleus was taken.

## Nuclear Membrane

A unique feature of the nuclear membrane or envelope is that it is composed of two membranes (Figure 3-6). The inner membrane surrounds and contains the nucleoplasm and its materials. The outer membrane is continuous with the endoplasmic reticulum (ER), an organelle discussed later. The electron microscope has revealed the presence of pores or openings in the double nuclear membrane. These pores have a very fine partition to hinder the free transport or leakage of materials of the nucleoplasm but which allow the passage of materials from the nucleoplasm, which must gain access to the cytoplasm. For example, when protein

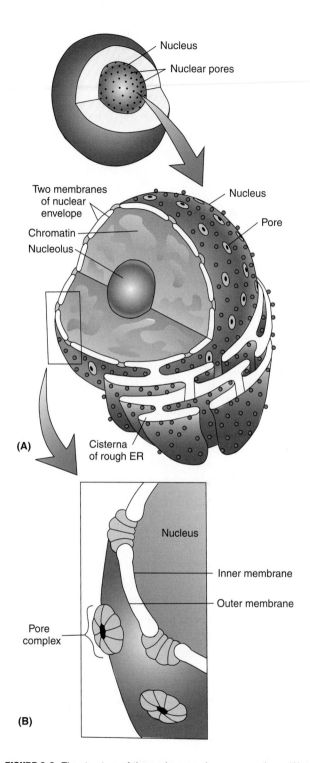

**FIGURE 3-6.** The structure of the nuclear membrane or envelope. (A) Diagrammatic view of the internal anatomy of the nucleus and the connection of the outer nuclear membrane with rough endoplasmic reticulum. (B) Diagrammatic view of the pore complex.

synthesis must take place, the code to make the protein is on the DNA in the nucleus but the protein is made at a ribosomal site in the cytoplasm. The code is copied from the DNA by a special molecule called messenger RNA (m RNA), which leaves the nucleus through a pore to go to the ribosome. We shall discuss this process in more detail later in the chapter. The structure of the nuclear membrane is the same fluid mosaic pattern as the cell or plasma membrane.

## Nucleoplasm

The fluid medium of the nucleus is called the nucleoplasm. It consists of a colloidal suspension of proteins, the nucleic acids DNA, **deoxyribonucleic acid** (dee-ock-see-rye-boh-noo-**KLEE**-ik **ASS**-id), and RNA, **ribonucleic acid** (rye-boh-noo-**KLEE**-ik **ASS**-id), enzymes, and other chemicals of the nucleus. Many chemical reactions occur in the nucleoplasm and are essential to cellular function and survival, including cellular reproduction.

## Chromatin

When the cell is stained, fine dark threads appear in the nucleus. This material is called **chromatin** (**KROH**-mah-tin) and is the genetic material of the cell. The cells of the human body contain 46 chromosomes (22 pairs of autosomes and one pair of sex chromosomes: one member of each pair comes from the father and one member from the mother). The egg cell and the sperm cell contain one half that number or 23 chromosomes. Chromosomes are made of DNA molecules and proteins. When the DNA molecules duplicate during cell division, they shorten and thicken and become visible. We now call the DNA chromosomes. When the cell is not dividing, the DNA molecules are long and thin and visible only as chromatin. All of the above terms are used to describe the different levels of chromosomal organization (Figure 3-7). We shall discuss this in greater detail in Chapter 4. DNA controls *all* of the functions of the cell.

## Nucleolus

The **nucleolus** (noo-**KLEE**-oh-lus) is a spherical particle within the nucleoplasm that does not have a covering membrane around it. It is composed of primarily DNA, RNA, and proteins. A cell may have more than one nucleolus. This structure is the site of ribosomal synthesis. It is involved in protein syn-

thesis because it makes the ribosomes and ribosomes are the sites of protein synthesis.

## The Mitochondria

A **mitochondrion** (singular) or mitochondria (my-toh-**KON**-dree-ah) (plural) are small oblong-shaped structures composed of two membranes (Figure 3-8). The outer membrane gives a mitochondrion its capsule shape; the inner membrane

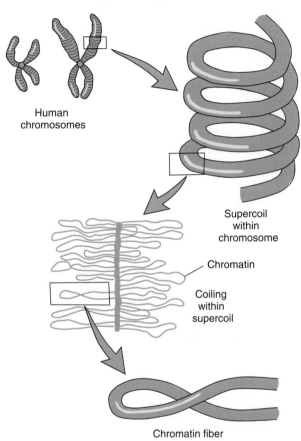

**FIGURE 3-7.** Some different levels of chromosomal organization.

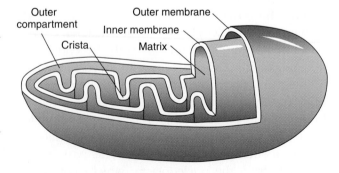

**FIGURE 3-8.** The membrane structure of a typical mitochondrion.

folds on itself to provide a surface on which the energy-releasing chemical reactions of the cell occur. When viewed under a light compound microscope, mitochondria appear only as small dark granules in the cytoplasm. It is the electron microscope that has revealed to us the true nature of the mitochondria. The folds of the inner membrane are called **cristae** (**KRIS**-tee). It is on the cristae that cellular respiration occurs, where food (chemical energy) is converted into another usable form of chemical energy, ATP. For this reason, the mitochondria are known as the powerhouses of the cell.

In its most simple expression, cellular respiration can be stated as follows:

Food (like glucose) + oxygen → energy + waste or $C_6H_{12}O_6 + 6O_2 \rightarrow ATP + 6CO_2 + 6H_2O$.

This chemical reaction will be discussed in greater detail in Chapter 4.

Most of the energy-producing reactions, which occur in the mitochondria, take place on the surface of the cristae. Cells with high energy requirements (like muscle cells), will have mitochondria with many folds or cristae. Cells with low energy requirements, like the lining of the cheek (epithelial cells), will have mitochondria with fewer folds or cristae. All cells will have approximately the same number of mitochondria.

## Lysosomes

**Lysosomes** (**LIGH**-so-sohmz) are small bodies in the cytoplasm that contain powerful digestive enzymes to enhance the breakdown of cellular components (Figure 3-1). The structure and size of lysosomes vary but they are generally spherical. They have three general functions:

1. They act in conjunction with stored food vacuoles. When a cell needs more energy, a lysosome will fuse with a stored food vacuole to break down the stored food into a more usable form that can go to a mitochondrion to be converted into ATP. For example, starch, a complex carbohydrate, will be broken down into simple sugars, protein into amino acids; and fats into fatty acids and glycerol.

2. Lysosomes also act in the maintenance and repair of cellular components. If a section of ER needs to be rebuilt, the lysosome will

break down the membrane into amino acids, fatty acids, glycerol, and so on and material that can be recycled to build new protein and phospholipids.

3. Lysosomes also act as suicide agents in old and weakened cells. This process is known as **autolysis** (aw-**TAHL**-ih-sis). The lysosome will expel all of its enzymes directly into the cytoplasm of the cell to destroy the cell and its organelles.

## Endoplasmic Reticulum

The **endoplasmic reticulum** (en-doh-**PLAZ**-mik re-**TIK**-you-lum) or ER is a complex system of membranes that forms a collection of membrane-bound cavities. These often interconnect into a membrane-bound system of channels within the cytoplasm. The shape and size of these cavities vary with the type of cell. When the cavities are sac-like or channel-like, they are called **cisternae** (sis-**TER**-nee) and are used to store and transport materials made by the cell. The ER is attached to the outer membrane of the nuclear membrane or envelope and ultimately connects with the cell membrane (Figure 3-9). With the use of the electron microscope, it was discovered that there are two types of ER, a rough ER, and a smooth ER.

### The Rough or Granular ER

All cells will have a **rough** or **granular ER**. It is called rough or granular because it has ribosomes attached to it. These are the granules on the ER. Because of the attached ribosomes, the rough ER is a site of protein synthesis. Proteins that will be secreted by the cell are synthesized there. The cavities and vesicles of the rough ER serve in the segregation and transport of these proteins in preparation for further discharge and processing. The rough ER may also be involved in the collection of digestive enzymes to form lysosomes.

### The Agranular or Smooth ER

Occasionally a **smooth** or **agranular ER** will be attached to a granular ER (Figure 3-9). Structurally the agranular form differs from the rough form. It does not have attached ribosomes. It also differs in function. Only certain cells have the agranular or smooth ER. It is found in the cells of the gonads in which sex hormones are being synthesized. One

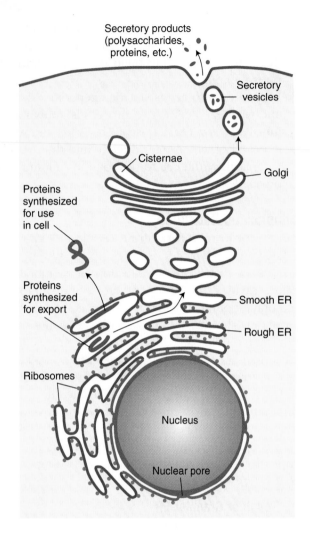

**FIGURE 3-9.** The structure and nature of the endoplasmic reticulum and the Golgi body.

function appears to be sex hormone synthesis. It is also found in the cells of the lacteals of the villi of the small intestine. Thus, it is also believed to be involved in the transportation of fats.

## The Golgi Apparatus

The **Golgi** (**GOHL**-jee) **apparatus** is also called the **Golgi body**. It consists of an assembly of flat saclike cisternae that resembles a stack of saucers or pancakes (Figure 3-9). Golgi bodies can differ in both size and compactness. They function as the points within the cell where compounds to be secreted by the cell are collected and concentrated. They may be seen attached to the ER. When the cell's secretions are a combination of both proteins and carbohydrates, the carbohydrates will be syn-

thesized in the Golgi apparatus and the complexes of carbohydrates and proteins are assembled there. In the pancreas, enzymes synthesized by the ribosomes are collected in the membranes of the Golgi apparatus and then are secreted. Lysosomes may also form at the Golgi body when digestive enzymes are collected there.

## Ribosomes

**Ribosomes** (**RYE**-boh-sohmz) are tiny granules distributed throughout the cytoplasm and are attached to the rough or granular ER. They are not surrounded by a membrane. Ribosomes are composed of ribosomal RNA and proteins. Messenger RNA attaches to ribosomes during proteins synthesis. There are many, many ribosomes in the cell because they are so essential to cell function. They are the sites of protein synthesis.

## Protein Synthesis

Proteins are essential to cellular function and structure. Proteins are part of membrane structures (proteins are embedded in the double phospholipid layer); enzymes are protein catalysts (all chemical reactions in the cell require enzymes); and our immune system functions through the production of antibodies (large proteins) that attack foreign proteins (antigens).

The code to make a particular protein lies on a DNA molecule in the nucleus. Genes on the DNA molecule constitute the code. However, proteins are made at the ribosomes. Therefore, this code must be copied and taken to the ribosomes. A special molecule called **messenger RNA** (mRNA) copies the code from the DNA molecule in the nucleus. This process is called **transcription** and occurs with the assistance of an enzyme called RNA polymerase. The mRNA then leaves the nucleus through a nuclear pore and goes into the cytoplasm to a ribosome or group of ribosomes. The ribosome will now assist in the assemblage of the protein because it now has the code or recipe to produce the protein. To make the protein, the ribosome now needs the ingredients, which are amino acids.

Another molecule will now go into the cytoplasm and collect the amino acids. This molecule is **transfer RNA** (tRNA). It is coded for a particular amino acid by means of three nitrogen bases at one end of the molecule known as the anti-codon. These three bases will fit or match with three bases on the mRNA molecule called the codon. In this way a series of tRNA molecules bring amino acids to certain sites on the mRNA molecule. This process is called **translation** (reading the code and bringing the appropriate amino acids in sequence along the mRNA). Now the ribosomes, with the assistance of enzymes, put the amino acids together by linking them up and forming a polypeptide chain (Figure 3-10). The numerous ribosomes found in the cell indicate the importance and significance of protein synthesis to the survival and function of the cell.

## Centrioles

Two **centrioles** (**SEN**-tree-olz) are found at right angles to each other near the nuclear membrane. The pair together is referred to as a **centrosome** (**SEN**-troh-sohm). They are composed of nine sets of triplet fibers (Figure 3-11). The inner fiber of each triplet is connected to the outer fiber of the adjacent triplet by a subfiber.

During cell division, the centrioles move to each side of the dividing cell and position themselves at a location called the opposite pole of the cell. They now form a system of **microtubules**, which are

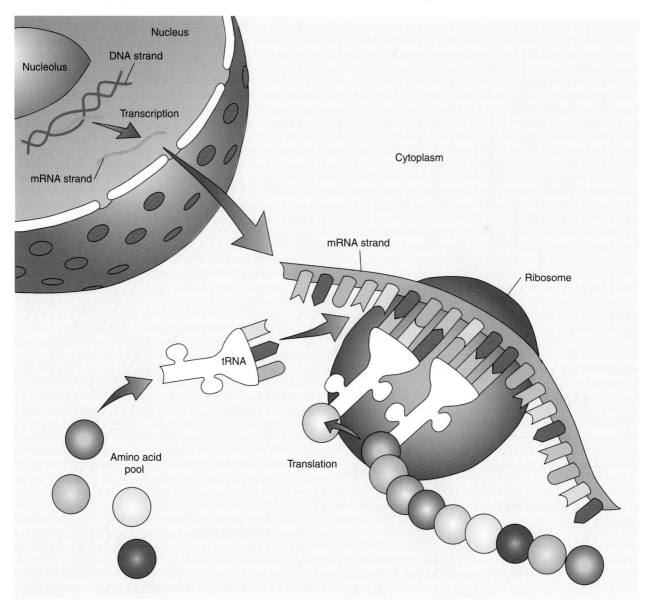

**FIGURE 3-10.** An overview of the process of protein synthesis.

Microtubule
triplet

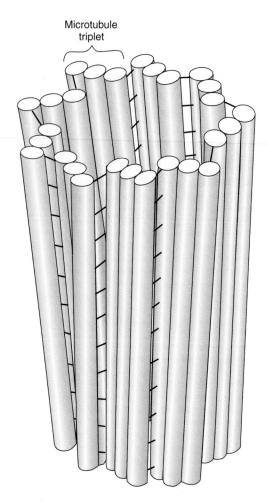

**FIGURE 3-11.** The structure of a centriole.

long, hollow cylinders made of a protein called **tubulin**. These fibers or microtubules redistribute the duplicated chromosomes during cell division into the appropriate new daughter cells.

### Cilia and Flagella

Cilia (**SIL**-lee-ah) and **flagella** (fla-**JELL**-ah) are cellular organelles located on the cell surface. They are composed of fibrils that protrude from the cell and beat or vibrate. Some single-celled organisms use these structures to move through a medium. For example, *Euglena* has a flagellum that propels it through the water; whereas a *Paramecium* is covered with row upon row of hundreds of cilia to allow it to swim in pond water. In the human body the male sperm cell is propelled by a single beating flagellum that assists it in reaching the female egg in the upper part of the fallopian or uterine tube where they unite in fertilization. Stationary cells,

like those that line our respiratory tract, are covered with cilia on their free edge to move the mucus-dust package upward across the cell surfaces to bring this material to the throat to be swallowed and then discharged from the body.

Although cilia and flagella are similar anatomically, a flagellum is considerably longer than a cilium. A cell with cilia will have row on row of cilia, but a cell with flagella will have one (like the sperm cell) or two or four like some single-celled protozoans.

Externally, these structures are hairlike protrusions from the cell membrane. Internally they are composed of nine double fibrils arranged in a cylindrical ring around two single, central fibrils (Figure 3-12). The microtubules or fibrils of the flagellum arise from a structure called the basal body found just below the area from which the flagellum protrudes from the surface of the cell membrane. The basal body or plate has a cylindrical structure like the centriole, that is, it is also composed of nine sets of triplet fibers.

### Plastids of Plant Cells

In our laboratory exercise on cells we will examine and compare plant cells with animal cells. Therefore, it is necessary to discuss these organelles found only in plant cells. There are three plastids found in plant cells. The most common and most numerous of these are the **chloroplasts** (**KLOR**-oh-plastz) that cause plants to look green.

Chloroplasts are large organelles found mainly in plant cells (Figure 3-13). They contain the green pigment chlorophyll. These organelles are the site of photosynthesis. It is here that the light energy of the sun is converted into chemical energy and food for use by both plants and animals. Without plants and their chloroplasts, animals could not survive on this planet. The process of photosynthesis occurs inside the chloroplast. This chemical equation is: $6CO_2 + 12H_2O \rightarrow C_6H_{12}O_6$ or glucose (sugar, food) $+ 6O_2$ (the air we breathe) $+ 6H_2O$

Chloroplasts are large enough to be easily seen with a light microscope. They are enclosed by a membrane but the internal membranous structure is complex. The inside contains many stacks of membranes called a **granum**. A granum is made of a stack of individual double membranes called a **thylakoid** (**THIGH**-lah-koid). The grana (plural) are

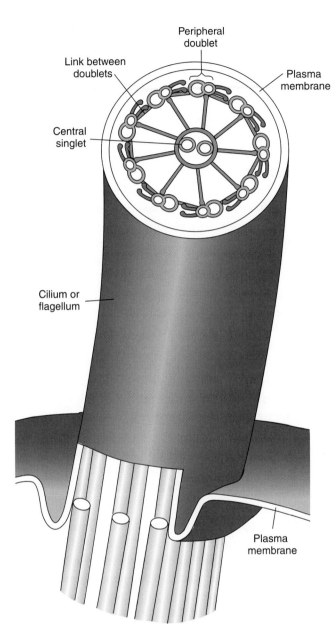

**FIGURE 3-12.** The internal anatomy of a cilius or a flagellum.

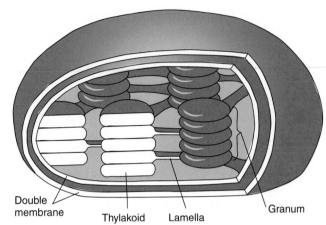

**FIGURE 3-13.** The internal anatomy of a chloroplast.

carotene (**KAR**-oh-teen), which produces a red/orange color (tomatoes and carrots). These pigments also produce the colors of flower petals and fruits. Another type of plastid is the **leucoplast** (**LOO**-koh-plast). Leucoplasts do not have any pigments—they are storage plastids. An onion bulb is full of leucoplasts where sugar is stored and a potato contains leucoplasts where starch is stored.

## The Cell Wall of Plant Cells
The cell membrane of plant cells is surrounded by a semirigid covering called the cell wall made of a complex carbohydrate called **cellulose** (**SELL**-you-lohs). Cellulose is synthesized by Golgi bodies by linking up glucose units. Animal cells do not have cell walls. This material is what we call fiber in our diet. It cannot be digested; thus, it keeps our stools soft. We eat fruits and vegetables to maintain a balance of fiber in our diet. This fiber may help prevent the development of colon cancer.

connected to one another by a different system of membranes called **lamella**. The grana are made of proteins, enzymes, chlorophyll, and other pigments arranged in a layered structure.

Plant cells also have two other types of plastids. **Chromoplasts** (**KROH**-moh-plastz) are similar in structure to chloroplasts but they contain other pigments like the carotenoid pigments. The carotenoid pigments are **xanthophyll** (**ZAN**-tho-fill), which produces a yellow color (the skin on a banana) and

## Summary Outline
### INTRODUCTION
1. The cell is the basic unit of biologic organization. It is composed of a fluid medium called protoplasm surrounded by a cell or plasma membrane. Structures within this protoplasm are called organelles.
2. The protoplasm inside the nucleus is called nucleoplasm; the protoplasm outside the nucleus is called cytoplasm.

## HISTORY OF THE CELL THEORY

1. Two Germans, Matthias Schleiden, a botanist, and Theodor Schwann, a zoologist, were the first biologists to propose the cell theory in the 1830s.
2. The modern cell theory states that cells are the basic units of organization of all organisms; all organisms are composed of one or more cells; cells arise from only preexisting cells through cell division; and all existing cells are the descendants of the first cells formed early in the evolutionary history of life on earth.

## THE CELL MEMBRANE

1. The cell membrane or plasma membrane is made up of a double phospholipid layer with proteins embedded in the phospholipid layer.
2. The phospholipid layer allows for the free passage of water molecules through the cell membrane via osmosis while the proteins act as channels, active transport areas, receptor sites, and identity markers for the cell.
3. This molecular arrangement of the cell membrane is referred to as a fluid mosaic pattern and is responsible for the selective permeability of the membrane. It is through the membrane that materials enter and exit the cell.

## CYTOPLASM OF THE CELL

1. The main constituent of cytoplasm is water. Chemical compounds like the mineral salts are dissolved in solution in this water; chemical compounds with the C-H bond (organic molecules) are in colloidal suspension.
2. In a solution, individual atoms or ions are distributed throughout the watery medium; in a colloid, clumps of atoms rather than individual atoms are distributed throughout the watery medium.
3. The water molecule has unique properties, which determines whether molecules will go into solution or a colloidal suspension. The oxygen atom in $H_2O$ has a stronger attraction for the electrons in the H-O bond than the hydrogen atoms; thus, the oxygen atom is slightly negative, whereas the two hydrogen atoms are slightly positive.

4. Polar compounds, such as the ionically bonded mineral salts, will dissolve in water and go into solution; nonpolar compounds, such as the covalently bonded molecules of proteins, carbohydrates, fats, and nucleic acids, will go into colloidal suspension.
5. The cytoplasm of the cell will also contain storage granules, fat droplets, and vacuoles.

## THE NUCLEUS

1. The nucleus is the control center of the cell. It is surrounded by a double nuclear membrane. The inner nuclear membrane surrounds the fluid part of the nucleus, called nucleoplasm, while the outer nuclear membrane connects with the endoplasmic reticulum.
2. The nuclear membrane is perforated with pores that allow materials like messenger RNA to leave the nucleus and go into the cytoplasm of the cell.
3. The genetic material inside the nucleoplasm is darkly stained threads of nucleic acids called chromatin. This chromatin will duplicate, shorten, and thicken during cell division and will become visible as chromosomes.
4. The nucleolus is a spherical particle within the nucleoplasm that does not have a covering membrane. It is the site where ribosomes are made.

## THE MITOCHONDRIA

1. The mitochondria are the powerhouses of the cell. Each mitochondrion is composed of two membranes. The outer membrane forms its capsular shape, and the inner membrane folds on itself to increase surface area.
2. The inner folds of the mitochondrion are called cristae. It is in the mitochondrion where the aerobic phase of cellular respiration occurs:

$$C_6H_{12}O_6 + 6O_2 \rightarrow ATP \text{ (energy)} + 6CO_2 + 6H_2O$$

3. Cells with higher energy requirements, like muscle cells, will have mitochondria with many cristae; those with lower energy requirements will have fewer cristae.

## LYSOSOMES

1. Lysosomes are small structures in the cytoplasm surrounded by a membrane and contain powerful digestive enzymes.

**2.** Lysosomes function in three different ways in the cell: they function with food vacuoles to digest stored food; they function in the maintenance and repair of cellular organelles; and they act as suicide agents in old and weakened cells.

## ENDOPLASMIC RETICULUM

**1.** The endoplasmic reticulum or ER is a complex system of membranes that makes up a collection of membrane-bound cavities or channels. These channels are called cisternae.

**2.** The ER connects with the outer nuclear membrane and with the cell membrane.

**3.** There are two types of ER. All cells have a rough or granular ER whose membranes have attached ribosomes. The funtion of rough ER is protein synthesis. Some cells also have a smooth or agranular ER, which does not have attached ribosomes. The function of a smooth ER can be the transportation of fats or the synthesis of the sex hormones.

## THE GOLGI APPARATUS

**1.** The Golgi body or apparatus is a collection of flat saclike cisternae that look like a stack of pancakes.

**2.** They function as points within the cytoplasm where compounds to be secreted by the cell are concentrated and collected. They act like storage warehouses of the cell.

**3.** If the cell is synthesizing carbohydrates and proteins, the carbohydrates will be synthesized in the Golgi apparatus.

## RIBOSOMES

**1.** Ribosomes are small granules distributed throughout the cytoplasm and attached to the rough ER. They are not covered by a membrane.

**2.** Ribosomes are the site of protein synthesis.

## PROTEIN SYNTHESIS

**1.** Proteins function in major and essential ways for cellular function and survival. They are part of the structure of membranes; they act as enzymes or catalysts that make chemical reactions occur in the cell; and they function in our immune response.

**2.** The code to make a particular protein is a gene on a DNA molecule. The DNA is found in the nucleus, whereas the protein is made at a ribosomal site in the cytoplasm.

**3.** A special molecule called messenger RNA copies the code from the DNA molecule in a process called transcription. The mRNA then leaves the nucleus through a nuclear pore and takes the code to a ribosome or group of ribosomes.

**4.** Other molecules called transfer RNAs go into the cytoplasm and pick up particular amino acids. Each tRNA molecule is coded for a particular amino acid by its anti-codon loop at the end of the molecule. The anti-codon loop will only match a particular site on the mRNA molecule called the codon. This process is called translation.

**5.** The ribosomes will now link up the amino acids brought to the mRNA molecule by the tRNA molecules and will construct the protein with the assistance of enzymes.

## CENTRIOLES

**1.** Two centrioles are found at right angles to each other near the nuclear membrane. The pair is referred to as a centrosome.

**2.** Each centriole is composed of nine sets of triplet fibers.

**3.** The centrioles form the spindle fibers during cell division and guide the duplicated chromosomes to their daughter cells.

## CILIA AND FLAGELLA

**1.** Cilia are short and flagella are long hairlike protrusions from the cell membrane. Internally they are composed of nine double fibrils arranged in a ring around two single central fibrils.

**2.** A cell with cilia will have row upon row of cilia. Cilia will move materials across the free surface of a cell, like respiratory tract cells, which move the mucous-dust package up to our throat.

**3.** A cell with a flagellum, like the sperm cell, will propel the cell through a medium.

## PLASTIDS OF PLANT CELLS

**1.** The most common plastid of plant cells is the chloroplast, which contains the green pigment chlorophyll that allows plant cells to perform photosynthesis.

2. Photosynthesis is the conversion of light energy (the sun) into chemical energy (food like glucose).
3. Chromoplasts are plastids that contain the carotenoid pigments, xanthophyll (yellow) and carotene (orange/red).
4. Leucoplasts are plastids that store food (e.g., sugar and starch). They contain no pigment and are colorless.

## THE CELL WALL OF PLANT CELLS

1. The cell membrane of plant cells is surrounded by a semirigid covering called the cell wall. It is composed of cellulose, synthesized by the Golgi apparatus, and secreted through the cell membrane.
2. Cellulose is the material in our diet that we call fiber.

## REVIEW QUESTIONS

1. Define a cell.
2. List the major points of the modern cell theory.
*3. Why is the molecular structure of a cell membrane referred to as a fluid mosaic pattern?
*4. Explain why some chemical compounds go into solution and others go into a colloidal suspension in the cytoplasm of a cell.
*5. Why is the nucleus considered the control center of the cell?
*6. Based on their structure why are mitochondria called the powerhouses of the cell?
7. List three functions of lysosomes.
8. What are the two types of endoplasmic reticulum and what are their functions in the cell?
9. What is the function of a Golgi apparatus?
*10. Why are ribosomes so numerous in the cytoplasm of a cell?
11. List three important functions of proteins in a cell.
12. What is a centrosome?
13. List the functions of cilia and flagella.
14. Name and define the three types of plastids found in plant cells.

*15. Why should plant cells be studied in a human anatomy and physiology class?

*Critical Thinking Questions

## Fill in the Blank
Fill in the blank with the most appropriate term.
1. The cell theory was first proposed in the 1830s by _____ and _____.
2. Modern details of cellular structure have been extensively studied because of the invention of the _____ microscope.
3. Cell membranes are made of layers, a double _____ with _____ embedded in this double layer.
4. The main component of cytoplasm is _____.
5. In a solution, _____ atoms or ions of a substance are distributed throughout the medium.
6. In a colloid, _____ of atoms are distributed throughout the medium.
7. Because the oxygen atom in $H_2O$ has a stronger attraction for the electrons in the H-O bond than the hydrogen atom does, the oxygen atom has a slightly _____ charge and the hydrogen atoms have a slightly _____ charge.
8. Ionically bonded molecules are called _____, whereas covalently bonded molecules are called non _____ molecules.
9. The nuclear membrane or envelope is composed of two membranes, the outer membrane is generally continuous with the _____, which often has ribosomes attached to it.
10. The fluid medium of the nucleus is specifically called _____.
11. During cell division, chromatin condenses into thick rodlike structures called _____, which become visible with a light microscope.
12. A spherical particle within the nucleus that does not have a covering membrane is the

_____; it is the site of ribosome synthesis.

13. The convolutions of the inner membrane of the mitochondrion are called _____.

14. _____ are small bodies in the cytoplasm that contain enzymes that enhance the breakdown of cellular components.

15. When the membrane-bound cavities of the endoplasmic reticulum are channel or saclike they are called _____.

16. The _____ seems to function as a point within the cell where compounds to be secreted by the cell are collected and concentrated and where carbohydrates are synthesized.

17. Protein synthesis occurs at the _____, which are composed of RNA and protein and are not surrounded by a membrane.

18. The interior of chloroplasts consists of many stacks of membranes called _____.

19. Internally a flagellum is composed of _____ double fibrils arranged in a cylindrical ring around _____ central single fibrils.

20. Centrioles form the _____, which distribute the daughter chromosomes during cell division to the daughter cells.

---

## Matching

Place the most appropriate number in the blank provided.

| | |
|---|---|
| ____ Mitochondrion | 1. Lysosomes |
| ____ Muscle cells | 2. Lacteals |
| ____ Enzymes | 3. Protein synthesis |
| ____ Sex hormone synthesized | 4. Redistribute chromosomes |
| | 5. Powerhouse of the cell |
| ____ Ribosomes | 6. Locomotion |
| ____ Chloroplasts | 7. Carotenoid pigments |
| ____ Centriole | 8. Cisternae |
| ____ Flagella | 9. Many cristae |
| ____ Cell wall | 10. Agranular endoplasmic reticulum |
| ____ Channels of the ER | 11. Cellulose |
| | 12. Site of photosynthesis |

## LABORATORY EXERCISE: CELL STRUCTURE

Materials needed: Compound light microscope; prepared microscope slides of the letter e, and colored threads, living *Elodea* plant and an onion bulb, living culture of *Paramecium*, flat-edged toothpicks and methylene blue stain, dissecting microscope and a moss plant, videotape or CD-ROM on "How to Use a Microscope."

### I.  USING A COMPOUND LIGHT MICROSCOPE

Your compound microscope is an expensive and delicate piece of equipment and must be handled carefully. Review the videotape or CD-ROM, provided by your instructor, on the operation and parts of your microscope. Figure 3-14 shows the parts of a compound light microscope.

### A.  PARTS OF A COMPOUND MICROSCOPE

1. Remove your assigned microscope from its storage area using two hands. Grab the *arm* with one hand and support the *base* with your other hand. Bring the microscope to your laboratory station and place it down gently. Unwind the electrical cord and plug it in.

2. Identify the *body tube*. At the top of the body tube is the *ocular lens* usually with a magnification of 10×. At the end of the body

(continues)

## LABORATORY EXERCISE: CELL STRUCTURE (continued)

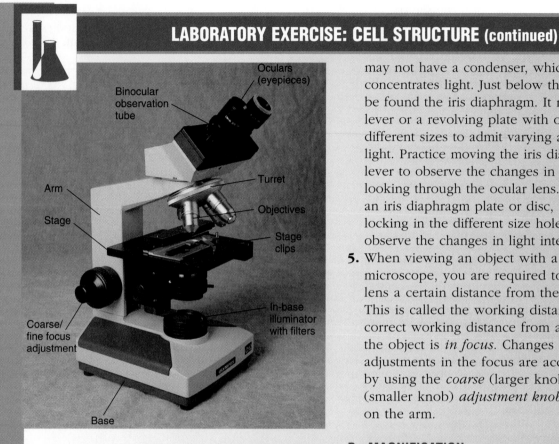

**FIGURE 3-14.** The parts of a compound light microscope.

tube are the other magnifying elements screwed into a *revolving nosepiece*. These elements are called the *objective lenses*. Although the number of objective lenses varies, there will usually be a low-power objective (10× magnification) and a high-power objective (40× magnification).

3. Underneath the body tube is the *stage*, a flat piece on which microscope slides are placed. The stage will have *stage clips* to hold the slide in place. There will be a hole in the stage to allow light to be reflected from its built in substage *lamp* through the stage opening. Light then passes through the specimen on the microscope slide into the body tube resulting in an image on the retina of your eye.

4. The importance of light makes necessary its careful adjustment. Your microscope may or may not have a condenser, which concentrates light. Just below the stage can be found the iris diaphragm. It may have a lever or a revolving plate with openings of different sizes to admit varying amounts of light. Practice moving the iris diaphragm lever to observe the changes in light by looking through the ocular lens. If you have an iris diaphragm plate or disc, practice locking in the different size holes to observe the changes in light intensity.

5. When viewing an object with a microscope, you are required to have the lens a certain distance from the object. This is called the working distance. At the correct working distance from an object, the object is *in focus*. Changes and adjustments in the focus are accomplished by using the *coarse* (larger knob) and *fine* (smaller knob) *adjustment knobs*, located on the arm.

### B. MAGNIFICATION

1. The magnifying power of most objectives and oculars is usually engraved. The ocular lens will be marked at the top edge. The objectives are engraved on the side of the objective cylinder.

2. The low-power objective will be engraved 10× which means that the objective marked will produce an image 10 times larger than the object on the microscope slide.

3. When using a compound microscope, you are using two sets of magnifiers. The ocular lens has a magnification of 10× and the lower power objective has a magnification of 10×. Under low power, the objective forms an image in the body tube ten times larger than the object on the microscope slide; the 10× ocular lens then magnifies that image another ten times. Thus the image that finally reaches your eye has a total magnification of 100 times.

## LABORATORY EXERCISE: CELL STRUCTURE (continued)

### C. USING THE MICROSCOPE

1. You are now ready to use the microscope, having reviewed its parts. Be sure the microscope is plugged into an electrical outlet; place the microscope at your lab table with the arm toward you. Turn on the illuminator lamp. Clean the ocular lens and the objectives with *lens paper* provided by your instructor.

2. Get a microscope slide with a letter e and place it on the stage over the stage opening. Be sure your letter e covered with a cover slip is in the center of the stage opening. Secure the slide with the stage clips. Place the low-power objective in place. It will click and lock into position. Lower the objective into place by turning the coarse adjustment knob. Your microscope should have an automatic stop so you will not crack the slide. Look through the eyepiece. Notice the appearance of the letter e under low power. Bring it into focus by slowly adjusting the coarse adjustment knob by raising it above the stopping point. Now look at the letter e on your microscope slide. It is upside down but when you look through the microscope it is right side up. Now move the slide to the right, the letter e moves to the left, now move the slide to the left, the letter e moves to the right. Move the slide away from you (up), the letter e moves toward you (down). Move the slide towards you (down) the letter e moves away from you (up). These phenomena are called *inversions*. Practice moving the slide around to get use to the inversions.

3. If you want to see more detail, you must switch to the high-power objective. Using your thumb and index finger unlock the low-power objective and move the high-power objective into position by rotating the nosepiece. Now use *only* the fine focus adjustment knob to bring that part of the letter e you are viewing into focus. Notice how the field of vision got smaller as the object to be viewed got bigger. Your magnification now under high power is 10× (ocular lens) × 40× high power objective = 400×. Remember to adjust the light if necessary.

### D. IMPORTANT CAUTIONS

1. Use only the fine focus adjustment knob to focus under high power, *never* use the coarse adjustment knob under high power.

2. Use only lens paper to clean the ocular lens and objectives, *never* use kim-wipes or other material. Other materials may scratch the delicate lens. Always clean your lenses before lab and at the end of lab.

3. Keep the stage of the microscope dry at all times to prevent corrosion of metal parts.

### E. DEPTH OF FOCUS

1. Get a microscope slide with three colored threads mounted together. Under low power focus where the three threads cross one over another. Now using the fine adjustment knob, slowly focus up and down. As you do this, notice how different parts of the threads and different threads become distinct. When one thread is in focus, the others above and below are blurred. By continually fine focusing up and down through the threads, you can perceive the depth dimension that is not evident when the focus is resting at one point.

2. Now turn to high power and notice that you can see much less depth than under low power. In fact you may not be able to distinguish one whole thread completely clearly under high power.

3. The vertical distance that will remain in focus at any particular time is called the depth of focus or depth of field. The

(continues)

## LABORATORY EXERCISE: CELL STRUCTURE (continued)

medium in which the threads are embedded between the cover slip and the microscope slide is like the water depth in a swimming pool. When the specimen is near the top close to the coverslip it is in focus, it will go out of focus if it swims down to the bottom of the microscope slide (if it is a live specimen like a *Paramecium* that you will observe later on).

### II. THE DISSECTING MICROSCOPE

1. Another common microscope in use in anatomy and other biology courses is the binocular dissecting microscope. Your instructor has set one up on demonstration at the front of the lab. This microscope has a pair of oculars, one for each eye. The distance between the oculars can be adjusted by pulling them together and by pushing them apart until you have adjusted them for the correct position of your eyes. The ocular pair has a magnification of 10×. The movable large single objective lens usually goes from 1× to 2×.

2. Place a small moss plant on the stage of the microscope (usually a large round glass plate). Move the plant around and change the objective lens to observe the arrangement of the small whorl of leaves on the stem.

### III. THE ELECTRON MICROSCOPE

Light microscopes can only magnify to about 2000×. Most of our knowledge of cellular fine structure has been derived from pictures taken with an electron microscope. Electron microscopy uses a beam of electrons rather than light and magnets instead of glass lenses. Electron beams have a much shorter wavelength than visible light, and refracting them with magnets yields resolutions thousands times greater than light. Special training is required to use an electron microscope.

Observe photographs taken of cellular details with an electron microscope. Your instructor will put on demonstration a number of electron micrographs.

### IV PREPARING YOUR OWN WET MOUNTS

Wet mounts are prepared by placing a drop of material on a *clean* microscope glass slide. If the material is dry, then place it in a drop of water on the center of the slide. A cover slip is then placed on top of the material by holding it at a 45° angle until the edge of the cover slip touches the drop of water. Then gently drop the cover slip on top of the material. The water will push air in front of it to prevent air bubbles.

### A. HUMAN EPIDERMAL CELLS

1. Gently scrape the inside of your cheek with a clean flat toothpick. Place the scrapings in a drop of water in the center of the slide. Add a small amount of Methylene blue stain to the drop of water by touching an eye droplet full of stain to the drop of water. Mix the stain, water, and cheek scrapings with your toothpick. Cover with a cover slip. This is the only slide we will use a stain on.

2. You have removed some of the protective epithelial cells that line your mouth. These cells are constantly being worn off and replaced by new cells. Therefore, these cells usually come off the cheek in masses.

3. Under low power of the microscope scan your slide until you find individual cells. Now turn to high power. Notice the cells are flat and irregular in shape. Locate the nucleus, the nucleolus, the nuclear membrane, the cytoplasm, and the cell membrane. The dark granules in the cytoplasm are probably mitochondria. You may also see some vacuoles.

## LABORATORY EXERCISE: CELL STRUCTURE (continued)

### B. PLANT CELLS

1. Cut an onion into quarters, with forceps strip a piece of thin epidermis from the inside of one of the leaves of the onion bulb. Make a wet mount by placing it in a drop of water; try to avoid folding of the epidermal tissue.

2. Compare this to the human epithelial cell. These plant cells have rigid cell walls, easily observable under low power. Switch to high power and observe the light nucleus with a number of nucleoli. Notice the large cell vacuole and clear cytoplasm. There are no chloroplasts in the onion bulb.

3. Take a young leaf from the top of an *Elodea* plant and make a wet mount of it to observe large green chloroplasts in the cells of this plant. Notice the large number of chloroplasts in the cytoplasm of the cells under low power. There are so many chloroplasts that any other cellular contents are obscured. In young leaves, the cytoplasm streams; thus, the chloroplasts will be moved in a current within the cell. Again note the rigid cell wall made of cellulose. The cell membrane is pushed up against the cell wall and so it is not visible as a separate entity.

### C. LIVING SINGLE-CELLED ANIMAL: PARAMECIUM

Make a wet mount of *Paramecium* by putting a drop of the culture (supplied by your instructor) onto a microscope slide covered with a glass cover slip. *Paramecium* is a single-celled ciliate animal (Figure 3-15). Examine your slide under low

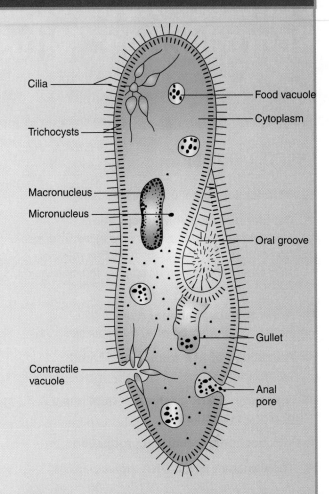

**FIGURE 3-15.** The structure of a *Paramecium*.

power because the *Paramecia* are large and actively swim in the watery medium. Observe the animal's structures, especially the beating cilia seen around the edge of the cell membrane, the large macronucleus, and the oral groove.

# 4

# Cellular Metabolism and Reproduction: Mitosis and Meiosis

## CHAPTER OUTLINE

- **Introduction to cellular metabolism**

- **Cellular metabolism or respiration:**
  *Glycolysis; The Krebs' citric acid cycle; The electron transport (transfer) system; Summary of ATP production during glycolysis, the citric acid cycle, and electron transport*

- **Anaerobic respiration:** *Fermentation; Anaerobic production of ATP by muscles*

- **Production of ATP from general food compounds**

- **Summary of ATP production from one glucose molecule**

- **Introduction to cellular reproduction**

- **The structure of the DNA molecule:** *The history of the discovery of DNA; The anatomy of the DNA molecule*

- **The cell cycle:** *Interphase; Mitosis:* Prophase, Metaphase, Anaphase, Telophase; *Cytokinesis*

- **Meiosis: a reduction division:** *The stages of meiosis:* Prophase I, Metaphase I, Anaphase I, Telophase I, Prophase II, Metaphase II, Anaphase II, Telophase II

- **Gametogenesis: the formation of the sex cells**

- **A comparison of mitosis and meiosis**

## CHAPTER OBJECTIVES

After studying this chapter, you should be able to:

1. Define metabolism.

2. Describe the basic steps in glycolysis and indicate the major products and ATP production.

3. Describe the Krebs' citric acid cycle and its major products and ATP production.

4. Describe the electron transport system and how ATP is produced.

5. Compare glycolysis with anaerobic production of ATP in muscle cells and fermentation.

6. Explain how other food compounds besides glucose are used as energy sources.

7. Name the discoverers of the anatomy of the DNA molecule.

8. Know the basic structure of the DNA molecule.

9. Name the nitrogen base pairs and how they pair up in the DNA molecule.

10. Define the stages of the cell cycle.

11. Explain the significance of mitosis in the survival of the cell and growth in the human body.

12. Understand the significance of meiosis as a reduction of the genetic material and for the formation of the sex cells.

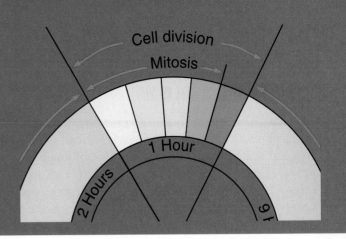

# KEY TERMS

# INTRODUCTION TO CELLULAR METABOLISM

For cells to maintain their structure and function, chemical reactions must occur inside the cell. These chemical reactions require an input of biologically usable energy. The most common and available form of energy within a cell is the chemical energy found within the structure of an ATP (adenosine triphosphate) molecule. We use the term **metabolism** (meh-**TAB**-oh-lizm) to describe the total chemical changes that occur inside a cell. There are two subcategories of metabolism: **anabolism** (an-**AB**-oh-lizm) is an energy-requiring process that builds larger molecules from combining smaller molecules and **catabolism** (ka-**TAB**-oh-lizm), which is an energy-releasing process that breaks down large molecules into smaller ones. These cellular metabolic processes are often called **cellular respiration** or **cellular metabolism**.

Molecules of ATP is made within the cell during a stepwise decomposition (catabolism) of organic molecules (carbohydrates, fats, and proteins). We measure the energy contained in food as **calories**. This decomposition releases the chemical energy (calories) stored in these organic foodstuffs and this energy is used to synthesize ATP (another form of chemical energy) from ADP (adenosine diphosphate) and $PO_4$ (inorganic phosphate). Thus, ATP is the energy source available to the cell to be used for all cell processes: chemical reactions use ATP as an energy source to maintain cellular structure and function.

Photosynthesis by plant cells is the ultimate source of the organic molecules (foodstuffs) that will be decomposed to form ATP. Photosynthesis requires $6CO_2 + 12H_2O$ in the presence of light and chlorophyll to produce $C_6H_{12}O_6$ (glucose) an organic molecule + $6O_2$ (oxygen) as a waste product + $6H_2O$ (water) as a waste product. The formation of ATP is the final step in the transformation of light energy into the chemical energy of a biologically usable form. This explains the significance of our dependence on plants to convert sun or light energy into food or chemical energy.

The most efficient cellular process by which ATP is formed during the breakdown of organic molecules requires molecular oxygen ($O_2$). This process

is called cellular or biochemical respiration or cellular metabolism. The overall chemical equation is: $C_6H_{12}O_6 + 6O_2 \rightarrow 6CO_2 + 6H_2O$ + energy in the form of ATP.

Respiration, therefore, requires an exchange of gases between the cell and its surroundings to allow the inflow of $O_2$ to the cell and the outflow of $CO_2$. Biochemical respiration is strictly the oxygen-requiring or **aerobic** process of ATP production. This biochemical meaning of respiration should not be confused with the everyday meaning of breathing. The most common substance decomposed aerobically in cells to produce ATP is glucose, $C_6H_{12}O_6$.

The breakdown of a glucose molecule into carbon dioxide gas and water is a continuous process. However we will discuss this process in three steps. The first step is called **glycolysis** (gligh-**KOL**-ih-sis). Because it does not require oxygen, it is also occasionally called **anaerobic** (without oxygen) **respiration**. This step occurs in the cytoplasm of the cell. The next two steps are called the **Krebs' citric acid cycle** and the **electron transfer** or **transport system**. These two steps require oxygen and they occur in the matrix and on the folds or cristae of the mitochondria of the cell.

# CELLULAR METABOLISM OR RESPIRATION

## Glycolysis

The first step in the biochemical respiration process is glycolysis. It is common to the aerobic breakdown of **glucose** and to the two different types of anaerobic breakdown of glucose molecules. One type of anaerobic glucose decomposition occurs in yeast cells (a type of fungus) and is called fermentation. The other type occurs in our muscle cells when we exercise and experience muscle fatigue and cannot get enough oxygen to our muscle cells. In the overall process of glycolysis, the $C_6$ (backbone chain of six carbon atoms) sugar glucose is slowly broken down by various enzymatic steps to two $C_3$ units of **pyruvic** (pye-**ROO**-vik) **acid**. Refer to Figure 4-1 as we discuss glycolysis.

The first step in glycolysis is the addition of a phosphate to the glucose. This process is called

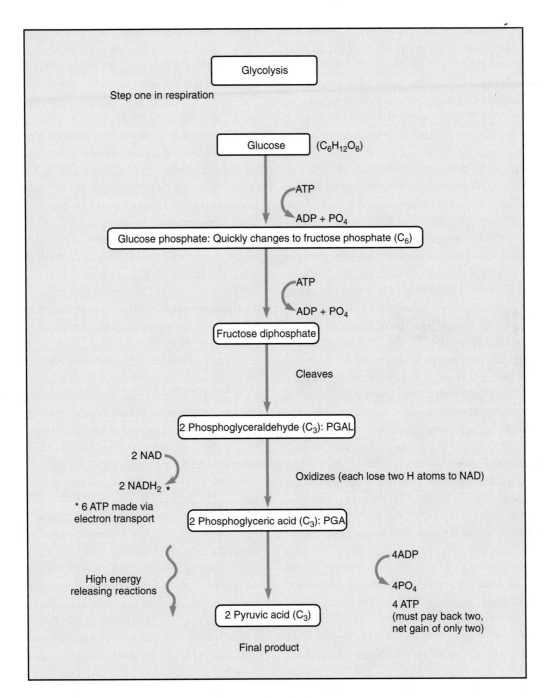

**FIGURE 4-1.** The basic steps in glycolysis, the first step in biochemical respiration.

**phosphorylation** (**fos**-for-ih-**LAY**-shun). The phosphate comes from the breakdown of an ATP molecule into ADP and $PO_4$, releasing the energy required to add the phosphate to the glucose. The glucose phosphate quickly changes to another $C_6$ sugar phosphate called fructose phosphate. In another ATP requiring reaction, the fructose phosphate is phosphorylated by breaking down another

ATP into ADP and $PO_4$. This phosphate is added to the fructose phosphate creating fructose diphosphate. So far we have not made any ATP but rather we have used up two ATP and these must be paid back from our final ATP production at the end of glycolysis.

In the next step of glycolysis, the fructose diphosphate splits or cleaves into two $C_3$ molecules of

**phosphoglyceraldehyde** (**fos**-foh-**GLISS**-er-**AL**-deh-hyde), abbreviated as **PGAL**. The PGAL is now oxidized (loses electrons) by the removal of two electrons and two H+ ions to form two **phosphoglyceric** (**fos**-foh-**GLISS**-er-ik) **acids**, abbreviated as **PGA**. The two hydrogen atoms that come off each of the two PGALs go to the electron transport system and get taken up by the electron carrier molecule **nicotinamide adenine dinucleotide** (**nik**-oh-**TIN**-ah-mide **ADD**-eh-neen dye-**noo**-klee-oh-tide) abbreviated as **NAD**. This step is actually part of the electron transport system and will result in the production of six ATP molecules. However this step occurs only if oxygen is present. In this process NAD gets reduced (gains electrons) to $NADH_2$. Because there were two PGALs, it happens twice. Each time an NAD gets reduced to $NADH_2$ and the electron transport system functions, three ATP molecules are made. Again because it happened twice, a total of six ATP are made in this aerobic step.

Next the two PGAs get broken down through a series of high-energy releasing enzymatic steps to two $C_3$ molecules of pyruvic acid. So much energy is given off in these steps that four ADP and four $PO_4$ get added to form four ATP molecules. The energy in the PGA molecules is converted to the high-energy four ATP molecules. In this step we make four ATP but it is from these ATP that we must pay back the two ATP used in the beginning of glycolysis. Therefore our net gain of ATP is only two ATP.

In summary, the glycolytic breakdown of one molecule of glucose produces two pyruvic acid molecules. It took two ATP to start the sequence and four ATP were produced. However to pay back the two ATP, our net gain is only two ATP. However we also produced two $NADH_2$ which are part of the electron transport system. When oxygen is present, we produce six more ATP via electron transport. Aerobic glycolysis produces six plus two or eight ATP molecules. Anaerobic glycolysis produces only two ATP.

## The Krebs' Citric Acid Cycle

In the presence of $O_2$, the two pyruvic acid molecules formed as a result of glycolysis are further broken down in the second step of biochemical respiration. This step is named after its discoverer, a German-born British biochemist, Sir Hans Krebs, who first postulated the scheme in 1937. This is the Krebs' citric acid cycle. We will explain this cycle using only one of the two pyruvic acid molecules produced in glycolysis. When finished we will multiply all products by two.

The $C_3$ pyruvic acid is first converted to **acetic acid** (ah-**SEE**-tic **ASS**-id) in a transition stage and then to the $C_2$ **acetyl-CoA** (ah-**SEE**-tal) by an enzyme called **CoA enzyme**. This causes the pyruvic acid molecule to lose a carbon and two oxygens in the form of $CO_2$ gas as a waste product. It also loses two hydrogens to NAD producing $NADH_2$ (thus via electron transport three ATP molecules are made in this step). The acetyl-CoA now enters the Krebs' citric acid cycle. This occurs on the cristae of the mitochondria (Figure 4-2).

The $C_2$ Acetyl-CoA reacts with a $C_4$ molecule **oxaloacetic** (**ok**-sah-low-ah-**SEE**-tik) **acid** to form the $C_6$ molecule **citric acid**, hence the name of the cycle. No ATP is produced in this step but an important event occurs. CoA enzyme is regenerated to react with another acetic acid to continue the cycle. Another enzyme now converts the citric acid to the $C_5$ **alpha-ketoglutaric** (**AL**-fah **KEY**-toh gluh-**TAYR**-ik) **acid**. This causes the citric acid to lose a carbon and two oxygens as $CO_2$ gas (waste product) and two hydrogens to NAD. Thus, NAD gets reduced via electron transport to $NADH_2$ and three ATP are made.

The $C_5$ alpha-ketoglutaric acid now gets broken down into the first $C_4$ molecule **succinic** (suk-**SIN**-ik) **acid**. It loses a carbon and two oxygens as $CO_2$ gas (waste product) and two hydrogens twice to NAD. Thus via electron transport six more ATP molecules are made. Succinic acid changes to another $C_4$ molecule **malic** (**MAH**-lik) **acid**. Finally the malic acid looses two hydrogens to **flavin adenine dinucleotide** (**FLAY**-vin **ADD**-eh-neen dye-**NOO**-klee-oh-tide), abbreviated as **FAD**. This is another electron carrier of the electron transport system and two more ATP molecules are made in this step. The malic acid now is converted to the oxaloacetic acid. Also going from alpha-ketoglutaric acid to oxaloacetic acid another ATP equivalent is made. This molecule is actually guanosine triphosphate (GTP).

In summary, for every pyruvic acid that enters the Krebs' citric acid cycle three $CO_2$, four $NADH_2$, one $FADH_2$, and one ATP (GTP) are produced. Because two pyruvic acids entered the cycle, we must multiply all of these products by two.

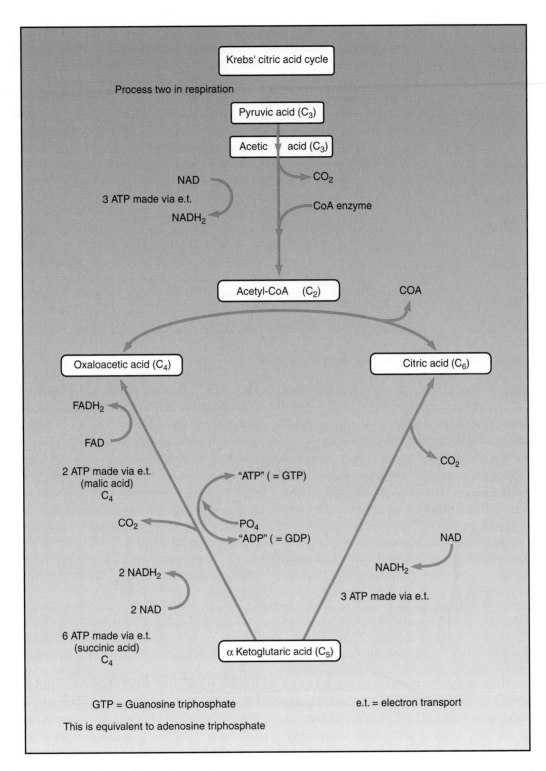

**FIGURE 4-2.** The Krebs' citric acid cycle and its products.

## The Electron Transport (Transfer) System

Most of the ATP produced during biochemical respiration is produced in the electron transport system (Figure 4-3). Two $NADH_2$ were produced in glycolysis. Two $NADH_2$ were produced during the acetyl-CoA formation. Then six $NADH_2$ and two $FADH_2$ were produced in the citric acid cycle. The NAD and FAD all donate the electrons of the

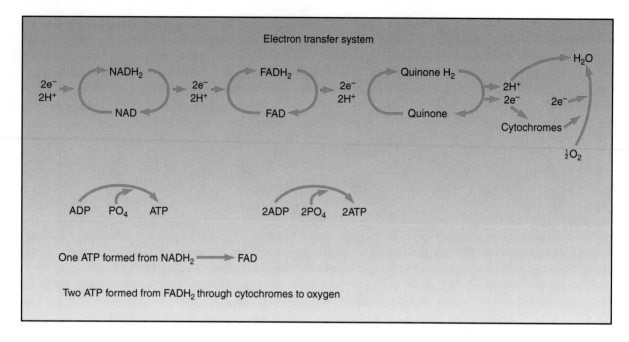

**FIGURE 4-3.** The electron transport or transfer system and ATP production.

hydrogen atoms that they captured in these reactions to the enzyme systems on the cristae of the mitochondria. Each of these electron carriers has a slightly different electron potential. As the electrons from the cofactor $NADH_2$ get transferred from one electron carrier to the next, they slowly give up their energy. This energy is used in the energy-requiring synthesis of ATP from ADP and inorganic phosphate.

The electron transport system functions as a series of reduction/oxidation reactions. When NAD accepts the two hydrogens, it gets reduced to $NADH_2$. When it gives up the two hydrogens to FAD, NAD gets oxidized while FAD becomes $FADH_2$ and gets reduced. This series of redox reactions continues until the electrons of the hydrogen atoms get ultimately donated to oxygen. Several kinds of electron carriers participate in this process: the cofactor NAD, the cofactor FAD, **quinone**, and the **cytochrome system**. There is some debate as to whether the hydrogen protons ($2H^+$) are transferred along with the electrons ($2e^-$) in this transport or not. A currently accepted scheme is shown in Figure 4-3.

This scheme illustrates why the breakdown of glucose requires oxygen ($O_2$). Oxygen is the ultimate electron acceptor for the electrons captured by the cofactors during glucose decomposition.

One ATP is formed during the first step of electron transfer from $NADH_2$ to FAD. During the following transfer from $FADH_2$ to quinone $H_2$ to the cytochrome system to $O_2$ (or $\frac{1}{2} O_2 = O$), two more units of ATP are formed. You will notice that the cytochrome system only accepts the two electrons and then transfers them to oxygen (O). Therefore, quinone $H_2$ must directly transfer the two hydrogen protons ($2H^+$) to oxygen (O), thus producing the waste product water ($H_2O$).

As we examine the electron transport system, we observe that when electrons are donated to NAD, three ATP units are formed during the entire electron transfer. However, when the electrons are donated directly to FAD and NAD is bypassed, only two ATP units are formed during the electron transfer.

## Summary of ATP Production During Glycolysis, the Citric Acid Cycle, and Electron Transport

The net products from glycolysis are two ATP units and two $NADH_2$ per glucose molecule. Because each $NADH_2$ molecule produces three ATP during electron transport, a total of eight ATP units result in glycolysis, which includes electron transport.

In the Krebs' citric acid cycle and transition stage, four $NADH_2$, one $FADH_2$, and one ATP (or GTP) are formed during the breakdown of each pyruvic acid. However, because each glucose molecule produces two pyruvic acid molecules, we actually form eight $NADH_2$, two $FADH_2$, and two ATP (or GTP) units. The number of ATP units formed during the citric acid cycle and electron transport then is 24 + 4 + 2 + or 30 ATP or 24 + 4 = 28 ATP and 2 GTP.

In total 30 ATP from the citric acid cycle and electron transport plus 8 ATP from glycolysis and electron transport produced a net gain of 38 ATP units per each glucose molecule or 36 ATP and 2 GTP. This represents a cellular capture of about 60% of the energy available from the breakdown of a single glucose molecule. This is very high efficiency compared to that of any man-made machine.

It is important to remember that cellular or biochemical respiration is a continuous process. Although we tend to discuss it in three "steps," these steps are not separate events. We have seen that electron transport is part of glycolysis when oxygen is available and that electron transport accounts for most of the ATP production in the Krebs' citric acid cycle.

# ANAEROBIC RESPIRATION

There are two situations when glucose is broken down in the absence of oxygen. One is when yeast cells (a type of fungus) feed on glucose and the process is called **fermentation**. The other situation occurs in our muscle cells when we overexercise and experience muscle fatigue and cannot get enough oxygen to the muscle cells. Then the muscle cells begin to break down glucose in the absence of oxygen, a much less efficient breakdown with less ATP produced. We will now look at these two anaerobic processes.

## Fermentation

Fermentation is the process by which yeast breaks down glucose anaerobically (in the absence of oxygen). The final products of fermentation are: carbon dioxide gas ($CO_2$), **ethyl alcohol** ($CH_3CH_2OH$), and ATP. In yeast cells, glucose breaks down, as in glycolysis, to produce two molecules of pyruvic acid, a net gain of two ATP, and two $NADH_2$. However, because oxygen is not used, the pyruvic acid molecules do not proceed to the citric acid cycle. Instead a yeast enzyme called a decarboxy-

lase breaks down the pyruvic acid to $CO_2$, and a $C_2$ compound **acetaldehyde** (ass-et-**AL**-deh-hyde) ($CH_3CHO$). It is the $CO_2$ gas that causes bread to rise and is the reason we add yeast to our flour (glucose), water, and eggs (which makes dough) when we bake bread. Because this process occurs without oxygen, the $NADH_2$ does not give its electrons to oxygen through the electron transport system as it does in aerobic respiration. Instead the $NADH_2$ donates its two hydrogen atoms to the acetaldehyde through the action of another yeast enzyme called an alcoholic dehydrogenase. This reaction regenerates the NAD and forms the final product ethyl alcohol. This product is what is produced in the beer, wine, and liquor industries to convert the sugars in grapes and the sugars in grains to alcohol.

In conclusion, the fermentation process produces only two ATP per glucose molecule. Obviously, this energy-capturing mechanism is much less efficient than aerobic respiration.

## Anaerobic Production of ATP by Muscles

The second situation that can occur in anaerobic respiration is the breakdown of glucose in human muscle cells when not enough oxygen becomes available due to muscle fatigue as when an athlete sprints. Again this process starts with glycolysis. However, the pyruvic acid formed undergoes a different fate. Again glycolysis yields two pyruvic acid molecules, a net gain of two ATP molecules, and two $NADH_2$ per glucose molecule. As it was in fermentation, the two $NADH_2$ cannot donate their electrons to oxygen. Instead the $NADH_2$ donates them to pyruvic acid to form **lactic** (**LAK**-tik) **acid**. It is the accumulation of lactic acid that causes the soreness in muscles that are overexercised. When muscles are overworked, the muscle cells need to produce extra energy in the form of ATP. Aerobic respiration produces much of this energy. However, if the muscle is worked more rapidly than oxygen ($O_2$) can be supplied to it from the bloodstream, the muscle cells will begin to produce the ATP anaerobically and lactic acid accumulates.

When we overexercise and our muscles get sore and we experience muscle fatigue, we notice that our heartbeat and breathing rate are accelerated. We sit down, breathe faster (to get more $O_2$ into our bodies), and the soreness slowly diminishes. When $O_2$ again becomes available, the lactic acid is converted back to pyruvic acid and aerobic respiration proceeds as normal. We note that anaerobic formation of ATP by muscles is much less efficient than aerobic respiration. Only two molecules of ATP are produced per glucose molecule.

## PRODUCTION OF ATP FROM GENERAL FOOD COMPOUNDS

Obviously we do not only eat glucose. So where do the other food compounds in our diet fit into the respiration cycle to produce ATP? If we think of the steps in biochemical respiration as parts of a very efficient cellular furnace where fuel (food) is converted to another form of chemical energy, ATP, then we can grasp a better understanding of how

other food molecules are "burned" to produce ATP (Figure 4-4).

Glucose is a simple carbohydrate. Other carbohydrates such as starch (plant carbohydrate) and glycogen (animal starch) as well as other types of sugars such as monosaccharides and disaccharides fit into the cellular furnace at the level where glucose enters the glycolytic sequence. If after digestion the food molecules are not needed immediately, they can be stored in the body (in food vacuoles or the liver, or converted to fat cells) until needed later to produce more ATP.

Digestion decomposes fat into fatty acids and glycerol. They too will enter the cellular furnace at a stage related to their chemical structure. Glycerol, a $C_3$ molecule, is similar to PGA and will enter at the PGA stage of glycolysis. Fatty acids enter the Krebs' citric acid cycle. Proteins are broken down by digestion into amino acids. Again they will enter the cellular furnace at a level related to their chemical struc-

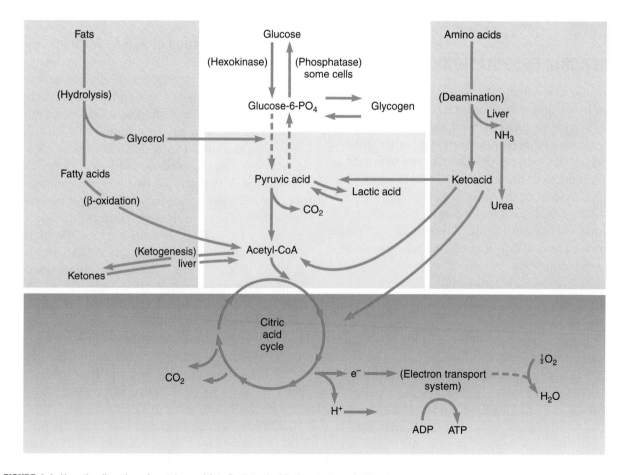

**FIGURE 4-4.** How the digestion of proteins and fats fits into the biochemical respiration process.

ture. Alanine, a $C_3$ amino acid, and lactic acid enter at the pyruvic acid stage. Glutamic acid, a $C_5$ amino acid, is similar to alpha-ketogluteric acid. Aspartic acid, a $C_4$ amino acid, resembles oxaloacetic acid. These amino acids enter into the citric acid cycle at different stages. So when you put that piece of chocolate into your mouth during class break to get some extra energy to finish class, you now will have a better understanding of how that carbohydrate is converted to ATP (Figure 4-5), the fuel that runs our cells. The simplest way of describing cellular or biochemical respiration is to begin the process with a glucose molecule (Figure 4-6). Glycolysis occurs in the cytoplasm of the cell and produces pyruvic acid. If oxygen is available, the pyruvic acid is eventually converted to acetyl-CoA, which then enters the citric acid cycle, eventually being converted to $CO_2$, $H_2O$, and 38 ATP. If oxygen is not available the pyruvic acid is converted to lactic acid and only two ATP molecules are produced.

## SUMMARY OF ATP PRODUCTION FROM ONE GLUCOSE MOLECULE

Table 4-1 summarizes products produced and the total ATP produced in the individual stages of the cellular metabolism of one glucose molecule. The stages are broken down into glycolysis, acetyl-CoA production, and the citric acid cycle.

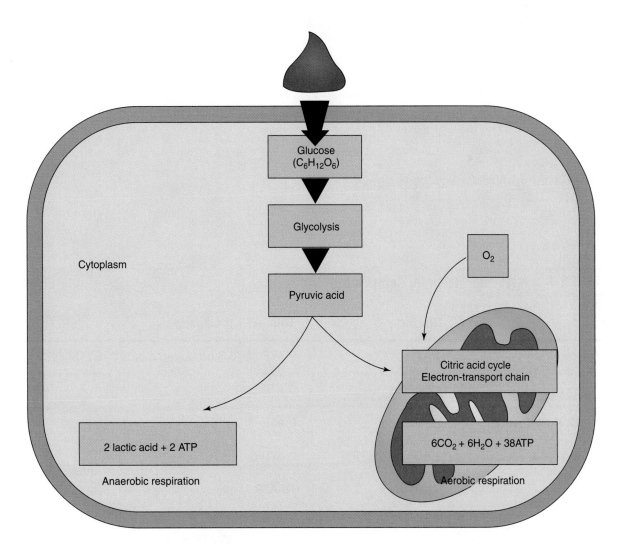

**FIGURE 4-5.** How a piece of chocolate gets metabolized to ATP.

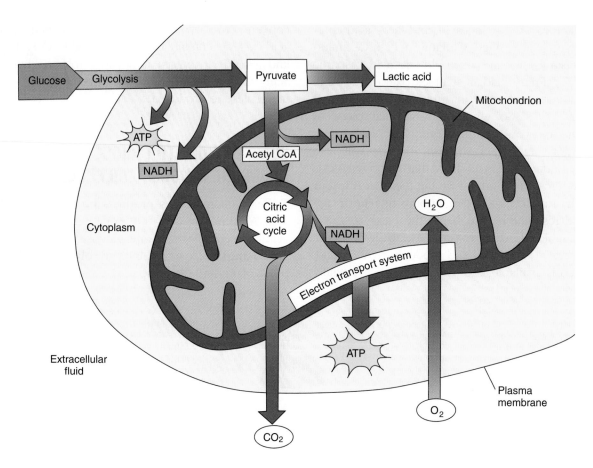

**FIGURE 4-6.** An overview of cellular respiration.

| TABLE 4-1 | ATP Production by Cellular Respiration | |
|---|---|---|
| **Step** | **Product** | **Total ATP Produced** |
| Glycolysis | 4 ATP | 2 ATP (4 ATP produced minus 2 ATP to start cycle) |
| | 2 NADH$_2$ | 6 ATP |
| Acetyl-CoA production | 2 NADH$_2$ | 6 ATP |
| Citric acid cycle | 2 ATP or 2 GTP | 2 ATP or 2 GTP |
| | 6 NADH$_2$ | 18 ATP |
| | 2 FADH$_2$ | 4 ATP<br>38 ATP or 36 ATP and 2 GTP |

# INTRODUCTION TO CELLULAR REPRODUCTION

Cellular reproduction is the process by which a single cell duplicates itself. In this process the genetic material in the nucleus is duplicated during interphase of the cell cycle followed by the process called **mitosis** (my-**TOH**-sis) when the nuclear material is replicated. This is followed by duplication of the cellular organelles in the cytoplasm called **cytokinesis**, (sigh-toh-kye-**NEE**-sis), which is the final event of mitosis leading to two new daughter cells. These processes, part of the cell cycle, allow our bodies to grow, repair themselves, and maintain our structures and functions. In other words, these processes allow us to maintain our life.

However, cellular reproduction is also the process by which our genetic material is passed on to our offspring from one generation to the next. In this process of cellular reproduction, special cells called sex cells, the egg and the sperm, are produced. In this type of cellular reproduction, the genetic material must not only be duplicated but it must also be reduced in half so that the female egg carries half of the genetic material or 23 chromosomes and the male sperm carries the other one half of the genetic material or the other 23 chromosomes. A special kind of cellular reduction division called **meiosis** (my-**OH**-sis), which occurs only in the gonads, allows this to occur. When a sperm and and egg unite in fertilization, the genetic material is returned to its full complement of 46 chromosomes.

Before we study these processes of cellular division, it is necessary to understand the basic structure of the DNA molecule, which constitutes the genetic material. We shall also examine the history of the discovery of the structure of DNA.

# THE STRUCTURE OF THE DNA MOLECULE

To better understand the structure of the DNA molecule, the history of the discovery of DNA and the anatomy of the DNA molecule will be discussed.

## The History of the Discovery of DNA

One of the most significant discoveries in biology of the 20th century was the discovery of the three-dimensional structure of the DNA molecule. A number of scientists made various contributions to our knowledge of the DNA molecule. The molecule itself was discovered in 1869 by a German chemist, Friedrich Miescher. He extracted a substance from the nucleus of human cells and the sperm of fish. He called it nuclein because it came from the nucleus. Because this material was slightly acid, it became known as **nucleic acid**.

It was not until the 1920s that any further discoveries were made. A biochemist, P. A. Levine, discovered that DNA contained three main components: phosphate ($PO_4$) groups, five carbon sugars; and nitrogen-containing bases called purines (adenine and guanine) and pyrimidines (thymine and cytosine).

The actual three-dimensional structure of DNA was discovered in the 1950s by three scientists. It was a British chemist, Rosalind Franklin, who discovered that the molecule had a helical structure similar to a winding staircase. This was accomplished when she conducted an x-ray crystallographic analysis of DNA. Her photograph was made in 1953 in the laboratory of another British biochemist, Maurice Wilkins. Two other researchers were also studying the DNA molecule at this time: James Watson, an American postdoctoral student, and an English scientist, Francis Crick, at Cambridge University in England. After learning informally of Rosalind Franklin's discovery, they worked out the three-dimensional structure of the DNA molecule. Rosalind Franklin's discovery of the helical nature of DNA was published in 1953 but Watson and Crick learned of her results before they were published. James Watson and Francis Crick won the Nobel Prize in 1962 after publishing their results. Rosalind Franklin, meanwhile, had tragically died of cancer prior to this event. Today, however, these three are given credit for discovering the structure of DNA, the molecule that contains all the hereditary information of an individual. An interesting account of the discovery of the nature of the molecule was published in 1968 by James Watson in his book *The Double Helix*. This discovery opened up a whole new field of research for the 20th century: recombinant DNA, the Human Genome Project, and genetic engineering to name just a few.

## The Anatomy of the DNA Molecule

DNA (**deoxyribonucleic acid**) is the hereditary material of the cell. It not only determines the traits an organism exhibits, but it is exactly duplicated during reproduction so that offspring exhibit their parent's basic characteristics. An organism's characteristics are due to chemical reactions occurring inside our cells. DNA governs these chemical reactions by the chemical mechanism of controlling what proteins are made.

Every DNA molecule is a double helical chain of **nucleotides** (noo-**KLEE**-oh-tides) (Figure 4-7). A nucleotide consists of a phosphate group ($PO_4$), a five-carbon sugar (deoxyribose), and an organic nitrogen-containing base, either a purine or a pyrimidine. There are two **purines** (**PYOO**-reenz), **adenine** (**ADD**-eh-neen) and **guanine** (**GWAHN**-een) and two **pyrimidines** (pih-**RIM**-ih-deenz),

A diagram of a short chain of DNA and its double helical structure

S = Deoxyribose, P = Phosphate, C = Cytosine,
G = Guanine, A = Adenine, T = Thymine

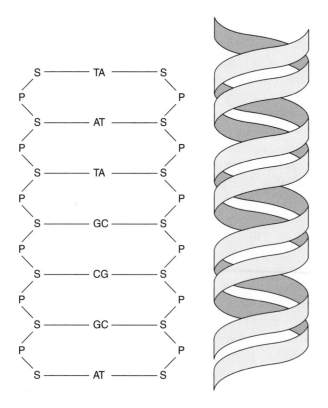

**FIGURE 4-7.** The double helical chain of nucleotides of a DNA molecule ( a very short section).

thymine (**THYE**-meen) and **cytosine** (**SYE**-toh-seen). Adenine always pairs up with thymine and guanine always pairs up with cytosine. Bonds form between the phosphate group of one nucleotide and the sugar of the next nucleotide. The organic nitrogen base extends out from the sugar of the nucleotide. It is easier to visualize the double helical nature of the DNA if we think of it as a spiral staircase. The handrails of the staircase are composed of the phosphate-sugar chain and the stairs of the staircase are the nitrogen base pairs.

If we look at Figure 4-8, we see that a pyrimidine always pairs with a purine. A pyrimidine is a single ring of six atoms (thymine and cytosine); a purine is a fused double ring of nine atoms (adenine and guanine). These organic nitrogen bases are a complex ring structure of carbon and nitrogen atoms. Because we know how the bases pair up in the double chain of nucleotides, if we only know one side of the helix, we can figure out the second side by matching bases. The two chains of the helix are held together by weak, hydrogen bonds between the base pairs. There are two hydrogen bonds between the pyrimidine thymine and the purine adenine, whereas there are three hydrogen bonds between the pyrimidine cytosine and the purine guanine. Because of the specific pairing of bases, the sequence of bases in one chain determines the sequence of bases in the other. We therefore refer to the two chains as complements of each other. A **gene** is a sequence of organic nitrogen base pairs that codes for a polypetide or a protein.

A major project of the 20th century that developed from Watson, Crick, and Franklin's discovery of DNA structure is the Human Genome Project. The objective of this project is to identify all the genes on all 46 chromosomes (DNA molecules). We know now that there are approximately three billion organic base pairs that code over 100,000 genes. We can think of the bases adenine (A), thymine (T), cytosine (C), and guanine (G) as the four letters of the alphabet of life. These base pairs determine all the characteristics of all the life we know on our planet—the basic structure of the DNA molecule is the same for all living organisms.

The DNA molecule must be duplicated before cell division. The molecule separates where the hydrogen bonds hold the two chains of nucleotides

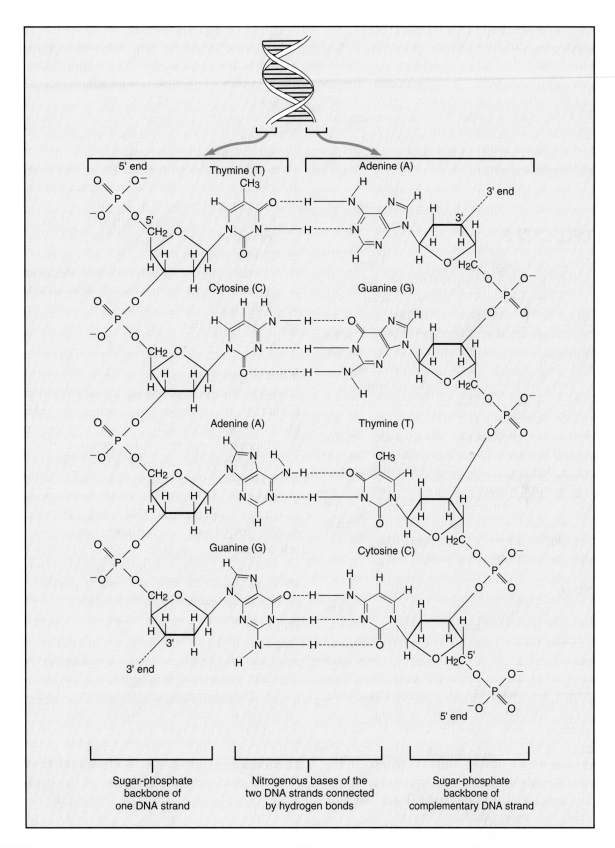

**FIGURE 4-8.** The hydrogen bonds between the purines and the pyrimidines and the chemical structure of a DNA molecule.

together and a new copy of the DNA chain is constructed (Figure 4-9). The first step is the unwinding of the molecule. This is accomplished by helicase enzymes that separate the hydrogen bonds between the base pairs and stabilize the nucleotide chains of the double helix. Then new nucleotides are added to the separated chains by DNA polymerase, another enzyme. In this way a copy of the DNA molecule is constructed.

# THE CELL CYCLE

All reproduction begins at the cellular level. The process by which a cell divides into two and duplicates its genetic material is called the **cell cycle** (Figure 4-10). The cell cycle is divided into three main stages: interphase (the stage in which great activity is occurring but this activity is not visible; thus, this stage used to be called a "resting stage"), mitosis, and cytokinesis. Two of these three stages have substages. We shall discuss all stages in detail. The time to complete a cell cycle will vary greatly among different organisms. Cells in a developing embryo will complete the cell cycle in less than 20 minutes. A dividing mammalian cell will complete the cycle in approximately 24 hours. Other cells in our bodies rarely duplicate and undergo the cell cycle, such as nerve cells and muscle cells. Human liver cells will divide only if damaged. They usually have cell cycles lasting a full year.

## Interphase

Refer to Figure 4-10 for illustrations of the stages of the cell cycle discussed below. A cell spends most of its time in the stage of the cell cycle known as **interphase.** This phase, the longest and most dynamic part of a cell's life, is not part of cell division. In fact, interphase means between phases. Yet during this time the cell is growing, metabolizing, and maintaining itself. During this time, the nucleus is seen as a distinct structure surrounded by its nuclear membrane. Inside the nucleoplasm the unwound strands of chromosomes are only visible as dark threads called **chromatin** (**KRO**-mah-tin). Interphase has three subphases: growth one ($G_1$), synthesis (S), and growth two ($G_2$). Some authors called the G phases gap one and gap two.

$G_1$ is the primary growth phase of the cell. It occupies the major portion of the life span of the cell. It is the time when the centrioles begin to make copies of themselves in animal cells. Plant cells do not have centrioles.

The synthesis or S phase is when the strands of DNA duplicate themselves. Each chromosome now consists of two sister **chromatids** attached to each other at a central region called the **centromere** but are not yet visible. Most chromosomes consist of 60% protein and 40% DNA.

The $G_2$ phase is the final phase for the preparation of cell division. In animal cells, the centrioles finish replicating and each cell now has two pairs. Mitochondria are replicated as the chromosomes now condense and coil into tightly compacted bodies. **Tubulin** is synthesized. This is the protein material that forms the microtubules and assembles at the spindle.

## Mitosis

Mitosis is the process of cellular reproduction that occurs in the nucleus and forms two identical nuclei. Because of the intricate movement of daughter chromosomes as they separate, this phase of the cell cycle has received a great deal of study by biologists. This phase can also be easily observed with a light microscope. Although mitosis is a continuous process, it is subdivided into four stages: **prophase**, **metaphase**, **anaphase**, and **telophase** (**TELL**-oh-faze). Refer to Figure 4-11 for an illustration of the stages of mitosis. The cells resulting from mitosis are exact duplicates or **clones** of the parent cell.

## Prophase

The coiled, duplicated, chromosomes have shortened and thickened and are now visible. Each chromosome consists of two sister or daughter chromatids. The sister chromatids remain attached to one another at the centromere (**SIN**-troh-meer). The centromere is a constricted or pinched-in area of the chromosome where a disk of protein called the **kinetochore** (kye-**NEE**-toh-kor) is found. In animal cells, the two centriole pairs begin to move apart to the opposite poles of the cell forming a group of microtubules between them called the **spindle fibers**. In plant cells, a similar group of spindle fibers forms even though there are no centrioles. As

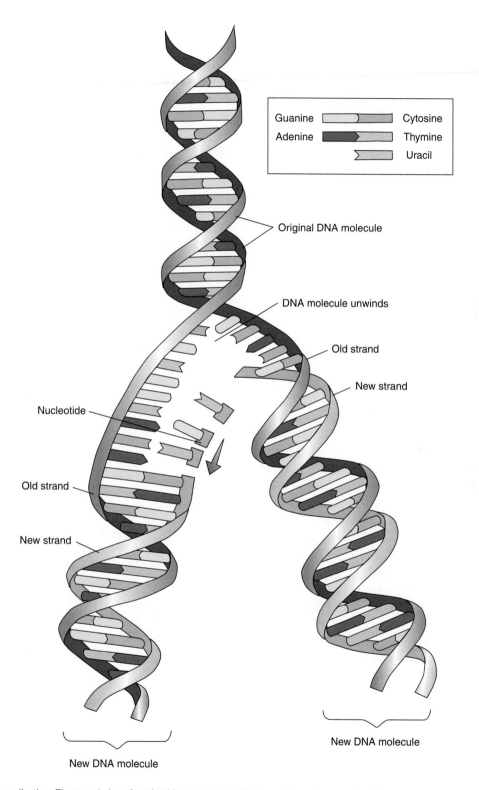

**FIGURE 4-9.** DNA replication. The two chains of nucleotides separate at the base pairs and are duplicated.

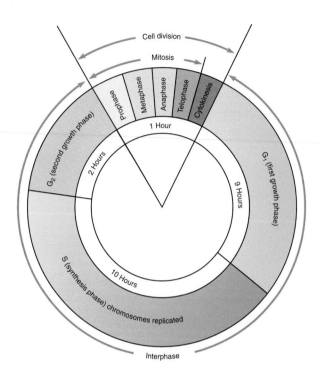

**FIGURE 4-10.** The stages of the cell cycle.

the centrioles move apart to the opposite poles of the cell, they become surrounded by a cluster of microtubules of tubulin that radiate outward looking like a starburst. This starburst form is called the **aster**. The spindle fibers form between the asters. As these fibers form, they push the centrioles to the opposite ends of the cell and brace the centrioles against the cell membrane. At this time the nuclear membrane breaks down and its components become part of the endoplasmic reticulum. The nucleolus is no longer visible.

Each chromosome has two kinetochores, one for each sister chromatid. As prophase continues, a group of microtubules grow from the poles to the centromeres of the chromosomes. The microtubules attach the kinetochores to the poles of the spindle. Because these microtubules coming from the two poles attach to opposite sides of the centromere, they attach one sister chromatid to one pole and the other sister chromatid to the other thus ensuring separation of the sister chromatids, each going to a different daughter cell.

## Metaphase

Metaphase is the second stage of mitosis and begins when the sister chromatids align themselves at the center of the cell. The chromosomes are lined up in a circle along the inner circumference of the cell called the equator of the cell. Held in place by the microtubules and attached to the kinetochore of their centromeres, the chromosomes become arranged in a ring at the equatorial or metaphase plate in the middle of the cell. At the end of metaphase each centromere now divides, separating the two sister chromatids of each chromosome.

## Anaphase

Anaphase is the shortest stage of mitosis and is one of the most dynamic stages to observe. The divided centromere, each with a sister chromatid, moves toward the opposite poles of the spindle. The motion is caused by the pulling of the microtubules on the kinetochore of each sister chromatid. The sister chromatids take on a V shape as they are drawn to their respective poles. At this time, the poles also move apart by microtubular sliding and the sister chromatids are drawn to opposite poles by the shortening of the microtubules attached to them. Cytokinesis, the division of the cytoplasm, may begin in anaphase.

## Telophase

The final stage of mitosis is telophase. The sister chromatids, which now can be called chromosomes, begin to decondense and uncoil. Their V-shaped or sausage form disappears into diffuse chromatin, becoming long and thin. The spindle apparatus is disassembled as the microtubules are broken down into units of tubulin to be used to construct the cytoskeleton of the new daughter cells. A nuclear membrane forms around each group of daughter chromosomes. Cytokinesis is nearly complete.

## Cytokinesis

The process of cell division is not yet complete because the actual separation of the cell into two new daughter cells has yet to occur. The phase of the cell cycle in which actual cell division occurs is called cytokinesis.

In animal cells, cytokinesis occurs as the cells separate by a furrowing in or pinching in of the cell membrane referred to as a **cleavage furrow**. The cell membrane indents to form a valley outside the spindle equator. This furrow first appears in late

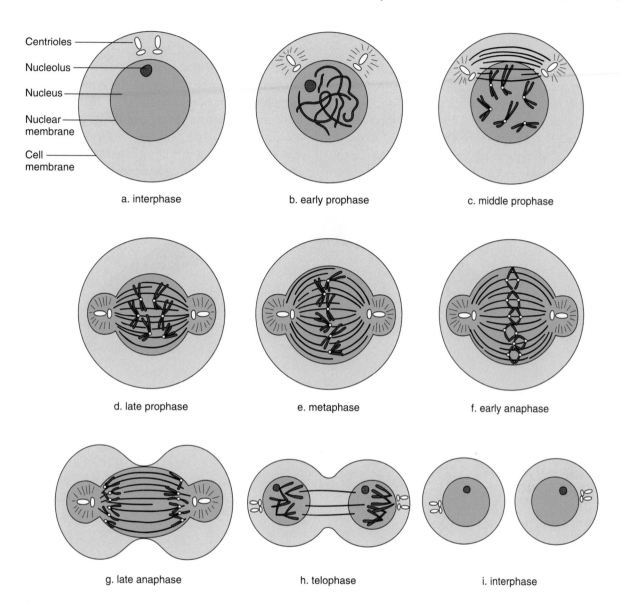

**FIGURE 4-11.** An illustration of interphase and the stages of mitosis.

anaphase and in telophase it is drawn in more deeply by the contraction of a ring of actin filaments that lie in the cytoplasm beneath the constriction points. As constriction proceeds, the furrow extends into the center of the cell and thus the cell is divided into two.

In plant cells, a **cell plate** forms at the equator. Small membranous vesicles form this cell plate, which grows outward until it reaches the cell membrane and fuses with it. Cellulose is then deposited in this new membrane forming a new cell wall that divides the cell in two.

Each new daughter cell now enters the interphase stage of the cell cycle. Each now begins its growth phase until it is ready to divide once more.

## MEIOSIS: A REDUCTION DIVISION

In sexual reproduction, two specialized cells (the sperm and the egg) known as gametes unite to form a **fertilized egg** or **zygote**. The advantage of sexual reproduction is the increased genetic variability that results from the uniting of the hereditary material of two different organisms. This results in a new individual, similar to but not identical to either parent. This new genetic variability gives the offspring a chance to adapt to a changing environment. To produce these special cells or gametes, a special kind of cellular division must occur. This special kind of division is called meiosis (mye-**OH**-sis) and it occurs only in special organs of the body, in the female gonads or ovaries and in the male gonads or testes.

Meiosis is a reduction division of the nuclear material so that each gamete contains only half as much hereditary material as the parent cell. When two gametes unite, the resulting zygote has the full complement of hereditary or DNA material. Humans have 46 chromosomes in our body cells; however, the human egg has only 23 and the human sperm has only 23 as a result of meiosis. This reduced number is called the **haploid** (**HAP**-loyd) (Greek

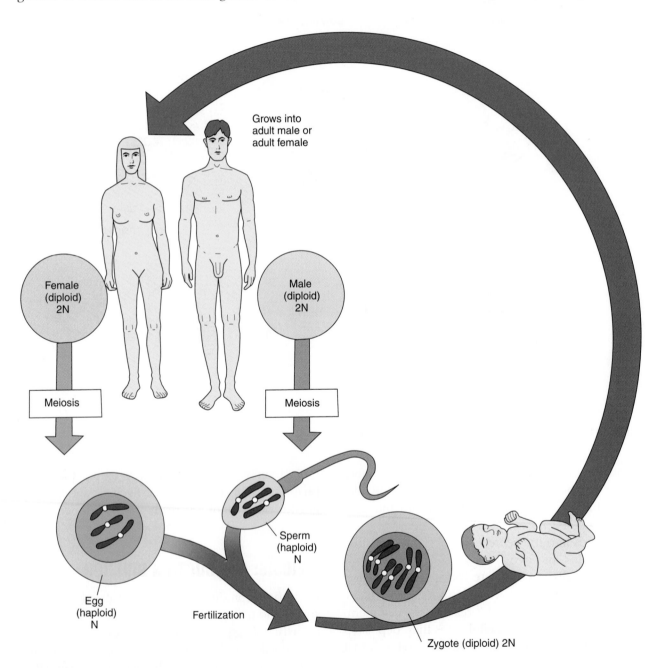

**FIGURE 4-12.** The sexual cycle.

haploos = one) or n number and the total or full complement of chromosomes is referred to as the 2n or **diploid** (**DIP**-loyd) (Greek di = two) number. Figure 4-12 illustrates the sexual cycle. We inherited 23 chromosomes from our mother through the egg fertilized at conception and 23 from our father's sperm.

Meiosis consists of two separate divisions where chromosomes are separated from one another but the DNA is duplicated only once. The first meiotic division is broken down into four substages: **prophase I**, **metaphase I**, **anaphase I**, and **telophase I**. It is in this first meiotic division that the chromosomes are reduced in half. The second meiotic division is also broken down into four substages: **prophase II**, **metaphase II**, **anaphase II**, and **telophase II**. In meiosis we end up with four daughter cells each containing only half the genetic material, whereas in mitosis we end up with two daughter cells each containing the full complement of genetic material.

## The Stages of Meiosis

The stages if meiosis are discussed below. Refer to Figure 4-13 to follow the discussion.

### Prophase I

The DNA has already duplicated before the onset of meiosis. Therefore, just like at the beginning of mitosis in interphase, each thread of DNA consists of two sister chromatids joined at their centromere. In prophase I the duplicated chromosomes shorten, coil, thicken, and become visible. It is here in meiosis that now something very different occurs. Each chromosome pairs up with its homologue. Remember that our 46 chromosomes exist as 23 pairs. One member of each pair was inherited from our mother and the other member of each pair from our father. In mitosis look-alike chromosomes did *not* pair up with one another. In meiosis homologous chromosomes are brought so close together that they line up side by side in a process called **synapsis**. We now have a pair of homologous chromosomes each with two sister chromatids. The visible pair of chromosomes is called a **tetrad** (Figure 4-14). The chromosomes are so close together that they may actually exchange genetic material in a process called **crossing-over**. Actual segments of DNA are exchanged between the sister

chromatids of the homologous chromosomes. Crossing-over is a common but random event and it occurs only in meiosis. Evidence of crossing-over can be seen with a light microscope as an X-shaped structure known as a chiasma or **chiasmata** (key-**AZZ**-mah-tah) (plural). The spindle forms from microtubules just as in mitosis; paired chromosomes separate slightly and orient themselves on the spindle attached by their centromere.

### Metaphase I

Spindle microtubules attach to the kinetochore only on the outside of each centromere and the centromeres of the two homologous chromosomes are attached to microtubules originating from *opposite* poles. This one-sided attachment in meiosis is in contrast to mitosis whose kinetochore on *both* sides of a centromere are held by microtubules. This ensures that the homologous chromosomes will be pulled to opposite poles of the cell. The homologous chromosomes line up on the equatorial plate. The centromeres of each pair lie opposite one another. The orientation on the spindle is random thus either homologue might be oriented to either pole.

### Anaphase I

The microtubules of the spindle shorten and pull the centromeres toward the poles, dragging both sister chromatids with it. Thus unlike mitosis, the *centromere does not divide* in this stage. Because of the random orientation of the homologous chromosomes on the equatorial plate, a pole may receive either homologue of each pair. Thus, the genes on different chromosomes assort independently.

### Telophase I

The homologous chromosome pairs have separated and now a member of each pair is at the opposite ends of the spindle. Now at each pole is a cluster of "haploid" chromosomes. The number has been reduced from 46 to 23 at each pole. However, each chromosome still consists of two sister chromatids attached by a common centromere. This "duplication condition" will be corrected in the second meiotic division. Now the spindle disappears, the chromosomes uncoil and become long and thin, and a new nuclear membrane forms around each cluster of chromosomes at the opposite poles. Cytokinesis occurs and we have two new cells formed at the end of the first

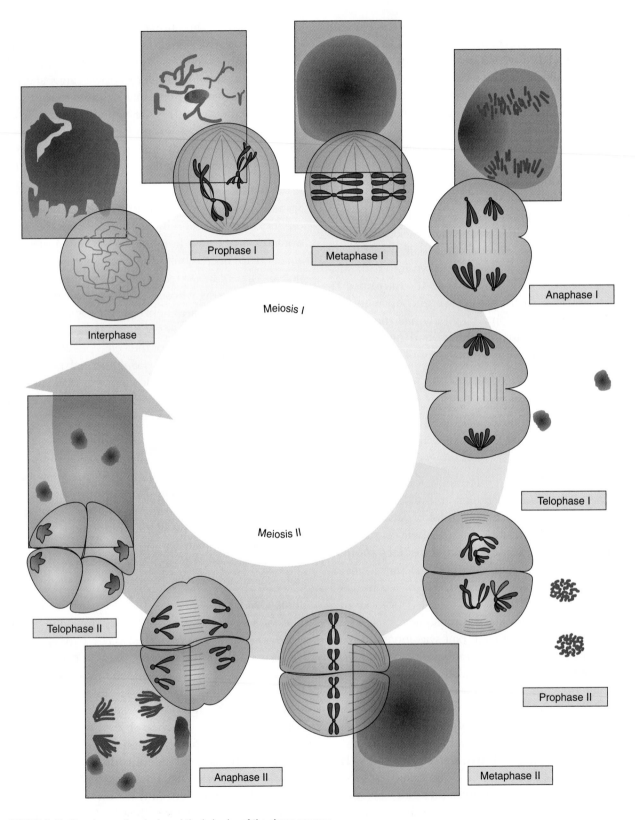

**FIGURE 4-13.** The stages of meiosis and the behavior of the chromosomes.

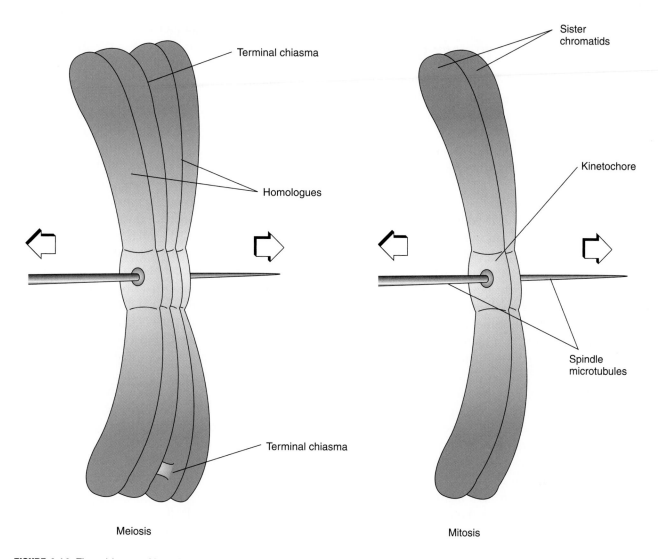

**FIGURE 4-14.** The pairing up of homologous chromosomes in prophase I of meiosis produces figures called tetrads. When crossing-over occurs, it is visible and called chiasmata.

meiotic division. The second meiotic division closely resembles the occurrences in mitosis.

### Prophase II

In each of the two daughter cells produced in the first meiotic division, a spindle forms, the chromosomes shorten, coil, and thicken. The nuclear membrane disappears but *no duplication of DNA occurs*.

### Metaphase II

In each of the two daughter cells, the chromosomes line up on the equatorial plate. Spindle fibers bind to *both* sides of the centromere. Each chromosome consists of two sister chromatids and one centromere.

### Anaphase II

The *centromeres* of the chromosomes *divide*. The spindle fibers contract, pulling the sister chromatids apart and moving each one to an opposite pole. Now each chromosome is truly haploid, consisting of one chromatid and one centromere.

### Telophase II

New nuclear membranes form around the separated chromatids, the spindle disappears, and the chromosomes uncoil and decondense. The result is four haploid daughter cells each containing one half the genetic material of the original parent cell or in our case each cell having 23 chromosomes instead of 46.

# GAMETOGENESIS: THE FORMATION OF THE SEX CELLS

The four haploid cells produced by meiosis are not yet mature sex cells. Further differentiation must now occur. This is known as **gametogenesis** (**gam**-eh-toh-**JEN**-eh-sis). The process occurring in the semiferous tubules of the testes is called **spermatogenesis** (**sper**-mat-oh-**JEN**-eh-sis) (Figure 4-15). The cytoplasm of each of the four cells produced, called spermatids, becomes modified into a tail-like flagellum. A concentration of mitochondria collect in the middle piece or collar. The mitochondria will produce the ATP necessary to propel the flagellum, which causes the sperm to swim. The nucleus of each cell becomes the head of the sperm. The genetic material is concentrated in the head of the sperm. The sperm cell will penetrate an egg and fuse with the genetic material of the egg in the process called fertilization, producing a fertilized egg or zygote.

The formation of the female egg, called **oogenesis** (oh-oh-**JEN**-eh-sis), occurs in the ovary (Figure 4-16). However, only one functional egg is produced. In the first meiotic division, there is an unequal distribution of the cytoplasm so that one cell is larger than the other. The larger cell in the second meiotic division also has unequal distribution of the cytoplasm. The three smaller cells produced are called **polar bodies** and eventually die. They have contributed cytoplasm to the single larger cell that will become the functional egg. The union of sperm and egg is called fertilization and restores the diploid number of chromosomes to 46.

# A COMPARISON OF MITOSIS AND MEIOSIS

The two types of cellular division consisting of mitosis and meiosis are easy to confuse. They have similarities but they also have differences. In both mitosis and meiosis the chromosomes duplicate or replicate in the phase of the cell cycle called interphase. However, in mitosis the end result is *two* daughter cells each with exactly the same number of chromosomes as the parent cell, whereas in meiosis the end result is *four* daughter cells each with only half the number of chromosomes as the parent cell. Mitosis consists of one division, whereas meiosis consists of two divisions.

In mitosis, when the genetic material duplicates, the homologous chromosomes are scattered in the nucleus and do *not* seek one another out. In meiosis, after duplication, the homologous pairs of chromosomes line up together and come so close that they entwine. Crossing-over or exchange of segments of DNA may occur. Crossing-over occurs only in prophase I of meiosis. This results in a recombination of existing genes, thus producing new genetic characteristics. In mitosis the centromere divides in anaphase. In meiosis the centromere does not divide in anaphase I. The centromere divides only in anaphase II. Figure 4-17 provides a summary comparison of mitosis and meiosis.

Mitosis occurs in all cells of our bodies on a regular basis (except nerve, muscle, and liver cells). After the egg is fertilized, the embryo develops by mitosis. After birth, we grow and mature by mitosis. When we cut our finger or bruise our tissues, the cells are repaired and replaced by mitosis. Liver cells divide only if damaged; muscle cells and nerve cells rarely divide by mitosis. Cells produced by mitosis can live for as long as necessary once produced. These cells all contain the same genetic information as the parent cell. In special sections of our gonads, the seminiferous tubules of the testes of the male and in the ovaries of the female, another kind of cell division occurs. Meiosis occurs only in these special cells of the gonads. It is a reduction division. The genetic material is reduced in half. This process begins at puberty in the male and in the embryo of the female. It will continue at puberty in the female. The cells produced cannot live on their own. They live for only a short time and eventually die unless they fuse in fertilization inside the female reproductive tract.

In each type of cellular division, the genetic material is exactly duplicated during interphase. Sometimes, however, the genetic material may be damaged by x-rays, radiation, or certain chemicals. When this happens, the cells' damaged genetic material may cause the cells not to go into interphase. They divide continuously, forming masses of tissues. This is cancer.

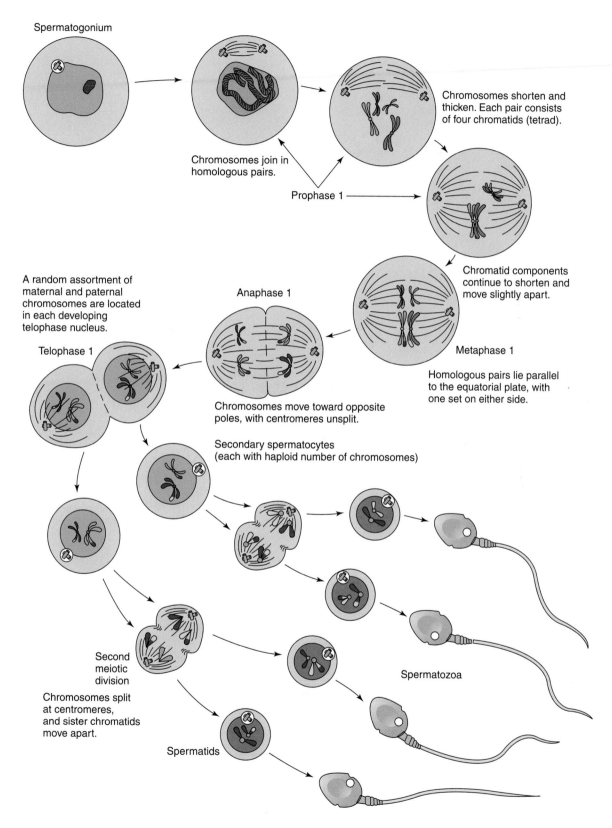

**FIGURE 4-15.** Spermatogenesis occurring in the seminiferous tubules of the testes.

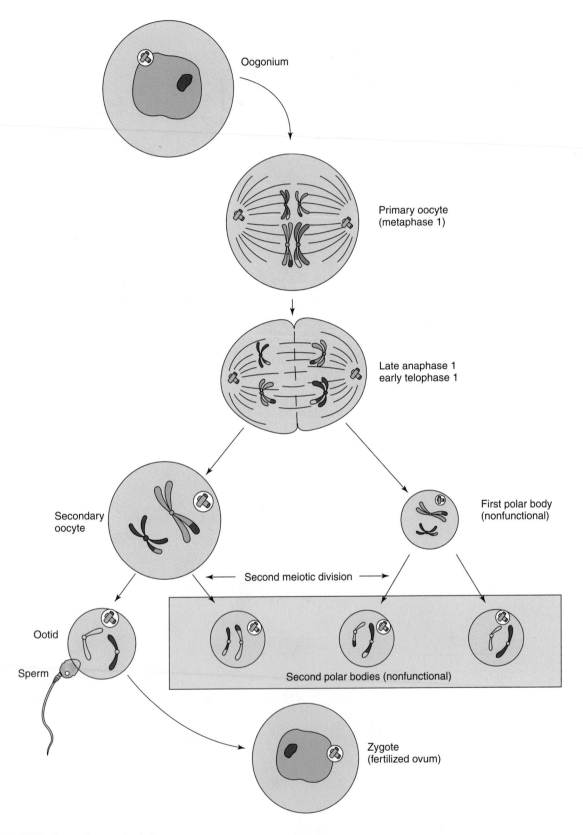

Oogonium

Primary oocyte
(metaphase 1)

Late anaphase 1
early telophase 1

Secondary
oocyte

First polar body
(nonfunctional)

Second meiotic division

Ootid

Sperm

Second polar bodies (nonfunctional)

Zygote
(fertilized ovum)

**FIGURE 4-16.** Oogensis occurring in the ovary.

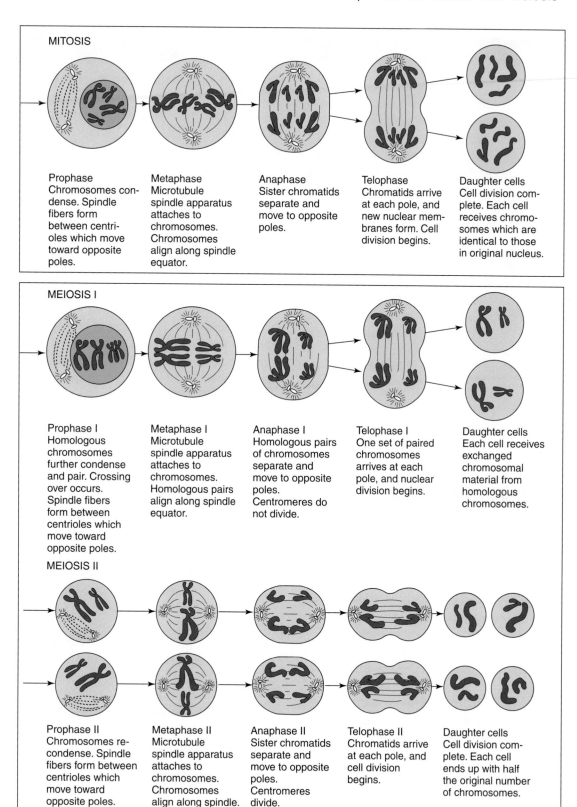

**FIGURE 4-17.** A comparison of mitosis and meiosis.

---

**Common Disease, Disorder or Condition**

## ■ CANCER

Cancer has a number of causes. One of these is incorrect information in the genetic material of a cell. When a cell duplicates its genetic material during the interphase S (synthesis) stage, rarely, a mistake can occur. The exact copying of the code can be disrupted by external factors such as excessive exposure to certain chemicals (smoke, asbestos), radiation (radioactive materials), x-rays, and even some viruses. This is called a **mutation**.

When the genetic code governing cell division is affected, cells continue to grow and do not go into interphase. They keep dividing uncontrollably. This results in a cluster of cells called a **tumor**. All the cells of the tumor contain the same genetic misinformation and some leave the tumor and travel to other parts of the body. They go to other sites and produce more tumors. We call these other tumors

at different sites **metastases** (meh-**TASS**-tah-seez) and when the defective cells spread they **metastasize** (meh-**TASS**-tah-size) to other parts of the body.

Cancer can occur in any tissue and a number of terms have developed to define these cancers. Tumors devloping from epithelial tissue are called **carcinomas** (kar-sin-**NOH**-mahz); those coming from connective tissue, like bone, are called **sarcomas** (sar-**KOM**-ahz). Cancer-causing agents are called **carcinogens** (kar-**SIN**-oh-jenz). Some of the most serious cancers in humans are lung cancer resulting from cigarette smoking, colorectal cancers caused by excessive red meat in the diet, and breast cancer. The cause of breast cancer appears to be related to a gene located on chromosome number 17, which is responsible for hereditary susceptibility to the disease.

---

## Summary Outline

### INTRODUCTION TO CELLULAR METABOLISM

1. The most common form of chemical energy that maintains cellular structure and function is the molecule ATP (adenosine triphosphate).
2. Metabolism is a general term that describes the total chemical changes that occur in cells. There are two subcategories: anabolism is the energy-requiring process that builds larger molecules by combining smaller molecules, and catabolism is the energy-releasing process that breaks down larger molecules into smaller ones. These cellular metabolic processes are often called cellular respiration.
3. ATP is made in a stepwise catabolism (decomposition) of food molecules like glucose. The chemical energy in food (calories) is released and used to put together ADP (adenosine diphosphate) and $PO_4$ (phosphate) to make ATP.
4. The overall chemical equation for cellular respiration is:

$$C_6H_{12}O_6 + 6O_2 \rightarrow 6CO_2 + 6H_2O + 38 \text{ ATP or}$$
36 ATP and 2 GTP

5. Cellular respiration consist of three processes or steps: glycolysis, Krebs' citric acid cycle, and electron transport.

### GLYCOLYSIS

1. Glycolysis occurs in the cytoplasm of the cell and does not require oxygen.
2. We must use two ATP molecules to start glycolysis and these must be "paid back" from our production of ATP.
3. The main products of glycolysis are fructose diphosphate, which splits into two phosphoglyceraldehyde molecules that oxidize to two phosphoglyceric acids, which convert to the final product of two pyruvic acid molecules.
4. When oxygen is present two hydrogens from each of the two phosphoglyceraldehydes go to the electron transport system beginning with the cofactor NAD. This produces six ATP.
5. When phosphoglyceric acid is decomposed to pyruvic acid four ATP are made, but we must

pay back the two that started the sequence. Thus, we produce only a net gain of two ATP.

6. In glycolysis we produce a total net gain of eight ATP. In anaerobic glycolysis in muscle cells and in fermentation only two ATP are produced.

## THE KREBS' CITRIC ACID CYCLE

1. The citric acid cycle is named for the British biochemist Sir Hans Krebs who first proposed the scheme in 1937.
2. The two pyruvic acid molecules produced in glycolysis are converted to acetic acid and then to acetyl-CoA through the action of CoA enzyme. Acetyl-CoA now enters the cristae of the mitochondria to go through the citric acid cycle.
3. The major chemical products in the cycle are citric acid, alpha-ketogluteric acid, succinic acid, malic acid, and oxaloacetic acid.
4. Most of the ATP is made by electron transport. For each of the two pyruvic acid molecules broken down, 14 ATP are made via electron transport for a total production of 28 ATP. In addition 2 ATP or GTP are produced in the citric acid cycle for a total of 30 ATP or 28 ATP and 2 GTP.
5. For each pyruvic acid molecule broken down three $CO_2$ are given off as waste products for a total of six $CO_2$ molecules produced.

## THE ELECTRON TRANSPORT SYSTEM

1. The electron transport system functions as a series of redox (reduction-oxidation) reactions.
2. There are several kinds of electron carriers in the electron transport system: NAD (nicotinamide adenine dinucleotide), FAD (flavin adenine dinucleotide), quinone, and the cytochrome system.
3. If the system begins with NAD, then three ATP are produced. If the system begins with FAD, then only two ATP are produced.
4. Oxygen is necessary for respiration because oxygen is the ultimate electron acceptor in the system.
5. When oxygen accepts the electrons from the two hydrogen atoms and the two hydrogen protons, water ($H_2O$) is produced as a waste product.

## SUMMARY OF ATP PRODUCTION

1. Glycolysis produces a total net gain of eight ATP.
2. The Krebs' citric acid cycle produces for each of the two pyruvic acid molecules 14 ATP via electron transport and one ATP or GTP. Thus the total ATP production in the cycle is 28 ATP and two GTP or 30 ATP.
3. The eight ATP from glycolysis and the 30 ATP from the citric acid cycle yield a total of 38 ATP from each glucose molecule.

## ANAEROBIC RESPIRATION

1. Fermentation is the process by which yeast cells break down glucose in the absence of oxygen. This process produces only two ATP and is much less efficient than glycolysis.
2. The other products of fermentation are carbon dioxide gas, which causes bread dough to rise, and ethyl alcohol, which is used in the beer, wine, and liquor industries.
3. When we overwork our muscles and cannot get enough oxygen to the muscle cells, they begin to break down glucose in the absence of oxygen. The total net gain of ATP is only two ATP molecules and pyruvic acid is converted to lactic acid.
4. The buildup of lactic acid in the muscle cells is what causes the soreness in overworked muscles. Our breathing and heartbeat rates accelerate to get more $O_2$ to the cells. Eventually the soreness goes away as lactic acid is converted back to pyruvic acid when oxygen again becomes available.

## PRODUCTION OF ATP FROM GENERAL FOOD COMPOUNDS

1. The cellular furnace that "burns" food to produce ATP consists of glycolysis, the Krebs' citric acid cycle, and electron transport.
2. Carbohydrates feed into the furnace at the level of glucose in glycolysis.
3. Fats are digested into glycerol, which feeds into the furnace at the phosphoglyceric acid stage of glycolysis, and fatty acids, which feed into the citric acid cycle.
4. Proteins are digested into amino acids. They feed into the furnace at different stages of glycolysis and the citric acid cycle based on their chemical structure.

5. Carbohydrates, fats, and proteins are all potential sources of cellular energy because they can all be broken down and their chemical energy can be converted into another form of chemical energy, ATP, which runs the cell's machinery.

## INTRODUCTION TO CELLULAR REPRODUCTION

1. Cellular reproduction is the process by which a single cell duplicates itself. Mitosis is duplication of the genetic material in the nucleus. Cytokinesis is the duplication of the organelles in the cytoplasm. Meiosis is a special kind of reduction division that occurs only in the gonads.

## THE STRUCTURE OF THE DNA MOLECULE

### The History of the Discovery of DNA

1. DNA was first discovered in 1869 by a German chemist, Friedrich Miescher.
2. In the 1920s P. A. Levine discovered that DNA contained phosphates, five-carbon sugars, and nitrogen-containing bases.
3. Rosalind Franklin, British, discovered the helical structure of DNA via x-ray crystallography studies.
4. James Watson, an American, and Francis Crick, British, won the 1962 Nobel Prize for working out the three-dimensional structure of the molecule.

### The Anatomy of the DNA Molecule

1. A DNA molecule is a double helical chain of nucleotides.
2. A nucleotide is a complex combination of a phosphate group ($PO_4$), a five-carbon sugar (deoxyribose), and a nitrogen-containing base, either a purine or a pyrimidine.
3. A pyrimidine consists of a single ring of six atoms of carbon and nitrogen. There are two pyrimidines in the molecule: thymine and cytosine.
4. A purine consists of a fused double ring of nine atoms of carbon and nitrogen. There are two purines in the molecule: adenine and guanine.
5. In the chain of nucleotides, bonds form between the phosphate group of one nucleotide and the sugar of the next nucleotide. The base extends out from the sugar.

6. Adenine of one chain always pairs with thymine of the other chain. Cytosine of one chain always pairs with guanine of the other chain. The bases are held together by hydrogen bonds.
7. A gene is a sequence of organic nitrogen base pairs that codes for a polypetide or protein.
8. In our 46 chromosomes there are billions of organic base pairs that encode over 100,000 genes.

## THE CELL CYCLE

1. The cell cycle is the process by which a cell divides into two and duplicates its genetic material.
2. A cell cycle is divided into three stages: interphase, mitosis, and cytokinesis.

### Interphase

1. Interphase is the time between divisions. It is divided into three sub-tages: $G_1$ (growth one), S (synthesis), and $G_2$ (growth two).
2. The major portion of the life of the cell is spent in $G_1$. During $G_1$, the primary growth phase, the two centrioles of animal cells begin to duplicate.
3. During the S phase, the genetic material or DNA duplicates itself.
4. During the $G_2$ phase, the two centioles complete duplication, mitochondria replicate, and the chromosomes condense and coil. Tubulin is synthesized.

### Mitosis

1. Mitosis, cellular division in the nucleus, has four stages: prophase, metaphase, anaphase, and telophase.

### Prophase

1. The duplicated chromosomes shorten, thicken, and become visible as two sister chromatids held together at a middle area called the centromere.
2. The two kinetochores are found at the centromere.
3. The centrioles move to opposite poles of the cell and form the spindle and asters in animal cells.
4. The nuclear membrane breaks down and the nucleolus disappears.
5. The microtubules attach the kinetochores to the spindle.

## Metaphase

1. The sister chromatids align themselves in a circle at the equator of the cell held in place by the microtubules attached to the kinetochores of the centromere.
2. The centromere divides.

## Anaphase

1. Each divided centromere pulls a sister chromatid to an opposite pole.
2. Cytokinesis begins.

## Telphase

1. The chromosomes begin to uncoil and decondense.
2. The spindle apparatus breaks down.
3. A new nuclear membrane forms around the cluster of chromosomes at each pole.
4. Cytokinesis is nearly complete.

## Cytokinesis

1. In animal cells a cleavage furrow forms by a pinching in of the cell membrane, resulting in two daughter cells.
2. In plant cells, a cell plate forms at the equator and grows outward effectively dividing the cell in two. The cell plate becomes a new cell wall.

## MEIOSIS: A REDUCTION DIVISION

1. Meiosis is a reduction division of the nuclear material; it occurs only in the gonads. It reduces the genetic material from 46 (diploid or 2n) to 23 (haploid or n) chromosomes.
2. Meiosis consists of two divisions resulting in four cells. The first meiotic division reduces the number of chromosomes in half. The second meiotic division corrects their duplicated nature.

## The Stages of Meiosis

## Prophase I

1. Homologous chromosomes pair and crossing-over may occur.
2. Spindle fibers form, the nuclear membrane breaks down, and the chromosomes are attached to the spindle by their centromeres.

## Metaphase I

1. Microtubules attach to the kinetochore on one side of the centromere. Homologous pairs of chromosomes align along the equator of the spindle.

## Anaphase I

1. The centromeres do *not* divide. The microtubules of the spindle shorten and pull the centromeres of the chromosomes to opposite poles, one member of each pair to a pole.

## Telophase I

1. A member of each pair of homologous chromosomes is at each pole. The number of chromosomes have been reduced in half. They are now haploid, but still duplicated.
2. The spindle disappears and a new nuclear membrane forms around each group of chromosomes at the pole.
3. The chromosomes uncoil and decondense.
4. Cytokensis occurs and two new daughter cells are formed.

## Prophase II

1. In each daughter cell a spindle forms, centrioles move to opposite poles, and the chromosomes coil and thicken.
2. The nuclear membrane disappears.

## Metaphase II

1. The chromosomes line up at the equator of the cell attached by the microtubules of the spindle.
2. Microtubules bind to *both* kinetochores of the centromere.

## Anaphase II

1. The centromeres divide.
2. The spindle fibers contract pulling the sister chromatids apart, one to each pole of the spindle.

## Telophase II

1. The chromatids arrive at each pole, where they uncoil and decondense.
2. A new nuclear membrane forms around the chromatids, and the spindle disappears.
3. Four haploid cells are formed as cytokinesis is completed.

## GAMETOGENESIS: THE FORMATION OF THE SEX CELLS

1. Spermatogenesis occurs in the seminiferous tubules of the testes. Each of the four cells produced by meiosis develops into sperm.
2. The cytoplasm of each cell develops into a tail-like flagellum and a concentration of mitochondria forms the collar or middle piece.

The head of the sperm is formed by the nucleus of the cell.

3. Oogenesis occurs in the ovary. Of the four cells produced only one becomes the functional egg. The other three are called polar bodies and contribute their cytoplasm to the functional egg.

## A COMPARISON OF MITOSIS AND MEIOSIS

1. Mitosis produces two daughter cells with the exact same genetic material as the parent cell.
2. Meiosis produces four daughter cells, each with half the genetic material of the parent cell.
3. In meiosis, homologous pairs of chromosomes line up in prophase I and exchange genetic material in a process called crossing-over.
4. Mitosis is a process of cellular division by which we grow, maintain, and repair ourselves. Most cells of our body undergo mitosis. Nerve and muscle cells rarely divide and liver cells divide only when damaged.
5. Meiosis occurs only in the gonads. Unlike the cells produced by mitosis, meiotic cells cannot live on their own. They must unite in fertilization in the female reproductive tract.
6. Cancer is uncontrolled cellular growth caused by damaged genetic material. Cells never go into interphase; they divide continuously.

## REVIEW QUESTIONS

1. Diagram glycolysis, the first step in the biochemical decomposition of a glucose molecule. Indicate where and how many ATP are produced.
2. Diagram the Krebs' citric acid cycle beginning with one molecule of pyruvic acid. Indicate where and how many ATP are produced.
3. Diagram the electron transport system with its electron carriers. Indicate where and how many ATP are produced.
*4. Why are fermentation and anaerobic production of ATP by muscle cells less efficient than glycolysis?
*5. Name some practical applications of the fermentation process for human advancement.

6. Name the four kinds of organic bases found in a DNA molecule and indicate how they pair up in linking the two helical chains of the molecule. Include a linear diagrammatic drawing of a short segment of DNA.
7. Name the three main stages of the cell cycle.
8. Name and explain what happens during the three substages of interphase.
*9. Why was interphase once called a "resting stage"?
10. Name and briefly describe the stages of the two meiotic divisions of meiosis.
*11. Why is meiosis called a reduction division?
*12. Compare the major differences between mitosis and meiosis.

*Critical Thinking Questions

## True or False

1. The breakdown of glucose requires oxygen because oxygen is the ultimate electron donor for the electrons used by the cofactors in the electron transport system.          T    F
2. The anaerobic decomposition of glucose by yeast cells yields one ATP, ethyl alcohol, $CO_2$, and NAD.          T    F
3. Lactic acid produced in the muscles during anaerobic respiration accumulates there and is never broken down or ever converted to other products.          T    F
4. The formation of lactic acid regenerates NAD for use in the glycolytic sequence.     T    F
5. Each molecule of glucose undergoing glycolysis yields one molecule of pyruvic acid.     T    F
6. One molecule of glucose undergoing aerobic respiration yields 34 molecules of ATP.  T    F
7. The overall chemical equation for respiration is $C_6H_{12}O_6 + 6O_2 \rightarrow 6CO_2 + 6H_2O +$ energy in the form of ATP.          T    F
8. When nicotine adenine dinucleotide gets reduced in electron transport, two molecules of ATP are produced.          T    F
9. Fermentation is as effective as glycolysis.          T    F
10. All foods taken into the body must be broken down to glucose before respiration can proceed.          T    F

## Fill in the Blank

Fill in the blank with the most appropriate term.

1. _____ discovered the helical nature of the DNA molecule via x-ray crystallography studies in England.

2. _____ and _____ won the Nobel Prize in 1962 for determining the three-dimensional structure of the DNA molecule.

3. The DNA molecule consists of a double helical chain of _____.

4. In the DNA molecule, every phosphate group is bonded to a _____.

5. The two types of nitrogen bases in the DNA molecule are: _____, a single ring of six atoms and _____, a fused double ring of nine atoms of carbon and nitrogen.

6. Adenine always pairs with _____, and cytosine always pairs with _____.

7. The nitrogen base pairs of the two chains of the DNA molecule are held together by _____ bonds.

8. Cellular division in the nucleus producing two identical nuclei is known as _____.

9. _____ is a reduction division of the nuclear material so that each gamete contains only half as much genetic material as the parent.

10. Exchange of genetic material between homologous chromosomes occurring in prophase I of meiosis is called _____.

11. The number of cells produced after a mitotic division is _____ whereas the number of cells produced after meiosis is _____.

12. Meiosis occurs only in the _____ of the human body.

---

## LABORATORY EXERCISE: CELLULAR METABOLISM

The author recommends students view the videotape "Cellular Respiration: Energy for Life" in lab. This videotape is produced by Human Relations Media, 175 Tompkins Ave., Pleasantville, NY 10570-3156. It runs 22 minutes and comes with a teacher's guide and student worksheets.

---

## LABORATORY EXERCISE: CELLULAR REPRODUCTION

1. Your instructor will show you a videotape or a CD-ROM on cell division. Two suggestions are: Carolina Biological Supply Company's video filmstrip "Cell Division" and The Center for Humanities videotape "Mitosis and Meiosis: How Cells Divide."

2. Set up your compound light microscope and observe the stages of mitosis by looking at slides of the whitefish blastula (animal) and an onion root tip (plant). Draw and label cells showing the following stages: interphase, prophase, metaphase, anaphase, and telophase.

3. Examine a prepared slide of human sperm. Draw and label the parts of a sperm cell.

4. Examine a prepared slide of the chromosomes of a fruit fly, *Drosophila*, from a smear of the fly's salivary gland.

5. Construct a portion of a DNA molecule from a kit supplied by your instructor.

# 5

# Tissues

## CHAPTER OUTLINE

- **Introduction**
- **Epithelial tissue:** *Classification based on shape; Classification based on arrangement; Classification based on function*
- **Connective tissue:** *Loose connective tissue; Dense connective tissue; Specialized connective tissue; Connective tissue functions*
- **Muscle tissue**
- **Nervous tissue**

## CHAPTER OBJECTIVES

After studying this chapter, you will be able to:

1. Classify epithelial tissue based on shape and arrangement and give examples.

2. Name the types of glands in the body and give examples.

3. Name the functions of connective tissue.

4. Compare epithelial tissue with connective tissue in terms of cell arrangement and interstitial materials.

5. Name the three major types of connective tissue and give examples.

6. List the functions of epithelial tissue.

7. List the three types of muscle and describe each based on structure and function.

8. Describe the anatomy of a neuron and the function of nervous tissue.

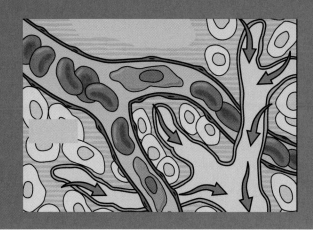

# KEY TERMS

# INTRODUCTION

The basic units of **tissue** (**TISH**-you) are groups of cells. These cells will have a similar function and a similar structure. Tissues are classified based on how these cells are arranged and what kind and how much material is found between the cells. Cells are either tightly packed or separated by interstitial material. The study of tissue is called **histology** (hiss-**TALL**-oh-jee).

The four basic types of tissue are epithelial, connective, muscle, and nervous. Each type is further subdivided into specific examples. These tissues combine to form organs. The various organs make up the systems of the body that allow us to function and survive in our complex world.

# EPITHELIAL TISSUE

**Epithelial** (ep-ih-**THEE**-lee-al) **tissue** functions in four major ways.

1. It protects underlying tissues. Our skin is epithelial tissue and protects us from the harmful rays of the sun and certain chemicals. The lining of our digestive tract is made of epithelial tissue and protects underlying tissue from abrasion as food moves through the tract.
2. It absorbs. In the lining of the small intestine nutrients from our digested food enter blood capillaries and get carried to the cells of our body.
3. It secretes. All glands are made of epithelial tissue; the endocrine glands secrete hormones, the mucous glands secrete mucus, and our intestinal tract contains cells that secrete digestive enzymes in addition to the pancreas and the liver, which secrete the major portions of digestive enzymes.
4. Epithelial tissue excretes. Sweat glands excrete waste products such as urea.

When epithelial tissue has a protective or absorbing function, it is found in sheets covering a surface, like the skin or intestinal lining. When it has a secreting function, the cells involute from the surface into the underlying tissues to form glandular structures. Only a minimal, if any, amount of inter-cellular material is found in epithelial tissue. The cells are very tightly packed together and thus this tissue is not as easily penetrated as other tissues.

Epithelial cells are anchored to each other and to underlying tissues by a specialized membrane called the **basement membrane**. This membrane acts like the adhesive on a tile floor, the tiles being the epithelial cells. It is very important because it acts as an anchor for the attached side of the epithelial cells and it provides protection for other underlying tissue like connective tissue.

Epithelial tissue can be named according to shape and structures that might be on the free or outer edge of the cells. This surface can be plain or it can have rows of cilia (those that line the respiratory tract), a flagellum (the sperm cell), microvilli (folds), and secretory vesicles (those that line the small intestine). Epithelial tissue can be one layer or several layers thick.

## Classification Based on Shape

Epithelial cells are classified as either squamous, cuboidal, or columnar. **Squamous** (**SKWAY**-mus) cells are flat and slightly irregular in shape (Figure 5-1). They serve as a protective layer. They line our mouth, blood and lymph vessels, parts of kidney tubules, our throat and esophagus, the anus, and our skin. If exposed to repeated irritation like the linings of ducts in glands, other epithelial cells can become squamous in appearance.

**Cuboidal** (**KYOO**-boyd-al) cells look like small cubes (Figure 5-2). They are found in glands and the lining tissue of gland ducts (sweat and salivary), the germinal coverings of the ovaries, and the pigmented layer of the retina of the eye. Their function can be secretion and protection. In areas of the kidney tubules, they function in absorption.

**Columnar** cells are tall and rectangular looking (Figure 5-3). They are found lining the ducts of certain glands (e.g., mammary glands) and the bile duct of the liver. They are also found in mucous-secreting tissues such as the mucosa of the stomach, the villi of the small intestine, the uterine tubes, and the upper respiratory tract. Many of these cells are ciliated.

## Classification Based on Arrangement

The four most common arrangements of epithelial cells are simple, stratified, pseudostratified, and

| Characteristics and Location | Morphology |
| --- | --- |

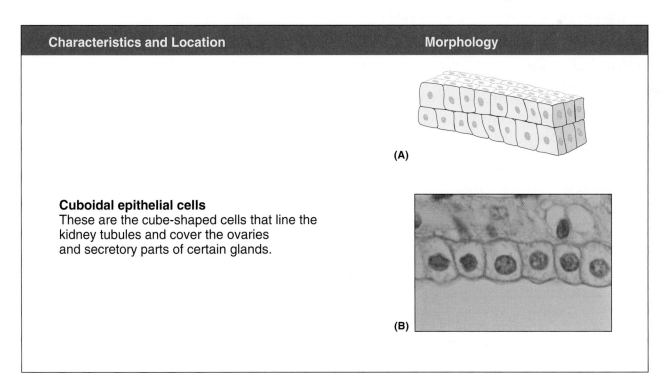

**(A)**

**Squamous epithelial cells**
These are flat, irregularly shaped cells. They line the heart, blood and lymphatic vessels, body cavities, and alveoli (air sacs) of lungs. The outer layer of the skin is composed of stratified and keratinized squamous epithelial cells. The stratified squamous epithelial cells on the outer skin layer protect the body against microbial invasion.

**(B)**

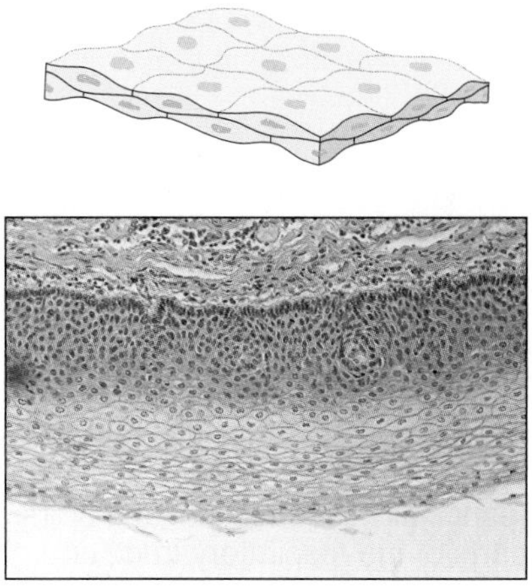

**FIGURE 5-1.** Views of squamous epithelium.

| Characteristics and Location | Morphology |
| --- | --- |

**(A)**

**Cuboidal epithelial cells**
These are the cube-shaped cells that line the kidney tubules and cover the ovaries and secretory parts of certain glands.

**(B)**

**FIGURE 5-2.** Views of cuboidal epithelium.

| Characteristics and Location | Morphology |
|---|---|
| **Columnar epithelial cells**<br>Elongated, with the nucleus generally near the bottom and often ciliated on the outer surface; they line the ducts, digestive tract (especially the intestinal and stomach lining), parts of the respiratory tract, and glands. | 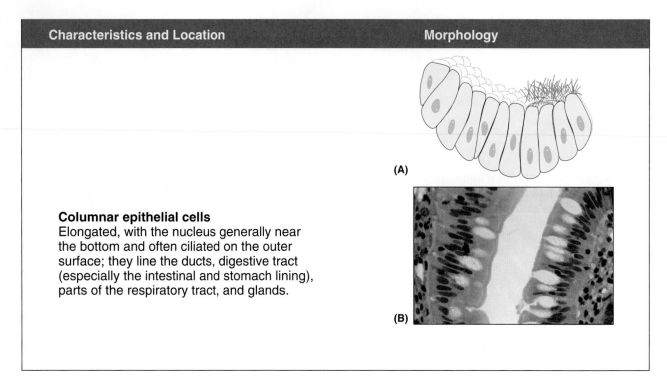<br>(A)<br><br>(B) |

**FIGURE 5-3.** Views of columnar epithelium.

transitional. As epithelial cells are named, a combination of the classification of both shape and arrangement is used. The **simple** arrangement is one cell layer thick. It is found in the lining of blood capillaries, the alveoli of the lungs, and in the loop of Henle in the kidney tubules. Refer to Figure 5-2 for simple cuboidal epithelium found in the lining of glandular ducts. Refer to Figure 5-3 for simple columnar epithelium found in the villi of the small intestine and the lining of the uterus. The **stratified** arrangement is several layers of cells thick. Refer to Figure 5-1B for stratified squamous epithelium found lining our mouth and throat and as the outer surface of our skin. Stratified cuboidal epithelium is found lining our sweat gland ducts and salivary gland ducts. Stratified columnar epithelium is found as the lining of the ducts of the mammary glands and in parts of the male urethra.

The **pseudostratified** arrangement appears to consist of several layers but in actuality, all cells extend from the basement membrane to the outer or free surface of the cells. This arrangement is usually seen with columnar cells. Figure 5-4A is an example of pseudostratified ciliated, columnar epithelium. We find this tissue in the throat, trachea, and bronchi of the lungs. **Transitional** epithelium consists of several layers of closely packed, flexible, and easily stretched cells (Figure 5-4B). When the surfaces of the cells are stretched, as in a full bladder, the cells appear squamous or flat but when the tissue is relaxed, as in an empty bladder, the layers of cells look ragged like the teeth of a saw. This type of epithelium lines the pelvis of the kidney, the ureters, the urinary bladder, and the upper part of the urethra.

## Classification Based on Funtion

Epithelial tissue can also be named or classified based on its function. The terms mucous membrane, glands, endothelium, and mesothelium all refer to epithelial tissue.

**Mucous (MYOO-kus) membrane** lines the digestive, respiratory, urinary, and reproductive tracts. It lines all body cavities that open to the outside. It is usually ciliated. Its most obvious function is to produce mucus, but it also concentrates bile in the gallbladder. It secretes enzymes for the digestion of food and nutrients before absorption. Mucous membrane protects, absorbs nutrients, and secretes mucus, enzymes, and bile salts.

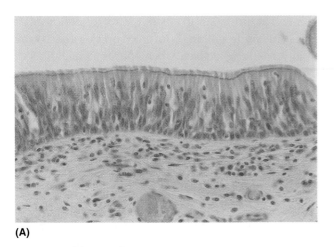

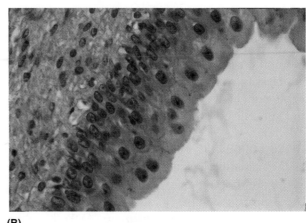

(A)                                                    (B)

**FIGURE 5-4.** Examples of (A) pseudostratified ciliated, columnar epithelium and (B) transitional epithelium.

**Glandular epithelium** forms glands. Glands are involutions of epithelial cells specialized for synthesizing special compounds. The body has two types of multicellular glands. **Exocrine** (**EKS**-oh-krin) **glands** have excretory *ducts* that lead the secreted material from the gland to the surface of a lumen (passageway) or the skin. There are two types of exocrine glands. **Simple exocrine glands** have single unbranching ducts. Some examples of simple exocrine glands are the sweat glands, most of the glands of the digestive tract, and the sebaceous glands. The other type of exocrine gland is the **compound exocrine gland**. These glands are made of several component lobules each with ducts that join other ducts. Thus, the ducts are branching. Examples of compound exocrine glands are the mammary glands and the large salivary glands. **Endocrine glands** are the second type of multicellular glands in the body. They are ductless and secrete hormones; examples are the thyroid and pituitary glands. **Goblet cells** are unicellular glands that secrete mucus. They are interspersed among the epithelial cells that make up mucous membranes.

**Endothelium** (**en**-doh-**THEE**-lee-um) is a special name given to the epithelium that lines the circulatory system. This system is lined with a single layer of squamous-type cells. Endothelium lines the blood vessels and the lymphatic vessels. The endothelium that lines the heart gets another special name and is called **endocardium**. A blood capillary consists of only one layer of endothelium. It is through this single layer of cells that oxygen,

carbon dioxide, nutrients, and waste are transported by the blood cells to the various cells of our bodies.

Our final type of epithelial tissue based on function is **mesothelium** (mezo-**THEE**-lee-um). This tissue is also called **serous** (**SEER**-us) **tissue**. It is the tissue that lines the great cavities of the body that have no openings to the outside. These membranes consists of a simple squamous cell layer overlying a sheet of connective tissue. Special names are associated with this type of epithelial tissue also. The **pleura** (**PLOO**-rah) is the serous membrane or mesothelial tissue that lines the thoracic cavity. The **pericardium** is the serous membrane that covers the heart; the **peritoneum** (**pair**-ih-toh-**NEE**-um) is the serous membrane lining the abdominal cavity. This tissue protects, reduces friction between organs, and secretes fluid. The term **parietal** refers to the walls of a cavity and **visceral** refers to the covering on an organ.

## CONNECTIVE TISSUE

The second major type of tissue is **connective tissue**. This type of tissue allows movement and provides support for other types of tissue. In this tissue, unlike epithelial, there is an abundance of intercellular material called **matrix** (**MAY**-trikz). This matrix is variable in both type and amount. It is one of the main sources of differences between the different types of connective tissue. There are also fibers of **collagen** (**KOL**-ah-jen) and **elastin** (ee-**LASS**-tin) embedded in this matrix. Sometimes the fibers are very apparent under the microscope, as in a tendon, whereas in other tissues the fibers are not very apparent as in certain cartilage. We can classify connective tissue into three subgroups: loose connective tissue, dense connective tissue, and specialized connective tissue.

## Loose Connective Tissue

As the name implies, the fibers of loose connective tissue are not tightly woven among themselves. There are three types of loose connective tissue: **areolar** (ah-**REE**-oh-lah), **adipose** (**ADD**-ih-pohz), and **reticular** (reh-**TIK**-you-lar). Loose connective tissue fills spaces between and penetrates into organs.

Areolar is the most widely distributed of the loose connective tissue. It is easily stretched yet resists tearing. This tissue has three main types of cells distributed among its delicate fibers: fibroblasts, histiocytes, and mast cells. **Fibroblasts** (**FYR**-broh-blastz) are small flattened cells with large nuclei and reduced cytoplasm; they are also somewhat irregular in shape. The term fibroblast (blast meaning geminal or embryonic) refers to the ability of these cells to form fibrils (small fibers). They are active in the repair of injury. **Histiocytes** (**HISS**-tee-oh-sightz) are large, stationary **phagocytic** (fag-oh-**SIH**-tik) cells that eat up (phago = to eat) debris and microorganisms outside the blood circulatory system. They function like some white blood cells (the leukocytes) do in the blood. When they are motile they are called **macrophages** (**MACK**-roh-fay-jez). A macrophage of loose connective tissue is specifically called a histiocyte. Histiocytes, as stated above, are stationary or fixed in tissue. **Mast cells** are roundish or polygonal in shape and are found close to small blood vessels. Mast cells function in the production of **heparin** (an anticoagulant) and **histamine** (an inflammatory substance produced in response to allergies). Areolar tissue is the basic support tissue around organs, muscles, blood vessels, and nerves (Figure 5-5). It forms the delicate membranes around the spinal cord and brain. It attaches the skin to its underlying tissues.

| Function | Characteristics and Location | Morphology |
|---|---|---|
| **Areolar (loose) connective** This tissue surrounds various organs and supports both nerve cells and blood vessels which transport nutrient material (to cells) and wastes (away from cells). Areolar tissue also (temporarily) stores glucose, salts, and water. | It is composed of a large, semifluid matrix, with many different types of cells and fibers embedded in it. These include fibroblasts (fibrocytes), plasma cells, macrophages, mast cells, and various white blood cells. The fibers are bundles of strong, flexible white fibrous protein called collagen, and elastic single fibers of elastin. It is found in the epidermis of the skin and in the subcutaneous layer with adipose cells. | 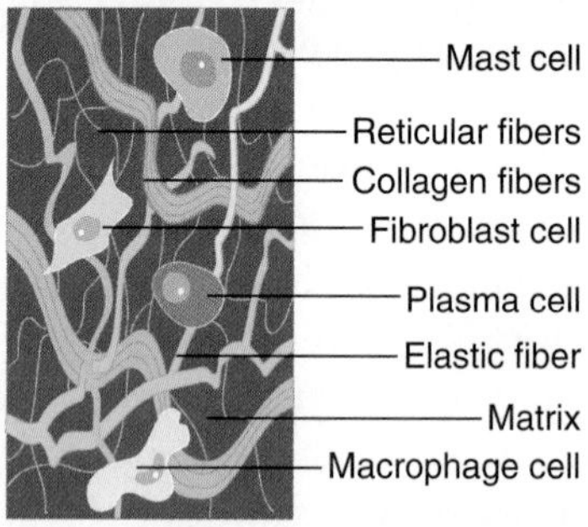 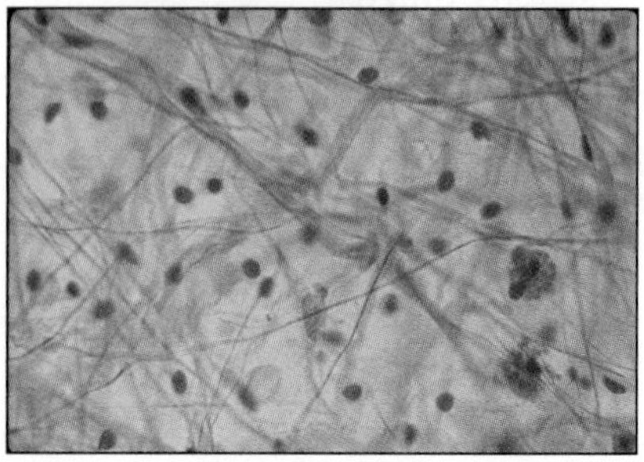 |

**FIGURE 5-5.** Views of areolar or loose connective tissue.

Adipose tissue is the second type of loose connective tissue (Figure 5-6). It is loaded with fat cells. Fat cells are so full of stored fat that their nuclei and cytoplasm are pushed up against the cell membrane. In a histologic section under a microscope, they look like large soap bubbles and are very easy to recognize. Adipose tissue acts as a firm, protective packing around and between organs, bundles of muscle fibers, and nerves, and it supports blood vessels. The kidneys have a surrounding layer of adipose tissue to protect them from hard blows or jolts. In addition, because fat is a poor conductor of heat, adipose tissue acts as insulation for the body, protecting us from excessive heat losses or excessive heat increases in temperature. Think of the animals in the Arctic and Antarctic. They can live there because of their layers of blubber, which is adipose tissue. The camel's hump is not a water storage organ but a thick hump of fat containing adipose tissue to protect the animal's internal organs from the heat of the desert.

Reticular tissue is the third type of loose connective tissue. It consists of a fine network of fibers that form the framework of the liver, bone marrow, and lymphoid organs such as the spleen and lymph nodes.

## Dense Connective Tissue

Again as the name implies, dense connective tissue is composed of tightly packed protein fibers. It is further divided into two subgroups based on how the fibers are arranged and the proportions of the tough collagen and the flexible elastin fibers. Examples of dense connective tissue having a *regular* arrangement of fibers are **tendons**, which attach muscle to bone, **ligaments**, which attach bone to bone, and **aponeuroses** (**ap**-oh-noo-**ROH**-sis), which are wide flat tendons (Figure 5-7). Tendons have a majority of tough collagen fibers, whereas ligaments (e.g., the vocal cords), have a combination of tough collagen and elastic elastin fibers.

Example of dense connective tissue having an *irregular* arrangement of these fibers are muscle sheaths, the dermis layer of the skin, and the outer coverings of body tubes like arteries. Capsules that are part of a joint structure also

| Function | Characteristics and Location | Morphology |
|---|---|---|
| **Adipose tissue**<br>This tissue stores lipid (fat), acts as filler tissue, cushions, supports, and insulates the body. | A type of loose, connective tissue composed of sac-like adipose cells; they are specialized for the storage of fat. Adipose cells are found throughout the body: in the subcutaneous skin layer, around the kidneys, within padding around joints, and in the marrow of long bones. | 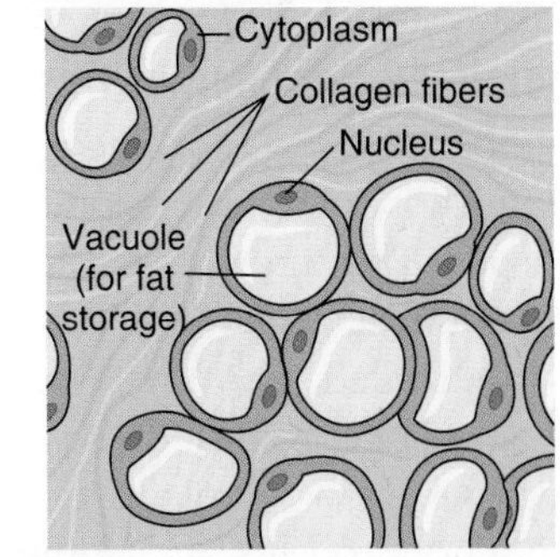 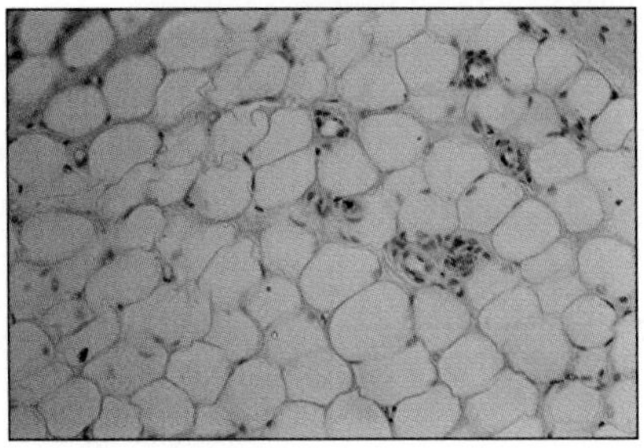 |

**FIGURE 5-6.** Views of adipose tissue. It surrounds the lobules of mammary glands. The amount of adipose tissue determines a woman's breast size.

| Function | Characteristics and Location | Morphology |
|---|---|---|
| **Dense fibrous**<br>This tissue forms ligaments, tendons and aponeuroses.<br>**Ligaments** are strong, flexible bands (or cords) which hold bones firmly together at the joints.<br>**Tendons** are white, glistening bands attaching skeletal muscles to the bones. **Aponeuroses** are flat, wide bands of tissue holding one muscle to another or to the periosteum (bone covering).<br>**Fasciae** are fibrous connective tissue sheets that wrap around muscle bundles to hold them in place. | Dense fibrous tissue is also called white fibrous tissue, since it is made from closely packed white collagen fibers. Fibrous tissue is flexible, but not elastic. This tissue has a poor blood supply and heals slowly. | 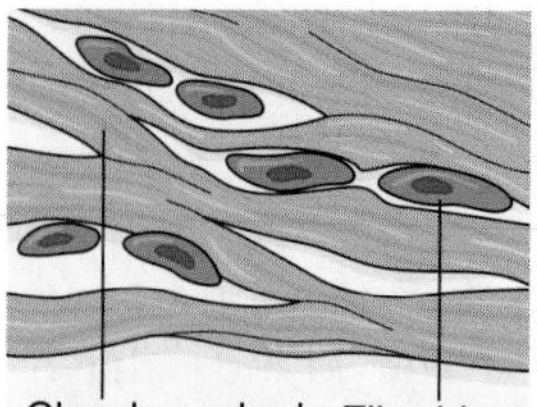 <br>Closely packed collagen fibers    Fibroblast cell |

**FIGURE 5-7.** Examples of dense connective tissue with a regular arrangement of fibers are tendons, ligaments, and aponeuroses. Those with an irregular arrangement of fibers are fascia.

have dense irregular connective tissue as do **fascia** (**FASH**-ee-ah), the connective tissue covering a whole muscle.

## Specialized Connective Tissue

A number of types of connective tissue have specialized functions. Cartilage is one of these special kinds of tissues. The three types of cartilage found in the body are hyaline, fibrous, and elastic. Cells of cartilage are called **chondrocytes** (**KON**-droh-sightz); they are large round cells with spherical nuclei. When we view cartilage under the microscope, these chondrocytes are found in cavities called **lacunae** (lah-**KOO**-nee). The lacunae are cavities in a firm matrix composed of protein and polysaccharides. Depending on the type of cartilage, various amounts of collagen and elastin fibers are embedded in the matrix causing the cartilage to be either flexible or very strong and resistant.

**Hyaline cartilage**, when viewed under the microscope, has a matrix with no visible fibers in it, hence the name hyaline, which means clear (Figure 5-8). As the fetus forms in the womb, the skeletal system is made entirely of hyaline cartilage and is visible after the first 3 months of pregnancy. Most of

this hyaline cartilage is gradually replaced by bone over the next 6 months through a process called ossification. However, some hyaline cartilage remains as a covering on the surfaces of the bones at joints. In our bodies, the costal cartilages that attach the anterior ends of our upper seven pair of ribs to the sternum is hyaline cartilage. The trachea and bronchi are kept open by incomplete rings of hyaline cartilage. The septum of our nose is also made of hyaline cartilage.

**Fibrocartilage** has a majority of tough collagenous fibers embedded in the matrix (Figure 5-9). These fibers make this type of cartilage dense and very resistant to stretching. The intervertebral disks that surround our spinal cord and act as shock absorbers between our vertebrae are made of this strong cartilage. It also connects our two pelvic bones at the pubic symphysis. Thus, we can flex our vertebral column and bend within a particular range of movement. During delivery, a minimal range of expansion of the birth canal can occur at the pubic symphysis due to the fibrocartilage.

The third type of cartilage is **elastic cartilage**. This type of cartilage has a predominance of elastin fibers embedded in the matrix. These fibers must be

| Function | Characteristics and Location | Morphology |
| --- | --- | --- |
| **Cartilage–** Provides firm but flexible support for the embryonic skeleton and part of the adult skeleton. **Hyaline–** Forms the skeleton of the embryo. | Hyaline cartilage is found upon articular bone surfaces, and also at the nose tip, bronchi and bronchial tubes. Ribs are joined to the sternum (breastbone) by the costal cartilage. It is also found in the larynx and the rings in the trachea. | 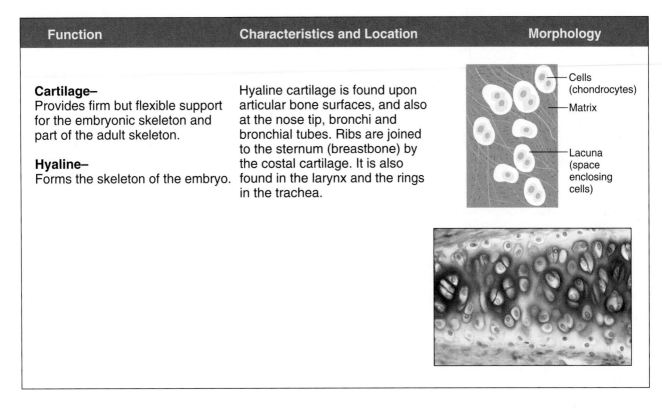 |

**FIGURE 5-8.** The anatomy of hyaline cartilage.

| Function | Characteristics and Location | Morphology |
| --- | --- | --- |
| **Fibrocartilage–** A strong, flexible, supportive substance, found between bones and wherever great strength (and a degree of rigidity) is needed. | Fibrocartilage is located within intervertebral discs and pubic symphysis between the pubic bones. | 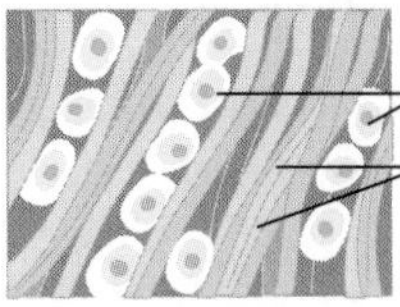 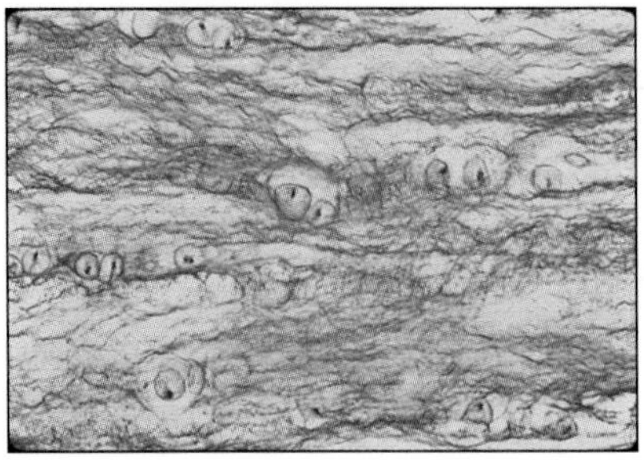 Chondrocytes Dense white fibers |

**FIGURE 5-9.** The anatomy of fibrocartilage.

specially stained to view under a microscope (Figure 5-10). These fibers permit this type of cartilage to be easily stretched and flexible while being capable of returning to its original shape. Elastic cartilage makes up our external ear or auricle, our ear canals or auditory tubes, and our epiglottis.

**Bone** is very firm specialized connective tissue. We will be covering bone in great detail in Chapter 7. If we section a bone we see that it is composed of two types of bone tissue: **compact bone**, which forms the dense outer layer of bone and looks solid, and **cancellous bone**, which forms the inner spongy-looking tissue underneath the compact bone. When viewed under a microscope, the bone cells called **osteocytes** (**OSS**-tee-oh-sightz) are also found in cavities or lacunae as we saw in cartilage. However, the matrix of bone is impregnated with mineral salts, particularly calcium and phosphorous, which give bone its firm, hard appearance (Figure 5-11).

Another specialized connective tissue is **dentin**, the material that forms our teeth. Dentin is closely related to bone in structure but is harder and denser. The crown of the tooth is covered with another material, enamel, which is white in appearance. Dentin is light brown. If you ever chipped a tooth, the brown material you saw under the white enamel was the dentin. The enamel is secreted onto the dentin of a tooth by special epithelial cells that make up the enamel organ. This secretion occurs just before the teeth break their way through the gums.

**Blood** and **hematopoietic** (hee-**MAT**-oh-poy-eh-tik) **tissue** are other examples of specialized connective tissue. Blood is unique connective tissue in that it is composed of a fluid portion (the plasma) and the formed elements of blood: the **erythrocytes** (eh-**RITH**-roh-sightz) or red blood cells and **leukocytes** (**LOO**-koh-sightz) or white blood cells (Figure 5-12). We will discuss blood in more detail in Chapter 13. Blood cells are formed in red bone marrow and some white blood cells are also formed in lymphoid organs. Marrow and lymphoid organs are referred to as hematopoietic tissue. Blood is liquid tissue circulating through the body. It transports oxygen, nutrients, hormones, enzymes, and waste products such as carbon dioxide gas and urea. It also protects the body through its white blood cells and helps to regulate body temperature.

| Function | Characteristics and Location | Morphology |
|---|---|---|
| **Elastic cartilage–** The intercellular matrix is embedded with a network of elastic fibers and is firm but flexible. | Elastic cartilage is located inside the auditory ear tube, external ear, epiglottis, and larynx. | 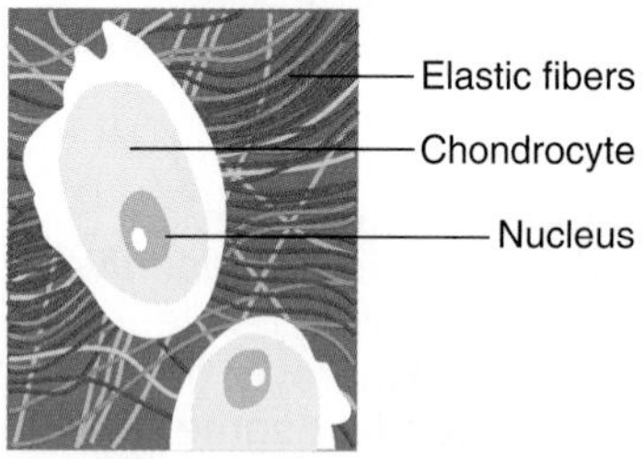 Elastic fibers / Chondrocyte / Nucleus |

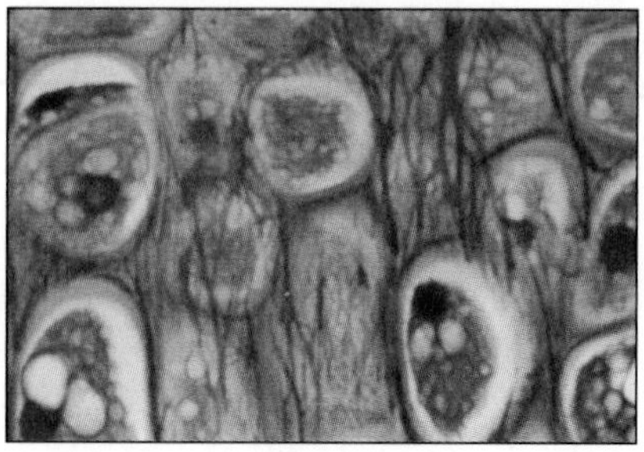

**FIGURE 5-10.** The anatomy of elastic cartilage.

| Function | Characteristics and Location | Morphology |
|---|---|---|
| **Bone (osseus) tissue–** Comprises the skeleton of the body, which supports and protects underlying soft tissue parts and organs, and also serves as attachments for skeletal muscles. | Connective tissue whose intercellular matrix is calcified by the deposition of mineral salts (like calcium carbonate and calcium phosphate). Calcification of bone imparts great strength. The entire skeleton is composed of bone tissue. | 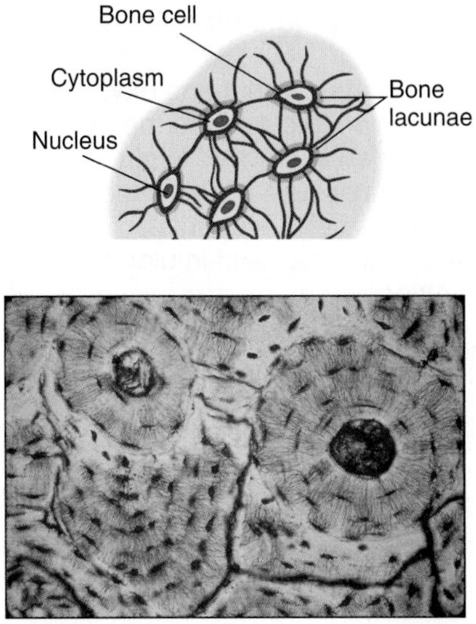 |

**FIGURE 5-11.** Views of compact bone.

**Lymphoid tissue** is another specialized connective tissue (Figure 5-13). Lymphoid tissue is found in the lymph glands or nodes, the thymus gland, the spleen, the tonsils, and the adenoids. Lymph tissue manufactures plasma cells like the B lymphocytes. This tissue's main role is antibody production and protects us from disease and foreign microorganisms.

The **reticuloendothelial** (reh-**tik**-you-loh-**in**-doh-**THEE**-lee-al) or **RE system** consists of those specialized connective tissue cells that do phagocytosis. Three types of cells fit into this category. The first type are the RE cells that line the liver (they get another special name: **Kupffer cells**), and those that line the spleen and bone marrow. The second type are the macrophages. These cells are also referred to as histiocytes or "resting-wandering" cells, because they are fixed in tissue until they must wander to an invader and devour it. Any phagocytic cell of the RE system can be called a macrophage. The third type of cell is a **neurolgia** (noo-roh-**GLEE**-ah) or **microglia** (my-**KROG**-lee-ah) cell. This is a phagocytic cell found in the central nervous system.

**Synovial membranes** line the cavities of freely moving joints and are also classified as specialized connective tissue. These membranes also line bursae, which are small sacs containing synovial fluid found between muscles, tendons, bones, and skin and underlying structures. They prevent friction where one organ overlies or moves over another.

## Connective Tissue Functions

Connective tissue has many and varied functions:

1. Support. Bones support other tissues of the body. On top of bones we find muscle, nerves, blood vessels, fat, and skin. Cartilage supports our nose and forms the bulk of the structure of our ear.
2. Nourishment. Blood carries nutrients to the cells of our body. Synovial membranes in joint capsules nourish the cartilage found on top of bones.
3. Transportation. Blood transports gases, enzymes, and hormones to cells.
4. Connection. Tendons connect muscles to bone and ligaments connect bone to bone.
5. Movement. Muscles pull on bones and bones move our bodies through our environment.
6. Protection. Bones protect vital organs of the body like the heart, lungs, brain, and spinal cord. Blood cells, especially the white blood

| Function | Characteristics and Location | Morphology |
|---|---|---|

**Vascular (liquid blood tissue) Blood–**
Transports nutrient and oxygen molecules to cells, and metabolic wastes away from cells (can be considered as a liquid tissue). Contains cells that function in the body's defense and in blood clotting.

Blood is composed of two major parts: a liquid called plasma, and a solid cellular portion known as blood cells (or corpuscles). The plasma suspends corpuscles, of which there are two major types: red blood cells (erythrocytes) and white blood cells (leukocytes). A third cellular component (really a cell fragment) is called platelets (thrombocytes). Blood circulates within the blood vessels (arteries, veins, and capillaries) and through the heart.

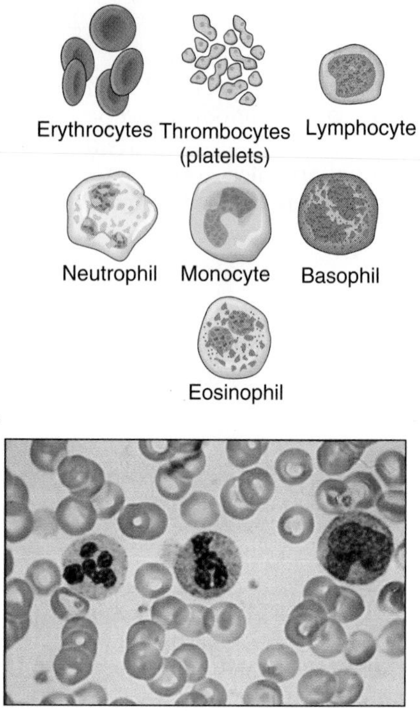

Erythrocytes  Thrombocytes  Lymphocyte
(platelets)

Neutrophil  Monocyte  Basophil

Eosinophil

**FIGURE 5-12.** Views of blood, a unique fluid connective tissue.

| Function | Characteristics and Location | Morphology |
|---|---|---|

**Lymph–**
Transports tissue fluid, proteins, fats and other materials from the tissues to the circulatory system. This occurs through a series of tubes called the lymphatic vessels.

Lymph is a fluid made up of water, glucose, protein, fats, and salt. The cellular components are lymphocytes and granulocytes. They flow in tubes called lymphatic vessels, which closely parallel the veins and bathe the tissue spaces between cells.

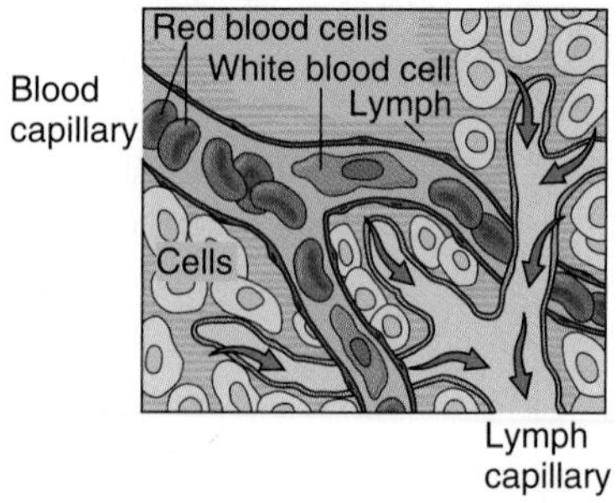

Red blood cells
Blood capillary
White blood cell
Lymph
Cells
Lymph capillary

**FIGURE 5-13.** A diagram of lymph tissue.

cells, protect us from foreign microorganisms and tissue injury.

7. Insulation. Adipose tissue (fat) insulates us from excessive heat loss and excessive increases in temperature.

8. Storage. Bone stores the mineral salts calcium and phosphorous. Adipose tissue stores the high-energy molecules of fat to be used and converted to adenosine triphosphate when necessary.

9. Attachment and separation. Connective tissue attaches skin to underlying muscle. It also forms layers around and between organs.

## MUSCLE TISSUE

The basic characteristic of **muscle tissue** is its ability to shorten and thicken or contract. This is due to the interaction of two proteins in the muscle cell: actin and myosin. We will discuss muscle cell contractility in greater detail in Chapter 9. Because a muscle cell's length is much greater than its width, muscle cells are frequently referred to as **muscle fibers**. The three types of muscle tissue are smooth, striated or skeletal, and cardiac.

**Smooth muscle** cells are spindle-shaped with a single nucleus (Figure 5-14). They are not striated (**STRYE**-ate-ed), that is, you do not see alternating dark and light bands when viewed under the microscope. This muscle tissue is involuntary; meaning we do not control its contraction. It is controlled by the autonomic nervous system. We find smooth muscle in the walls of hollow organs like those of the digestive tract, arteries, and veins. The muscle cells are arranged in layers: an outer longitudinal layer and an inner circular layer. Simultaneous contraction of the two layers pushes materials inside the hollow organs in one direction. Hence, food is pushed by contraction of the smooth muscles along the digestive tract, called **peristalsis** (pair-ih-**STALL**-sis), and blood is pushed along in arteries and veins. Urine is also pushed down the ureters from the kidneys by contraction of smooth muscle.

**Striated** or **skeletal muscle** is the muscle we normally think about when we mention muscle (Figure 5-15). It is the tissue that causes movement of our body by pulling on bones, hence the name skeletal muscle. The long thin cells of skeletal muscle are multinucleated and striated. We can see alternating light bands of the thin protein filaments of actin and dark bands of the thick protein filaments of myosin. When we eat "meat" of animals and fish, it is usually muscle that we are consuming. Muscle makes up about 40% of our total weight and mass. Striated muscle is voluntary and is under the control of the central nervous system.

**Cardiac muscle** is found only in the heart. Like skeletal muscle it is striated and like smooth muscle it is uninucleated and under the control of the autonomic nervous system (Figure 5-16). The cells

| Function | Characteristics and Location | Morphology |
|---|---|---|
| **Smooth (nonstriated involuntary)** These provide for involuntary movement. Examples include the movement of materials along the digestive tract, controlling the diameter of blood vessels and the pupil of the eyes. | Smooth muscle is nonstriated because it lacks the striations (bands) of skeletal muscles; its movement is involuntary. It makes up the walls of the digestive, genitourinary, respiratory tracts, blood vessels, and lymphatic vessels. | 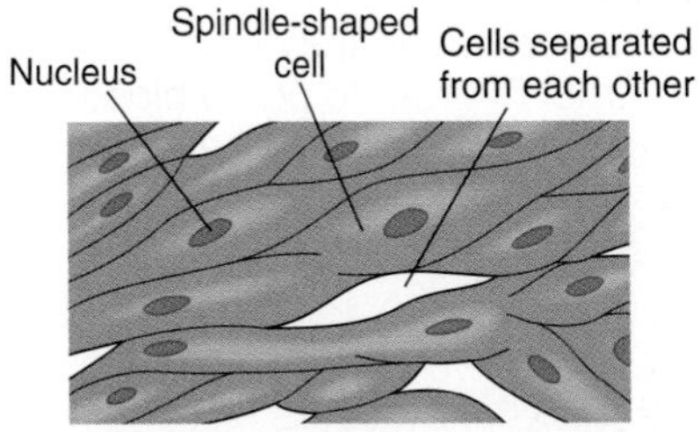 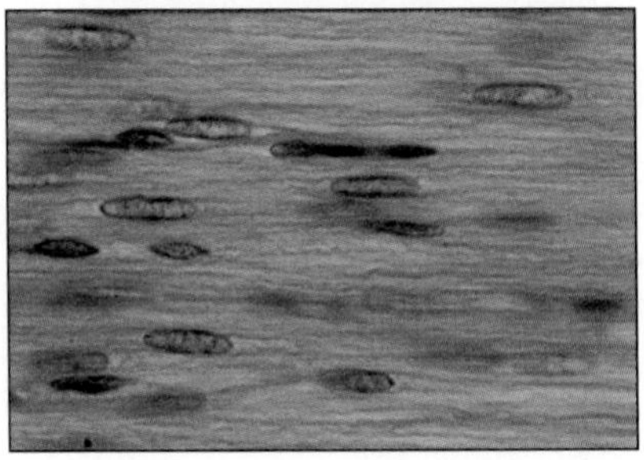 |

**FIGURE 5-14.** Views of smooth muscle cells.

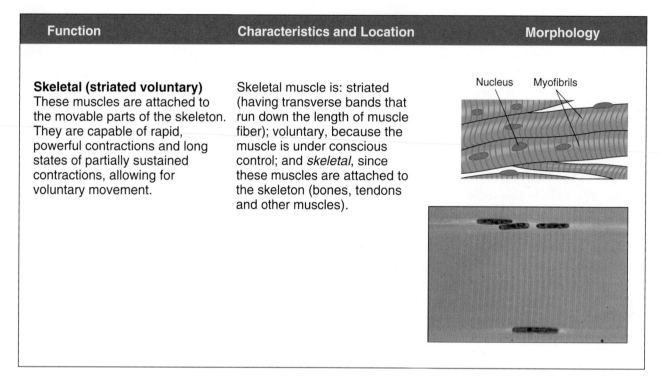

| Function | Characteristics and Location | Morphology |
| --- | --- | --- |
| **Skeletal (striated voluntary)** These muscles are attached to the movable parts of the skeleton. They are capable of rapid, powerful contractions and long states of partially sustained contractions, allowing for voluntary movement. | Skeletal muscle is: striated (having transverse bands that run down the length of muscle fiber); voluntary, because the muscle is under conscious control; and *skeletal*, since these muscles are attached to the skeleton (bones, tendons and other muscles). | Nucleus    Myofibrils |

**FIGURE 5-15.** Views of skeletal muscle cells.

| Function | Characteristics and Location | Morphology |
| --- | --- | --- |
| **Cardiac** These cells help the heart contract in order to pump blood through and out of the heart. | Cardiac muscle is a striated (having a cross-banding pattern), involuntary (not under conscious control) muscle. It makes up the walls of the heart. | 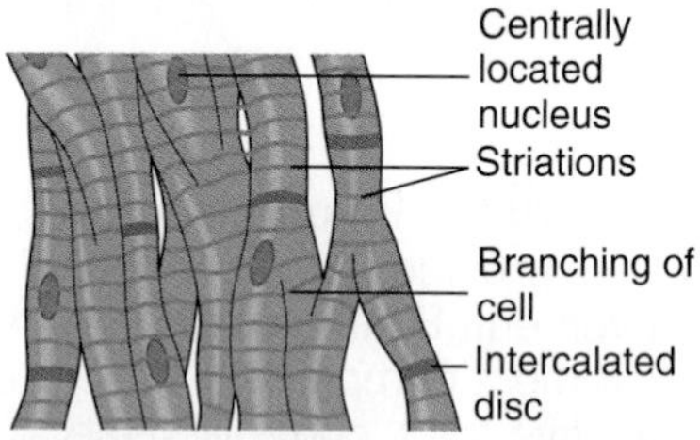 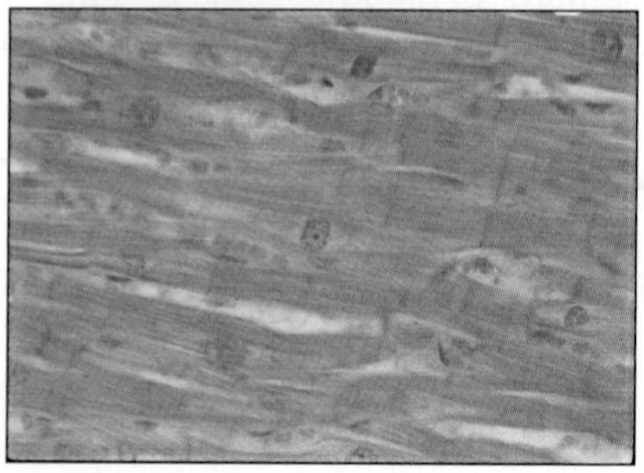 Centrally located nucleus Striations Branching of cell Intercalated disc |

**FIGURE 5-16.** Views of cardiac muscle cells.

of cardiac muscle are cylindrical in shape with branches that connect to other cardiac cells. These branches connect with one another through special areas called **intercalated** (in-**TER**-kah-**lay**-ed) **disks**. The cells are much shorter than either skeletal or smooth muscle cells. This is the muscle that causes contraction or beating of the heart; thus, it pumps the blood through our body. The interconnected branches of cardiac muscle cells guarantee coordination of the pumping action of the heart (to be discussed further in Chapter 14).

## NERVOUS TISSUE

The basic unit of organization of nervous tissue is the nerve cell or **neuron** (**NOO**-ron) (Figure 5-17). Actually the neuron is a conducting cell, whereas other cells of the system called neuroglia are supporting cells. These different types of nerve cells are discussed in greater detail in Chapter 10. Neurons are very long cells, so like muscle cells, they are called nerve fibers. It is basically impossible to view an entire neuron even under low power of the microscope due to their length. However, we can view the parts of a neuron as we scan a microscope slide. The **cell body** contains the nucleus. It also has rootlike extensions called **dendrites** (**DEN**-drytz) that receive stimuli and conduct them to the cell body. **Axons** (**AK**-sonz) are long thin extensions of the cell body that transmit the impulse towards the **axon endings**.

Nervous tissue makes up the brain, spinal cord, and various nerves of the body. It is the most highly organized tissue of the body. It controls and coordinates body activities. It allows us to perceive our environment and to adapt to changing conditions. It coordinates our skeletal muscles. Its special senses include sight, taste, smell, and hearing. It controls our emotions and our reasoning capabilities. It allows us to learn through the memory process.

---

## Summary Outline
### INTRODUCTION
1. Histology is the study of tissues.
2. The four kinds of tissue are epithelial, connective, muscle, and nervous.

| Function | Characteristics and Location | Morphology |
|---|---|---|
| **Neurons (nerve cells)** These cells have the ability to react to stimuli. **1. Irritability–** Ability of nerve tissue to respond to environmental changes. **2. Conductivity–** Ability to carry a nerve impulse (message) | Nerve tissue is composed of *neurons* (nerve cells). Neurons have branches through which various parts of the body are connected and their activities coordinated. They are found in the brain, spinal cord, and nerves. | 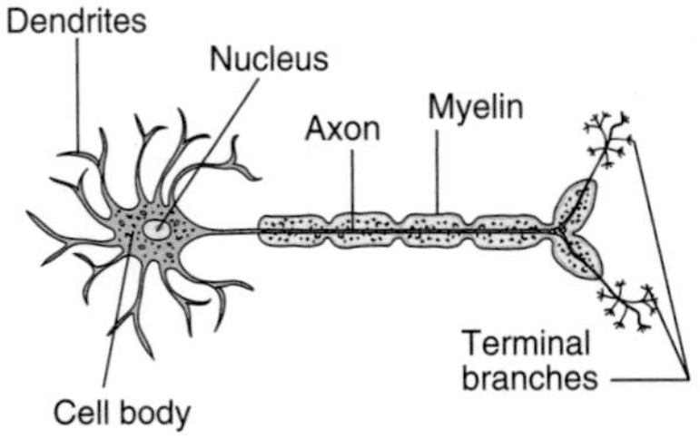 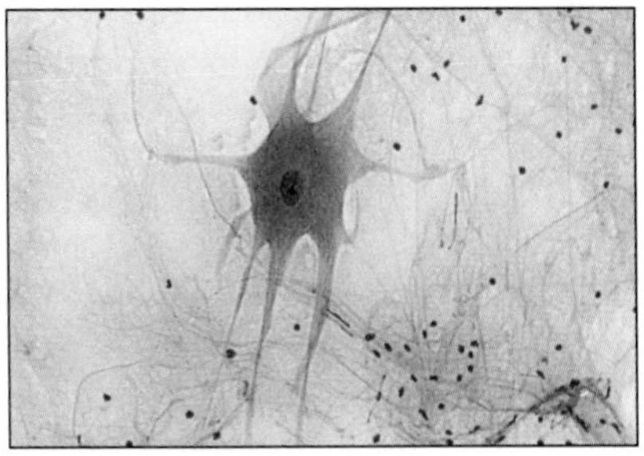 |

**FIGURE 5-17.** Views of a neuron (multipolar, motor neuron).

## EPITHELIAL TISSUE

1. Epithelial tissue functions in four ways: it protects underlying tissues; it absorbs nutrients; it secretes hormones, mucus, and enzymes; and it excretes waste like urea in sweat.
2. The basement membrane acts as an anchor and adhesive for epithelial cells.
3. Epithelial tissue can be named according to shape, arrangement, or function.
4. Epithelial tissue is made of cells closely packed together with very little intercellular material.

### Classification Based on Shape

1. Squamous epithelial cells are flat and serve a protective function like the lining of our mouths and our skin.
2. Cuboidal epithelial cells are shaped like cubes and function in protection and secretion.
3. Columnar epithelial cells are tall and rectangular. They function in secretion and absorption.

### Classification Based on Arrangement

1. Simple epithelium is one cell layer thick.
2. Stratified epithelium is several layers of cells thick.
3. Pseudostratified epithelium looks like it is several layers thick but, in reality, all cells extend from the basement membrane to the outer surface.
4. Transitional epithelium consists of several layers of closely packed, easily stretched cells. When stretched they appear flat, when relaxed they look ragged or saw-toothed.

### Classification Based on Function

1. Mucous membrane produces mucus. It protects, absorbs nutrients, and secretes enzymes and bile salts in addition to mucus.
2. Simple exocrine glands such as sweat and sebaceous glands have single unbranching ducts.
3. Compound exocrine glands are made of several branching lobules with branching ducts. Examples are the mammary glands and the large salivary glands.
4. Endocrine glands are ductless and secrete hormones directly into the bloodstream.
5. Endothelium lines the blood and lymphatic vessels. The endothelium of the heart is called the endocardium.
6. Mesothelium or serous tissue lines the great cavities of the body. The pleura lines the thoracic cavity. The peritoneum lines the abdominal cavity. The pericardium covers the heart.

## CONNECTIVE TISSUE

1. Connective tissue is made of cells with lots of intercellular material called matrix.
2. Fibers of tough collagen or fibers of flexible elastin can be embedded in this matrix.
3. The three subgroups of connective tissue are loose connective tissue, dense connective tissue, and specialized connective tissue.

### Loose Connective Tissue

1. The three types of loose connective tissue are areolar, adipose, and reticular.
2. Loose connective tissue fills space between and penetrates into organs.
3. Areolar is the most widely distributed type of loose connective tissue. It contains three types of cells: fibroblasts, which make fibrils for repair; histiocytes or macrophages, which do phagocytosis; and mast cells, which produce the anticoagulant heparin and histamine, an inflammatory substance.
4. Adipose tissue is loose connective tissue with fat stored in its cells. It protects and insulates.
5. Reticular tissue forms the framework of the liver, spleen, lymph nodes, and bone marrow.

### Dense Connective Tissue

1. Dense connective tissue having a regular arrangement of embedded fibers are tendons, ligaments, and aponeuroses.
2. Dense connective tissue having an irregular arrangement of embedded fibers are muscle sheaths, joint capsules, and fascia.

### Specialized Connective Tissue

1. The cells of cartilage are called chondrocytes. The three types of cartilage tissue are hyaline, fibrocartilage, and elastic.
2. Hyaline cartilage is found in the costal cartilages that attach the ribs to the sternum, in the septum of our nose, and the rings that keep our trachea and bronchi open.

3. Fibrocartilage is very strong; intervertebral disks are made of fibrocartilage.
4. Elastic cartilage is easily stretched and flexible. It is found in the ears, epiglottis, and auditory tubes.
5. The two types of bone tissue are compact or dense and cancellous or spongy. Bone cells are called osteocytes. They are embedded in a matrix of calcium and phosphorous, the mineral salts responsible for the hardness of bone.
6. Our teeth are made of dentin; the crown of the tooth is covered with enamel.
7. Blood is composed of a liquid portion called plasma and the blood cells. Blood cells are formed in red bone marrow, a hematopoietic tissue.
8. Lymphoid tissue makes up our lymph glands, thymus, spleen, tonsils, and adenoids. This tissue produces the plasma cells or B lymphocytes that produce antibodies.
9. The reticuloendothelial (RE) system is involved in phagocytosis in connective tissue. Kupffer cells line the liver; RE cells also line the spleen and bone marrow. Macrophage is a term for any phagocytic cell of the RE system. Neuroglia or microglia cells do phagocytosis in the nervous system.
10. Synovial membranes line joints and bursae. They produce synovial fluid, which lubricates joints and nourishes cartilage.

### Connective Tissue Functions

1. It supports other tissues.
2. It provides nourishment: blood carries nutrients.
3. It transports: blood transports enzymes and hormones.
4. It connects various tissues to one another.
5. It provides movement via bones.
6. It protects vital organs (bones of skull and thorax) and provides immunity (lymphoid tissue and white blood cells).
7. It insulates and maintains temperature (adipose tissue).
8. It provides storage areas: bone stores calcium and phosphorous, adipose tissue stores fat.
9. It attaches and separates other tissues of the body.

## MUSCLE TISSUE

1. The three types of muscle tissue are smooth, striated or skeletal, and cardiac.
2. Due to the interaction of two proteins, actin and myosin, muscle cells can shorten their length or contract. Some pull on bones and bring about movement.
3. Smooth muscle cells are long, unicellular, and nonstriated. They are involuntary and are arranged in two layers around hollow organs: an outer longitudinal layer and an inner circular one. They are found in the digestive tract, arteries and veins, and the ureters of the kidney.
4. Striated or skeletal muscle cells are long, multinucleated, and striated. They are voluntary and pull on bone causing movement.
5. Cardiac muscle cells are found only in the heart. They are striated, uninucleated, and cylindrical in shape with branches that connect to branches of other cardiac cells via intercalated disks. These cells are responsible for pumping blood through the heart.

## NERVOUS TISSUE

1. Nervous tissue is composed of two types of nerve cells: neurons are conducting cells and neuroglia are supporting cells.
2. A neuron is composed of a cell body with a nucleus, extensions of the cell body called dendrites, and a long axon with axon endings.
3. Nervous tissue controls and coordinates the activities of the body.

## REVIEW QUESTIONS

1. Name the three cell shapes of epithelial tissue.
2. Name the two types of exocrine glands and give an example of each.
3. Name four functions of epithelial tissue.
*4. Compare the structure of epithelial tissue with that of connective tissue.
*5. Why is adipose tissue considered a good insulator?
6. Name five functions of connective tissue and give examples.

**7.** Name the three types of muscle tissue.

**8.** Name the two types of nerve cells found in nervous tissue.

*\* Critical Thinking Questions*

## Fill in the Blank

Fill in the blank with the most appropriate term.

**1.** The three types of loose connective tissue are: _____, _____, and _____.

**2.** _____ are cells that form fibrils and are active in the repair of injury.

**3.** _____ are phagocytic cells that operate outside the vascular system—they are often fixed and are found in areolar tissue.

**4.** _____ cells function in the production of heparin and histamine.

**5.** _____ tissue is loose connective tissue with fat-containing cells.

**6.** Examples of dense connective tissue having a regular arrangement of fibers are _____, _____, and _____.

**7.** Examples of dense connective tissue having an irregular arrangement of fibers are _____, _____, _____, and _____ sheaths.

**8.** The three types of cartilage are _____, _____, and _____.

**9.** The two common types of bone tissue are _____ and _____.

**10.** A tooth is made up of _____, the crown of the tooth is covered by _____, the hardest substance in the body.

**11.** _____ membranes line the cavities of the freely moving joints and bursae.

**12.** The two types of protein fibers that can be found in the matrix of connective tissue are _____ and _____.

## Matching

Place the most appropriate number in the blank provided.

____ Heparin
____ Histamine
____ Chondrocytes
____ Ossification
____ Enamel
____ Marrow
____ Erythrocytes
____ Leukocytes
____ Neuron
____ Neuroglia

1. Cells of cartilage
2. Blood platelets
3. Hardest substance in the body
4. White blood cells
5. Blood-forming tissue
6. Anticoagulant
7. Red blood cells
8. Fat cells
9. Supports the neuron
10. Conducting cell
11. Inflammatory substance
12. Formation of bone

---

## LABORATORY EXERCISE: TISSUES

Materials needed: A compound microscope and prepared microscope slides.

### A. EPITHELIAL TISSUE

1. Examine a prepared slide of stratified squamous epithelial tissue. Two types of slides will be available. Slides made from the internal tissues of a human like the epiglottis will be nonkeratinized, that is, the cells will have nuclei. If the slide is of the skin, it will be keratinized, that is, the cells will not have nuclei. Refer to Figure 5-1 in the text as you do your microscope examination of this tissue.

2. Examine a prepared slide of simple cuboidal epithelium. This slide will be from a duct of a gland. Refer to Figure 5-2 in the text as

(continues)

## LABORATORY EXERCISE: TISSUES (continued)

you examine these cells shaped like cubes attached to a basement membrane.

3. Examine a prepared slide of simple columnar epithelium. The best slide of this type of tissue comes from the intestine. Refer to Figure 5-3 in the text as you examine these tall rectangular cells.

4. Examine a prepared slide of pseudostratified cilated, columnar epithelium. Notice how the cilia on the free edge of the cells looks like flames or waves. Try to see that each cell will extend from the basement membrane. Refer to Figure 5-4A in the text.

### B. CONNECTIVE TISSUE

1. Examine a prepared slide of hyaline cartilage. Notice how the chondrocytes are in a cavity or lacuna and that the matrix appears clear. No fibers are visible in the matrix. Refer to Figure 5-8 in the text as you view your slide.

2. Examine a prepared slide of elastic cartilage. This slide has been specially stained to show the elastin fibers embedded in the matrix surrounding the chondrocytes in their lacuna. Refer to Figure 5-10 in the text as you view this slide.

3. Examine a prepared slide of fibrocartilage. Notice how thick and wavy the fibers of collagen are arranged in the matrix. Note the fewer chondocytes in their lacunae compared to the other two types of cartilage. Refer to Figure 5-9 as you view this slide.

4. Examine a prepared slide of compact bone. Refer to Figure 5-11 of the text as you view this slide. Identify the central canal surrounded by rings of bone. The central canal contains a blood capillary. The rings of bone are formed by the mineralized matrix and are called lamellae. Note the lacunae which contain the osteocytes.

5. Examine a prepared slide of human blood stained with Wright's stain. First examine under low power. Look for an area where you see some dark-stained cells. These will be leukocytes with stained nuclei. Switch to high power. You will be able to identify the many erythrocytes without nuclei and various leukocytes with their stained nucleus that usually appears folded. Also notice the tiny stained specks in the plasma; these are thrombocytes or platelets. Refer to Figure 5-12 in the text.

### C. MUSCLE TISSUE

1. Examine a prepared slide of smooth muscle. Notice the spindle tapering cells of smooth muscle with no cross striations. They are uninucleated and under the microscope look like flowing water in a stream. Refer to Figure 5-14 in the text.

2. Examine a prepared slide of skeletal muscle. Notice that the cells are large, multinucleated with visible cross striations. They look like thick poles under the microscope. The cross striations are alternating bands of thick myosin protein filaments (dark) and thin actin protein filaments (light). Refer to Figure 5-15 in the text as you view this tissue.

3. Examine a prepared slide of cardiac muscle. Refer to Figure 5-16 in the text. Notice that the cells are striated and uninucleated. The cells have branches that look like splits in a pole. Notice the thick intercalated disks that connect the branches of the cardiac cells.

### D. NERVOUS TISSUE

1. Examine a prepared slide of a multipolar neuron. This slide comes from the spinal cord of an ox. Search under low power to identify a cell body with nucleus and dendrite extensions. Notice the very long axons and at the ends of axons the axon endings. Refer to Figure 5-17 in the text.

# 6

# The Integumentary System

## CHAPTER OUTLINE

## CHAPTER OBJECTIVES

After studying this chapter, you should be able to:

1. Name the layers of the epidermis.

2. Define keratinization.

3. Explain why there are skin color differences among people.

4. Describe the anatomic parts of a hair.

5. Compare the two kinds of glands in the skin based on structure and secretion.

6. Explain why sweating is important to survival.

7. Explain how the skin helps to regulate body temperature.

8. Name the functions of the skin.

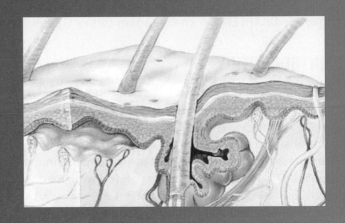

# KEY TERMS

## INTRODUCTION

The integumentary system is made up of the skin and its appendages. See Concept Map 6-1: Integumentary System. The appendages or modifications of the skin are hair, nails, sebaceous, ceruminous, and sweat glands. The word integument means a covering and the skin of an average adult covers well over 3000 square inches of surface area of the body. The skin weighs about 6 pounds (this is nearly twice the weight of the brain or the liver). It receives approximately one third of all the blood circulating through the body. It is flexible yet rugged, and under normal conditions can repair and regenerate itself. Our skin is almost entirely waterproof. It protects us from the harmful ultraviolet rays of the sun through special pigment-producing cells. It is an effective barrier to most harmful chemicals, keeping them from entering our internal environment. It participates in the dissipation of water through sweating and helps regulate our body temperature.

## THE LAYERS OF THE SKIN

Our skin consists of two main layers (Figure 6-1). The **epidermis** (ep-ih-**DER**-mis) is a layer of epithelial tissue that can further be divided into sublayers. It is found on top of the second layer of the skin call the **dermis**. This is a layer of dense connective tissue that connects the skin to tissues below it, like fat and muscle. Beneath the dermis is the subcutaneous layer.

### The Epidermis

The outermost or epidermal layer of the skin is composed of stratified, squamous, keratinized (no nucleus) epithelial cells. These cells are held together by highly convoluted, interlocking cellular links called **desmosomes** (**DEZ**-meh-somz). These desmosomes are responsible for the unique flexibility, entirety, and whole continuous structure of the skin. The epidermis is thickest where it receives the most abrasion and weight—on the palms of the hands and the soles of the feet. It is much thinner over the ventral surface of the trunk.

The epidermis rests on a basement membrane. The lowermost cells on this membrane divide by mitosis, so new cells push older cells up toward the surface. As they move up, they change shape and chemical composition because they lose most of their water and eventually die. This process is called **keratinization** (**kair**-ah-**tin**-ih-**ZAY**-shun) because the cells become filled with **keratin** (**KAIR**-ah-tin), a protein material. These dead, outermost cells are constantly being shed. This outermost layer forms an effective barrier to substances that would penetrate the skin and this layer is very resistant to abrasion.

The process of keratinization produces distinctive layers of the epidermis called **strata** (plural) or **stratum** (**STRAT**-um), singular (Figure 6-2). There are five layers from outermost to deep. They are the stratum corneum (**STRAT**-um **COR**-nee-um), commonly called the horny or leathery layer; the stratum lucidum (**STRAT**-um **LOO**-sid-um), commonly called the clear layer; the stratum granulosum (**STRAT**-um **gran**-you-**LOH**-sum), commonly called the granular layer; and the stratum spinosum (**STRAT**-um spye-**NOH**-sum), commonly called the spiny or prickly layer. The innermost layer and the most important is the stratum germinativum (**STRAT**-um jer-mih-**NAY**-tih-vum) or the regenerative layer.

### The Stratum Corneum

The **stratum corneum** forms the outermost layer of the epidermis. It consists of dead cells converted to protein. They are called keratinized cells because they have lost most of their fluid. The organelles of the cell are now just masses of the hard protein keratin that gives this layer its structural strength. These cells are also covered and surrounded with lipids to prevent any passage of fluids through this layer. These cells have only about 20% water as compared to cells in the lowermost layer that have about 70%. The cells resemble scales in shape and can consist of up to 25 layers. By the time cells reach this layer, the desmosomes have broken apart and, therefore, these cells are constantly being sloughed off. The shedding of these cells from the scalp produces what we call dandruff.

This layer also functions as a physical barrier to light and heat waves, microorganisms (e.g., like bacteria, fungi, protozoa, and viruses), and most chemicals. The thickness of this layer is determined by the amount of stimulation on the surface by abrasion or

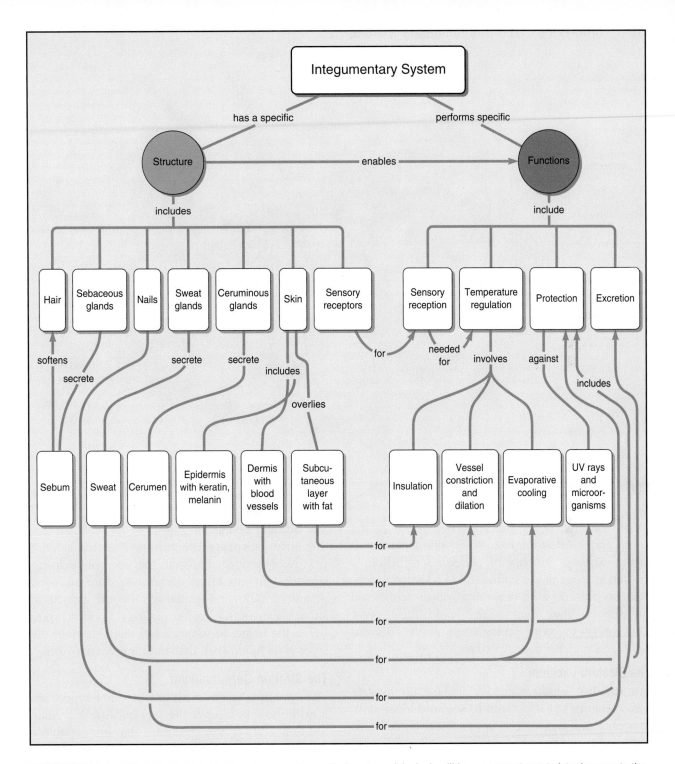

**CONCEPT MAP 6-1.** This is the first introduction of a concept map. Each system of the body will have a concept map to introduce you to the relationship between various structures of the system and how these structures enable the system to perform its functions. A concept map is basically an outline that allows major topics in a chapter to be observed on one page, and the reader sees an overview of those topics.

The concept map breaks up a topic into its major components. First the system of the body will be divided by connecting lines into its *structures* and *functions*. Then each of these two major topics will be further subdivided into smaller components. Connecting lines or arrows will be used to join related divisions for the purpose of showing relationships. Occasionally, a brief description or word may be used along with the connecting lines to reinforce the explanation of the relationship. Spend a few minutes examining the concept map before you read further in the chapter. It will set the stage for what you are about to read. When you go back to study the information in the chapter, referring back to the concept map will help you remember what you have read.

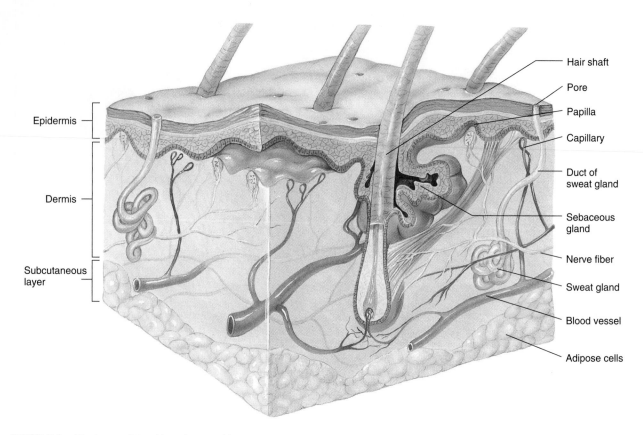

**FIGURE 6-1.** The layers of the skin and some of its appendages.

weight bearing, hence the thickened palms of the hands and soles of the feet. When skin is subjected to an excessive amount of abrasion or friction, a thickened area called a **callus** (**KAL**-us) will develop. Students who do a lot of writing will develop small calluses on their fingers that hold their pens. Abrasion on the bony prominences on the foot can produce structures we call **corns**.

### The Stratum Lucidum

The **stratum lucidum** lies directly beneath the stratum corneum but is difficult to see in thinner skin. It is only one or two cell layers thick. Its cells are transparent and flat.

### The Stratum Granulosum

The **stratum granulosum** consists of two or three layers of flattened cells. Because granules tend to accumulate in these cells, it was named the granular layer. These granules have nothing to do with skin color. This layer is very active in keratinization. In this layer the cells lose their nuclei and become compact and brittle.

### The Stratum Spinosum

The **stratum spinosum** consists of several layers of prickly or spiny-shaped cells that are polyhedron in structure. In this layer, desmosomes are still quite prevalent. The outline caused by the polyhedral shapes causes the cell's outlines to look spiny, hence the name. In some classification schemes, this layer is included with the stratum germinativum.

### The Stratum Germinativum

The **stratum germinativum** is the deepest and most important layer of the skin because it contains the only cells of the epidermis that are capable of dividing by mitosis. When new cells are formed they undergo morphologic and nuclear changes as they get pushed upward by the dividing cells beneath them. Therefore, these cells give rise to all the other upper layers of the epidermis. The epidermis will regenerate itself only so long as the stratum germinativum remains intact. Its basal layer, called the **stratum basale** (**STRAT**-um **BAY**-sil), rests on the basement membrane.

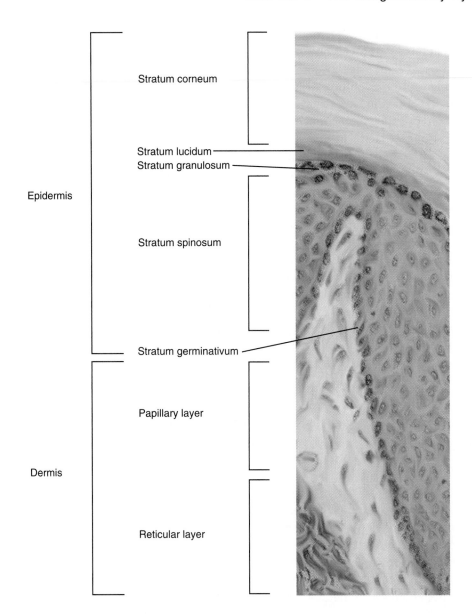

Stratum corneum

Stratum lucidum

Stratum granulosum

Epidermis

Stratum spinosum

Stratum germinativum

Papillary layer

Dermis

Reticular layer

**FIGURE 6-2.** The epidermal and dermal layers of the skin.

The stratum germinativum also contains cells called **melanocytes** (**MEL**-ah-no-sightz), which are responsible for producing skin color. Melanocytes are irregularly shaped with long processes that extend between the other epithelial cells of this layer. They produce a pigment called **melanin** (**MEL**-ah-nin); which is responsible for variations in skin pigmentation. All races have the same number of melanocytes but the different races have specific genes that determine the amount of melanin produced by the melanocytes. Darker skinned individuals have more active melanocytes that produce more melanin.

Melanocytes are activated to produce melanin by exposure to sunlight. We darken when we expose ourselves to the sun. All races get darker after exposure to the sun over a period of time. We call this getting a suntan.

Based on the discoveries and research done in anthropology by the Leakey family in Olduvai Gorge, Tanzania, scientists believe humans evolved in Africa. The first humanoids were probably very dark to protect themselves from the harmful ultraviolet rays of the sun. They had very active melanocytes like today's Africans. Over time, some humans migrated away from the equator and genetic recombinations and mutations governing the activity of their melanocytes occurred. Over long periods this led to the evolution of the different races, whose variations in skin color are determined by the amount of melanin produced and its distribution. The strongest factor in increasing pigmentation in the skin is the sun's stimulating effect on melanocytes. Melanin cross-links with protein to form a tough resistant compound. Hence, heavily pigmented skin is more resistant to external irritation. People who live closer to the equator, where there is maximum exposure to sunlight, will be darker than people who live in the north like the Baltic States of Norway, Sweden, Finland, and Denmark. This variation in melanin content is the principal factor responsible for the color differences among races. Individuals of darker-skinned races have more active melanocytes, while individuals of lighter-skinned races have less active melanocytes.

Larger amounts of melanin can occur in certain areas of the body producing the darkened areola area of the nipples, freckles, and moles, although other areas of the body's skin have less melanin, like the palms of the hands and the soles of the feet. Even though many genes are responsible for skin color, one mutation can cause the absence of skin color by preventing the production of melanin. This condition is called **albinism** (**AL**-bih-nizm) and results from a recessive gene that causes the absence of melanin. Albinos have no pigment in their skin and appendages of the skin. Their hair is white, their eyes pink, and their skin very fair. These individuals must be very careful to avoid overexposure to the sun.

## The Dermis

The dermis is also known as the **corium** (**KOH**-ree-um). It lies directly beneath the epidermis and is often referred to as the true skin. It is composed

---

### Common Disease, Disorder or Condition

### ■ BURNS

Burns are classified into three major categories: first-degree, second-degree, and third-degree. First- and second-degree burns can also be categorized as **partial-thickness burns**. These burns do not completely destroy the stratum germinativum's basal layer and regeneration of the epidermis will occur from both within the burn area or from the edges of the burn.

**First-degree burns** involve just the epidermis. They can be caused by brief contact with very hot or very cold objects. They can also be caused by sunburn, being overexposed to the harmful rays of the sun. Sunscreen should always be used to protect the skin from sunburn. Symptoms of first-degree burns are redness and pain. There may also be slight swelling or edema. These burns can heal in about 7 days with no scarring.

**Second-degree burns** involve both the epidermis and the dermis. With minor dermal involvement symptoms will include redness, pain, swelling, and

blisters. Healing can take up to 2 weeks with no scarring. If there is major dermal involvement the burn can take several months to heal and the wound might appear white. Scar tissue may develop.

In **third-degree burns**, also called **full-thickness burns,** the epidermis and the dermis are completely destroyed. Recovery can only occur from the edge of the burn wound. Interestingly third-degree burns are usually painless because the sensory receptors in the skin have been destroyed. The pain usually comes from the area around the third-degree burn where first- and second-degree burns surround the area. Third-degree burns usually require skin grafts because they take a long time to heal and will form disfiguring scar tissue. Skin grafts will prevent these complications and speed healing. Skin grafts use the epidermis and part of the dermis from another part of the body, usually the buttocks or thighs, and the graft is then placed on the burn. Interstitial fluid from the burn helps heal the area.

of dense connective tissue with tough white collagenous fibers and yellow elastin fibers. Blood vessels, nerves, lymph vessels, smooth muscles, sweat glands, hair follicles, and sebaceous glands are all embedded in the dermis.

The dermis can be divided into two portions (see Figure 6-2). The **papillary portion** is the area adjacent to the epidermis and the **reticular portion** is found between the papillary portion and the fatty subcutaneous tissue beneath. A sheet of areolar tissue, usually containing fat (adipose tissue), is known as the subcutaneous tissue or superficial fascia and attaches the dermis to underlying structures like muscle or bone. This subcutaneous tissue is sometimes referred to as the **hypodermis**. It is into this area that hypodermic injections are given. The pink tint of light-skinned individuals is due to blood vessels in the dermis. There are no blood vessels in the epidermis. When embarrassed, blood vessels in the dermis dilate. This causes "blushing" or the reddish tint seen in the facial area.

When a light-skinned individual suffocates or drowns, carbon dioxide in the blood causes the blood to take on a bluish tinge. This results in the bluish discoloration of skin or **cyanosis** (sigh-ah-**NOH**-sis) caused by lack of oxygen in the blood. When a dark-skinned individual suffocates or drowns, the same condition occurs but results in a grayish or ashy tinge to the skin rather than a bluish tinge.

# THE APPENDAGES OF THE SKIN

The appendages associated with the skin include hair, nails, sebaceous glands, ceruminous glands or wax glands in the ear canal, and sweat glands.

## Hair

**Hair**, in addition to mammary glands, is a main characteristic of all mammals. When the hair is very thick and covers most of the surface of the body, as on a dog or cat, it is called fur. Even on humans, hair covers the entire body except the palms of the hands, the soles of the feet, and certain portions of the external genitalia (e.g., the head of the penis). In some parts of the body, the hair is so small that it appears invisible, yet in other places it is very obvious as on the head, in the armpits, and around the genitalia. The amount of hair a person develops is related to complex genetic factors.

Each individual hair is composed of three parts (Figure 6-3): the **cuticle**, the **cortex**, and the **medulla**. The outermost portion is the cuticle, which consists of several layers of overlapping scalelike cells. The cortex is the principle portion of the hair. Its cells are elongated and united to form flattened fibers. In people with dark hair, these fibers contain pigment granules. The middle or central part of the hair is called the medulla. It is composed of cells with many sides. These cells frequently contain air spaces. There are other parts to the anatomy of a hair. The **shaft** is the visible portion of the hair. The **root** is found in an epidermal tube called the **hair follicle**. The follicle is made of an outer connective tissue sheath and an inner epithelial membrane continuous with the stratum germinativum.

Attached to the hair follicle is a bundle of smooth muscle fibers that make up the **arrector** (ah-**REK**-tohr) **pili** (**PIH**-lye) **muscle**. This muscle causes the goose flesh appearance on our skin when we get scared or when we get a chill. The muscle is involuntary and when it contracts it pulls on the hair follicle causing the hair to "stand on its end." We see the goose flesh appearance where hair is scarce. When dogs or cats get angry their hairs stand up on the nape of their necks. This is all the result of contraction of the arrector pili muscles.

## Hair Growth

Hair growth is similar to the growth of the epidermis. Note that the hair follicle is an involution of the epidermis. The deeper cell layers at the base of the hair follicle are responsible for the production of new cells by mitosis. The epithelial cells of the hair follicle divide by mitosis and get pushed upward because of the basement membrane. As the cells move upward, they keratinize and form the layers of the hair shaft. Hair growth begins in the hair bulb. Blood vessels in the hair bulb provide the nourishment to produce the hair. Hair grows in cycles. The duration of the cycle depends on the hair. Scalp hair grows for 3 years and rests for 1 or 2 years. Hair loss normally means the hair is being replaced because the old hair falls out of the follicle when a new hair begins to form. Some people, particularly men, have a genetic predisposition for

**(A)**

**(B)**

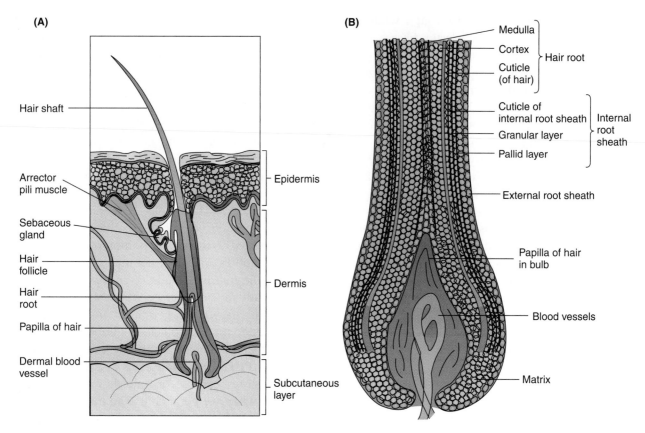

**FIGURE 6-3.** The anatomy of an individual hair.

what is called pattern baldness. These men suffer a permanent loss of hair because the hair follicles are also lost. This occurs because male sex hormones affect the hair follicles of men with this genetic trait and they become bald.

## Hair Texture

We classify hair texture as straight, curly, or tightly curly (kinky). This is due to genetic factors controlling the nature of the keratin of the hair. The keratin of the cortex of the hair is polymerized and cross-linked chemically in a characteristic folded configuration called alpha keratin making the fibers elastic. The alpha keratin chain in some individuals produces straight hair, in others curly, and in still others tightly curled. When stretched, the keratin chain gets drawn or pulled out into a more linear form called beta keratin. Unless the hair is greatly distended or altered by chemical agents, it will return immediately to its normal alpha configuration. When you wash your hair, it can be elongated

to one and one half its normal length due to the weight of the water on the hair. This is possible because the protein keratin can be readily stretched in the direction of the long axis of the molecular chains of amino acids.

Permanent waves act on this principle and people can change the texture of their hair by going to a beauty salon for treatment. The hair stylist will stretch and mold the hair into the desired new wave: big rollers for straighter hair, small tight rollers for curlier hair. Then a chemical reducing agent is placed on the hair to rupture the old disulfide bonds of the alpha keratin chain. Next a new chemical oxidizing agent is placed on the hair to re-establish new stabilizing cross-links in the new position of the beta chain. Remember the chemicals only affected the visible portion of the hair or the shaft. The new cells growing from the hair bulb will not have the new texture, and the permanent wave or new style will eventually "grow out." Another visit to the beauty salon must occur in a few months to redo the process.

## Hair Color

Hair color is also determined by complex genetic factors. For example, some people turn gray in their youth, yet others turn gray in their forties, fifties, or even as late as their sixties. We do know that gray hair occurs when pigment is absent in the cortex of the hair. White hair results from both the absence of pigment in the cortex plus the formation of air bubbles in the shaft.

Hereditary and other unknown factors determine the graying of hair. An interesting research project was done with black cats and gray hair. The hair of a black cat turned gray when its diet was deficient in pantothenic acid (an amino acid). Restoring this substance to its diet caused the gray hair to return to black. Unfortunately this only works with cats. So the hair coloring industry is still secure.

Great frights, like being in a serious plane or car accident, can cause people's hair to change color and go gray or white. We do not know what physiologic processes are triggered that cause this to occur, other than the trauma of such an experience.

## Nails

At the ends of fingers and toes, we have nails. (Figure 6-4). Other animals have claws (birds, reptiles, cats, and dogs) or hooves (horses, cows, deer, and elk). The nail is a modification of horny (leathery) epidermal cells composed of very hard keratin. Air mixed in the keratin matrix forms the white crescent at the proximal end of each nail called the **lunula** (**LOO**-noo-lah). Again the size of the lunula will vary from person to person and sometimes

from nail to nail due to genetic factors. The **nail body** is the visible part of the nail. The **nail root** is the part of the nail body attached to the **nail bed** from which the nail grows approximately 1mm per week unless inhibited by disease. The **cuticle** or eponychium is stratum corneum that extends out over the proximal end of the nail body.

Our fingernails grow faster than our toenails. Regeneration of a lost fingernail occurs in $3\frac{1}{2}$ to $5\frac{1}{2}$ months. Regeneration of a lost toenail occurs in 6 to 8 months as long as the nail bed remains intact. As we age, the rate of growth of nails slows.

## Sebaceous Glands

**Sebaceous** (see-**BAY**-shus) **glands** (Figure 6-1) develop along the walls of hair follicles and produce **sebum** (**SEE**-bum). This is an oily substance that is responsible for lubricating the surface of our skin, giving it a glossy appearance. Sebaceous secretions consist of entire cells containing the sebum. As the cells disintegrate, the sebum moves along the hair shaft to the surface of the skin where it produces a cosmetic gloss. Brushing hair causes the sebum to cover the shaft of our hair, making hair shiny. Remember how good your dog or cat looks after a good brushing. The coat of fur glistens and shines due to the sebum.

Sebaceous secretion is under the control of the endocrine system. It increases at puberty resulting in acne problems in adolescents and it decreases in later life resulting in dry skin problems. It also increases in late pregnancy.

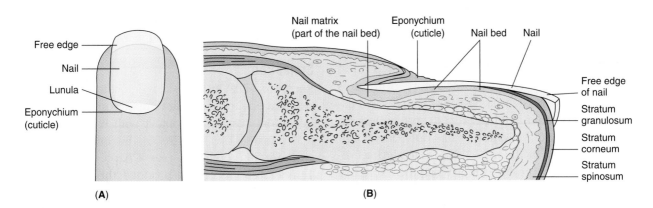

**FIGURE 6-4.**   The anatomy of a nail. (A) Posterior view of finger and (B) fingernail and underlying structures.

## ■ ACNE IN ADOLESCENTS

During puberty the sebaceous glands secrete an excessive amount of sebum. The opening of the gland can become clogged with this oily substance. Because so much is being secreted, it cannot make its way onto the surface of the skin. The fatty oil oxidizes in the presence of air and becomes discolored producing a "blackhead." The sebum retained in the gland can provide a growth medium for pus-producing bacteria. If the clog is near the surface of the skin, this results in a pimple. If the clog is deep in the gland along the shaft of the hair, the result is a boil. This must be lanced by a physician so that it can be drained of excess fluid and the bacterial infection.

To prevent blackheads and pimples, adolescents should frequently wash their faces on a regular daily basis. They should also use astringents like alcohols to dry the surface of their skin.

## Sweat Glands

**Sweat glands** (Figure 6-1) are simple tubular glands found in most parts of the body. They are not found on the margins of the lips and the head of the penis. They are most numerous in the palms of our hands and in the soles of our feet. It has been estimated that there are 3000 sweat glands per square inch on the palms of our hands. When you get nervous think about which area of your body gets sweaty first—your hands!

Each sweat gland consists of a secretory portion and an excretory duct. The secretory portion is located below the dermis, in the subcutaneous tissue, and is a blind tube twisted and coiled on itself. A blind tube is one that has only one opening, in this case at the top. From the coiled secretory portion that produces the sweat, the excretory duct spirals up through the dermis into the epidermis and finally opens on the surface of the skin.

Sweat contains the same inorganic materials as blood but in a much lower concentration. Its chief salt is sodium chloride, which is the reason sweat tastes salty. Its organic constituents include urea, uric acid, amino acids, ammonia, sugar, lactic acid, and ascorbic acid. Sweat itself is practically odorless. That may surprise you because many of us have been in a locker room at a gym. Actually the odor is produced by the action of bacteria feeding on the sweat. Remember the last time you did some strenuous exercise? You are sweating but there is no odor for the first 10 or 15 minutes. After that time odor developed because it took that long for the bacterial population to grow in the sweat and their effects to be smelled.

Sweating is also an important physiologic process that cools the body. Sweating leads to loss of heat in the body because heat is required to evaporate the water in sweat. Therefore sweating helps to lower body temperature. Some people are born without sweat glands—they have a congenital absence of these glands. These individuals can easily die of heat stroke if exposed to high temperatures even if only for a brief period of time. Other individuals have overactive sweat glands and must use stronger deodorants and antiperspirants. Due to hair in the armpits, sweat accumulates there. Because our armpits are usually covered while our arms are at our sides, the environment is ideal for bacteria to feed on the sweat, hence the need for deodorants.

# FUNCTIONS OF THE INTEGUMENTARY SYSTEM

The skin functions in sensation, protection, thermoregulation, and secretion.

## Sensation

Receptor sites in the skin detect changes in the external environment for temperature and pressure. Receptor sites are in contact with sensory neurons that transmit the impulse to the brain and spinal cord for interpretation (see Chapters 10 and 11). Temperature receptors produce the sensations of hot and cold. Pressure receptor sites allow us to interpret excessive pressure that results in the sensation of pain as when we get pinched. They also detect mild pressure that results in the sensation of pleasure as from a gentle massage or a petting stroke. Combinations of varying degrees of those stimulations at these receptor sites produce other sensations that we call burning, itching, or tickling. These receptor sites allow us to react to external stimuli and to interpret what is occurring in the outside world.

## Protection

The skin is an elastic, resistant covering. It prevents passage of harmful physical and chemical agents. The melanin produced by the melanocytes in the stratum germinativum protects us from the damaging ultraviolet rays of sunlight. Most chemicals cannot gain entry into the body through the skin but the chemicals that cause poison ivy and poison oak can penetrate this barrier.  Fat-soluble chemicals like DDT, a chlorinated hydrocarbon pesticide, can also get through the skin. If you put your hand in a can of gasoline, you will not be poisoned. However, if you put your hand in a can of DDT, you could be poisoned. People who work with certain insecticides must wear protective clothing to prevent the penetration of these chemicals through their skin.

The lipid content of the skin inhibits the excessive loss of water and electrolytes through the skin. Normal skin is impermeable to water, carbohydrates, fat, and protein. However, all true gases and certain volatile substances will pass through the epidermis like the organic pesticide mentioned above. The numerous openings around hair follicles can act as channels for absorption of these materials.

Skin also has an acid mantle. This acidity kills most bacteria and other microorganisms that make contact with our skin. Soaps and shampoos will often be labeled as pH balanced, which indicates that these cleansers will not destroy the acid mantle of the skin. Some skin diseases will destroy the acidity of certain areas of the skin, impairing the self-sterilizing capabilities of our skin. These diseases make the skin prone to bacterial infections.

Nails protect the ends of our digits. Fingernails can also be used in defense. Hair on our head acts as an insulator and helps prevent heat loss. Hairs in our nose filter out large foreign particles like soot. Eyelashes protect our eyes from foreign objects.

## Thermoregulation

Normal body temperature is maintained at approximately 98.6°F (37°C). Temperature regulation is critical to our survival because changes in temperature affect the functioning of enzymes. The presence of enzymes is critical for normal chemical reactions to occur in our cells. When people get high fevers they can die because the heat of a fever destroys the enzymes by breaking up their chemical structure. Without enzymes, chemical reactions cannot occur and our cellular machinery breaks down and death results.

When external temperatures increase, blood vessels in the dermis dilate to bring more blood flow to the surface of the body from deeper tissue beneath. In the skin the blood with its 98.6°F temperature or heat is then lost by radiation, convection, conduction, and evaporation. When we sweat, the water in sweat evaporates, which requires energy and thus carries away heat to reduce body temperature.

When external temperatures decrease, the first response is for blood vessels in the dermis to dilate to bring heat to the surface to warm our extremities. Light-skinned individuals will have rosy cheeks when they first go out during a cold wintery day.

### Health Alert

### ■ AGING

As we age many visible changes occur in our skin. A decrease in secretions of sebum results in drier skin. We hear and see advertisements for skin moisturizers, a big source of income for the cosmetic industry. Loss of collagen and elastin fibers in the dermis results in the skin sagging and wrinkling. Blood flow to the skin decreases with age and the skin becomes thinner and looks more translucent. The number of melanocytes decreases in certain areas causing the darkening appearance of other areas of the skin referred to as age spots. Lack of melanin also affects the graying and production of white hair with increased age.

Excessive exposure to the cold cannot be maintained for long, so blood vessels then constrict to bring the heat inside to preserve the vital organs of the body. Frostbite occurs when the skin of the extremities no longer gets a blood supply due to the maintained constriction of the blood vessels in the dermis to conserve heat. The tissues in the tips of these extremities die and turn black.

## Secretion

The skin produces two secretions: sebum and sweat. Sebum is secreted by the sebaceous glands. In addition to imparting a cosmetic gloss to our skin and moisturizing our skin, sebum has both antifungal and antibacterial properties. It helps prevent infection and maintains the texture and integrity of the skin. Sweat is produced by the sweat glands and is essential in the cooling process of the body. Sweat also contains waste products such as urea, ammonia, and uric acid and so can also be considered an excretion. A secretion is something beneficial whereas an excretion is something the body does not need and could be harmful.

The skin is actively involved in the production of vitamin D. Exposure to the ultraviolet rays of the sun stimulates our skin to produce a precursor molecule of vitamin D that then goes to the liver and kidneys to become mature vitamin D. Vitamin D is necessary for our bodies because it stimulates the intake of calcium and phosphate in our intestines. Calcium is necessary for muscle contraction and

bone development. Phosphorous is an essential part of adenosine triphosphate. Because we live indoors, and in colder climates wear heavy clothing, we sometimes do not get enough exposure to the sun to adequately produce enough vitamin D. We also should ingest vitamin D through our diets. Good sources of vitamin D are milk and fish oils.

## Body Systems Working Together To Maintain Homeostasis: The Integumentary System

### Skeletal System

- Vitamin D manufactured by the skin helps provide calcium for strong bones.

### Muscular System

- Vitamin D helps provide calcium for muscle contraction.
- Facial muscles produce facial expressions of body language.
- Shivering helps control body temperature by warming the body.

### Nervous System

- Receptor sites for temperature and pressure changes in the skin provide information to the nervous system so we can cope with our external environment.
- Nerves activate sweat glands.

## Common Disease, Disorder or Condition

### ■ SKIN CANCER

Skin cancer usually develops from excessive exposure to the ultraviolet rays of the sun, which in the reason sunscreens should be used when engaging in outdoor recreational activities or when one's occupation requires outdoor work. Common areas of development of skin cancers are the face, neck, and hands. There are three types of skin cancers, of which two can be lethal.

The most common type of skin cancer is **basal cell carcinoma**. This cancer produces an open ulcer and can be easily treated with radiation ther-

apy or surgical removal. This cancer rarely spreads. The first dangerous type of skin cancer is **squamous cell carcinoma,** which produces a nodular tumor that is highly keratinized and found in the epidermis. If untreated it can spread to the dermis, metastasize, and cause death. The most dangerous type of skin cancer is **malignant melanoma**. It is rare and associated with a mole on the skin. A mole is a grouping of melanocytes. They become cancerous and metastasis is common. The melanoma can appear as a dark nodule or a spreading flat lesion. Unless treated early, this cancer is fatal.

| Common Disease, Disorder or Condition |
|---|

## ■ DISORDERS OF THE INTEGUMENTARY SYSTEM

### Ringworm

**Ringworm** is caused by several species of fungus. Its symptoms include itchy, patchy scalelike lesions with raised edges. In earlier times, it was believed that this condition was caused by worms, hence its other name, tinea, which is Latin for worm. Ringworm on the feet is called athlete's foot; in the groin area it is called jock itch. Ringworm of the scalp is called tinea capitus and is most common in children. Untreated it can lead to hair loss and secondary bacterial infections.

### Psoriasis

**Psoriasis** (soh-**RYE**-ah-sis) is a common chronic skin disorder that may be genetic in orgin. The actual cause is unknown. It is characterized by red patches covered with thick, dry, and silvery scales that develop from excessive production of epithelial cells. These patches can develop anywhere on the body. When the scales are scraped away bleeding usually results. There is no known cure for this disease but it can be controlled with corticosteroids, ultraviolet light, and tar solution creams and shampoos.

### Warts

**Warts** are caused by human papillomavirus. The virus causes uncontrolled growth of epidermal tissue. The virus is transmitted by direct contract with an infected individual. The growths are usually benign and disappear spontaneously. They can also be removed surgically or with topical applications.

### Cold Sores

**Cold sores,** also known as **fever blisters,** are caused by a herpes simplex virus. Initial infections show no symptoms but the virus can remain dormant in the skin around the mouth and in the mucous membrane of the mouth. When activated it produces small, fluid-filled blisters that can be both painful and irritating. Stress seems to activate the virus.

### Impetigo

**Impetigo** (im-peh-**TYE**-go) is a highly contagious skin disease of children caused by the bacterium *Staphylococcus aureus*. The skin erupts with small blisters containing pus that rupture easily producing a honey-colored crust. The blisters usually develop on the face and can spread. The bacteria are spread by direct contact and enter the skin through abrasions. Treatment includes cleansing with antibacterial soaps and antibiotics.

### Shingles

**Shingles** is caused by the herpes zoster or chickenpox virus that develops after the childhood infection. The virus remains dormant within cranial or spinal nerves. Trauma or stress somehow activates the virus to travel through the nerve paths to the skin where it produces very painful, vesicular skin eruptions. Treatment is symptomatic with lotions to relieve itching and analgesics to control pain.

### Vitiligo

**Vitiligo** (vit-ill-**EYE**-go) is an acquired skin disease resulting in irregular patches of skin of various sizes completely lacking in any pigmentation. The depigmented white patches are often located on exposed areas of skin. The cause of the disease is unknown. It is said that the singer Michael Jackson suffers from this condition.

## Endocrine System

- Hormones control the secretion of sebum from the sebaceous glands.
- Hormones increase blood flow to the skin.
- Hormones control the amount of fat in subcutaneous tissue.

## Cardiovascular System

- Blood vessels in the dermis help regulate body temperature by dilating or constricting.
- Dilation of blood vessels in light skin produces blushing during embarrassing moments.

## Lymphatic System

- Skin is an effective barrier against invasion by microorganisms providing a first defense for the immune system.
- Sebum has antifungal and antibacterial properties.
- The acid mantle of the skin helps prevent most bacterial infections.

## Digestive System

- Vitamin D produced by the skin causes calcium and phosphorous to be absorbed in the intestine.
- Excess calories can be stored as fat in subcutaneous tissue.

## Respiratory System

- Receptor sites in the skin can bring about changes in breathing rates.

## Urinary System

- Kidneys can restore water and electrolytes lost during sweating.

## Reproductive System

- Stimulation of receptor sites in the skin can bring about sexual interest.
- Sucking on the nipple causes the pregnant female to produce milk from her mammary glands.

## Summary Outline

### INTRODUCTION

1. The integumentary system is made up of the skin, hair, nails, sebaceous glands, ceruminous

or wax glands in the ear canal, and sweat glands.
2. The skin is waterproof, it protects us from ultraviolet radiation, and through sweating it dissipates water and helps regulate body temperature.

### THE LAYERS OF THE SKIN

1. The skin is composed of two layers: the upper epidermis and the lower dermis or corium.

### The Epidermis

1. The epidermis is composed of stratified, squamous, keratinized epithelium.
2. As cells move up to the surface of the epidermis they lose water, and their nuclei and change chemically, a process called keratinization.
3. The five layers of the epidermis are from outermost to deep:
   stratum corneum or horny layer
   stratum lucidum or clear layer
   stratum granulosum or granular layer
   stratum spinosum or spiny layer
   stratum germinativum or regenerative layer.

### The Stratum Corneum

1. It consists of dead cells converted to protein or keratinized cells that constantly are being shed.
2. It is a barrier to light and heat waves, most chemicals, and microorganisms.

### The Stratum Lucidum

1. This layer is only one or two flat and transparent layers of cells thick. It is difficult to see.

### The Stratum Granulosum

1. This layer is two or three layers of cells very active in keratinization.

### The Stratum Spinosum

1. This layer consists of several layers of spiny-shaped polyhedron-like cells.
2. The interlocking cellular bridges or desmosomes are found in this layer.

### The Stratum Germinativum

1. This layer rests on the basement membrane. Its lowermost layer of cells is called the stratum basale.
2. This layer is the layer that produces new epidermal cells by mitosis.
3. Melanocytes of this layer produce melanin. This pigment is responsible for skin color and

protection from the harmful ultraviolet rays of the sun.

4. Dark-skinned individuals have more active melanocytes.

5. Albinism is a genetic condition that results in the absence of melanin.

### The Dermis

1. The dermis is also called the corium or true skin and is composed of dense connective tissue.

2. Blood and lymph vessels, nerves, muscles, glands, and hair follicles are found in the dermis.

3. It is divided into two portions: the papillary portion below the epidermis and the reticular portion above the subcutaneous tissue.

4. The subcutaneous tissue can be called the hypodermis.

### THE APPENDAGES OF THE SKIN

1. The appendages of the skin include hair, nails, sebaceous glands, ceruminous or wax glands, and sweat glands.

### Hair

1. Hair covers the entire body except the palms of the hands, the soles of the feet, and parts of the external genitalia.

2. Each individual hair is made of three parts: the outer cuticle, the cortex, which is the principle portion with pigment granules, and the inner medulla with air spaces.

3. The visible portion of a hair is called the shaft.

4. The root of a hair is in a hair follicle.

5. When the arrector pili smooth muscle contracts, it causes a hair to stand on end and produces "goose flesh."

### Hair Growth

1. Hair growth begins with the cells deep in the hair follicle at the hair bulb growing by mitosis and nourished by blood vessels.

2. Hair grows in cycles and rests between cycles.

### Hair Texture

1. Hair texture can be classified as straight, curly, or tightly curly and is due to genetic factors.

2. Hair in the alpha keratin chain is elastic; when stretched it is in the beta keratin chain.

### Hair Color

1. Hair color is determined by complex genetic factors.

2. Gray hair occurs when pigment is absent in the cortex.

3. White hair results from both the absence of pigment and air bubbles in the shaft.

4. Heredity and other unknown factors cause hair to turn gray.

### Nails

1. A nail is a modification of epidermal cells made of very hard keratin.

2. The lunula is the white crescent at the proximal end of a nail caused by air mixed with the keratin.

3. The nail body is the visible portion of a nail. The nail root is the part covered by skin.

4. The nail grows from the nail bed.

5. The cuticle is stratum corneum that extends over the nail body.

### Sebaceous Glands

1. Sebaceous glands produce sebum and are found along the walls of hair follicles.

2. Sebum, an oil, gives a cosmetic gloss to skin and moisturizes it.

3. Sebaceous secretion is controlled by the endocrine system, increasing during puberty and late pregnancy and decreasing with age.

### Sweat Glands

1. Sweat glands are most numerous in the palms of our hands and in the soles of our feet.

2. The secretory, blind tube portion, of a sweat gland is in the subcutaneous tissue. The excretory portion goes through the dermis to the surface.

3. The odor of sweat is produced by the action of bacteria feeding on the sweat.

4. Sweating is an important physiologic process that helps cool the body.

### FUNCTIONS OF THE INTEGUMENTARY SYSTEM

1. The skin functions in sensation, protection, thermoregulation, and secretion.

### Sensation

1. Receptor sites for changes in temperature (hot and cold) and pressure (pleasure and pain) are found in the skin.

2. Combinations of stimulations result in the sensations of itching, burning, and tickling.

### Protection

1. The skin prevents the entrance of harmful physical and chemical agents into the body.

2. Melanin protects us from the harmful ultraviolet rays of the sun.

**3.** The lipid content of skin prevents excessive water and electrolyte loss.

**4.** The acidic pH of skin kills most bacteria and microorganisms that come in contact with our skin.

**5.** Hair acts as an insulator, protects our eyes, and filters out foreign particles in our nose.

**Thermoregulation**

**1.** Normal body temperature is regulated by blood vessel dilation and constriction in the dermis of the skin.

**2.** Sweating is an evaporation process that cools the body.

**Secretion**

**1.** Sebum has antifungal and antibacterial properties.

**2.** Sweat contains waste products such as urea, uric acid, and ammonia so it is also an excretion.

**3.** The skin helps manufacture vitamin D through exposure to ultraviolet rays of the sun

## REVIEW QUESTIONS

**1.** List the five layers of the epidermis with their common names.

**2.** List and describe four functions of the integumentary system.

*__3.__ If all people have the same number of melanocytes in their skin, how do we explain the differences in color among the various races?

*__4.__ Why would a person born with an absence of sweat glands be very susceptible to death by exposure to heat?

**\*Critical Thinking Questions**

## Matching

Place the most appropriate number in the blank provided.

| | | |
|---|---|---|
| ____ Melanin | 1. | Central axis of hair |
| ____ Keratinization | 2. | Skin pigment |
| ____ Dermis | 3. | Visible portion of hair |
| ____ Cuticle | 4. | White crescent of nail |
| ____ Medulla | 5. | Desmosomes |
| ____ Shaft | 6. | Produces brittle dry cells without nuclei |
| ____ Cortex | 7. | Lubricates surface of skin |
| ____ Lunula | 8. | Blue or ashy color of skin |
| ____ Sebum | 9. | Arrector pili muscle |
| ____ Cyanosis | 10. | Principle portion of hair, cells are elongated |
| | 11. | Corium |
| | 12. | Outermost layer of hair, scalelike cells |

## LABORATORY EXERCISE: THE INTEGUMENTARY SYSTEM

Materials needed: A compound microscope and prepared microscope slides.

1. Examine a prepared slide of a section of skin from the palm of the hand. Try to distinguish the different layers of the epidermis. Note the basement membrane. Notice that the cells closest to the basement membrane are nonkeratinized but those farthest away in the stratum corneum are keratinized. Note the two layers of the dermis: the papillary portion and the reticular portion.

2. Examine a prepared slide of hair shafts from the human scalp. Note the structure of the hair follicle surrounding the shaft of hair.

3. Your instructor will show you a videotape or CD-ROM on "The Skin."

# 7

# The Skeletal System

## CHAPTER OUTLINE

■ **Introduction**

■ **The functions of the skeletal system**

■ **The growth and formation of bone:** *Deposition of bone; Types of ossification; Maintaining bone*

■ **The histology of bone:** *The haversian system of compact bone; Cancellous bone; Bone marrow*

■ **The classification of bones based on shape:** *Long bones; Short bones; Flat bones; Irregular bones; Sesamoid bones*

■ **Bone markings:** *Processes; Fossae*

■ **Divisions of the skeleton**

■ **The axial skeleton:** *The cranial bones; The facial bones; The orbits; The nasal cavities; The foramina of the skull; The hyoid bone; How to study the bones of the skull; The torso or trunk; The thorax; The sternum; The ribs*

■ **The appendicular skeleton:** *The bones of the upper extremities; The bones of the lower extremities*

■ **The arches of the foot**

■ **Body systems working together to maintain homeostasis: the skeletal system**

## CHAPTER OBJECTIVES

After studying this chapter, you should be able to:

1. Name the functions of the skeletal system.

2. Name the two types of ossification.

3. Describe why diet can affect bone development in children and bone maintenance in older adults.

4. Describe the histology of compact bone.

5. Define and give examples of bone markings.

6. Name the cranial and facial bones.

7. Name the bones of the axial and appendicular skeleton.

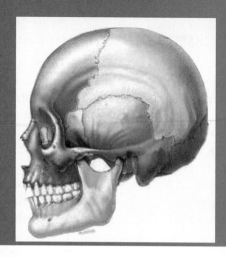

# KEY TERMS

## INTRODUCTION

The supporting structure of the body is the framework of joined bones that we refer to as the skeleton. It enables us to stand erect, to move in our environment, to accomplish extraordinary feats of artistic grace like ballet moves and athletic endeavors like the high jump, as well as normal physical endurance. The skeletal system allows us to move a pen and write and aids us in breathing. It is closely associated with the muscular system. The skeletal system includes all the bones of the body and their associated cartilage, tendons, and ligaments. Despite the appearance of the bones, they are indeed composed of living tissue. The hard, "dead" stonelike appearance of bones is due to mineral salts like calcium phosphate embedded in the inorganic matrix of the bone tissue. Leondardo da Vinci (1452–1519), the famous Italian Renaissance artist and scientist, is credited as the first anatomist to correctly illustrate the skeleton with its 206 bones. See Concept Map 7-1: Skeletal System.

## THE FUNCTIONS OF THE SKELETAL SYSTEM

The skeleton has five general functions:

1. It supports and stabilizes surrounding tissues such as muscles, blood vessels, nerves, fat, and skin.
2. It protects vital organs of the body such as the brain, spinal cord, the heart, and lungs and it protects other soft tissues of the body.
3. It assists in body movement by providing attachments for muscles that pull on the bones that act as levers.
4. It manufactures blood cells. This process is called **hematopoiesis** (**hem**-ah-toh-poy-**EE**-sis) and occurs chiefly in red bone marrow.
5. It is a storage area for mineral salts, especially phosphorous and calcium, and fats.

Associated with the bones are cartilage, tendons, and ligaments. **Cartilage**, a connective tissue, is the environment in which bone develops in a fetus. It is also found at the ends of certain bones and in joints in adults, providing a smooth surface for adjacent bones to move against each other. **Ligaments** are tough connective tissue structures that attach bones to bones like the ligament that attaches the head of the femur to the acetabulum of the pelvic bone in the hip joint. **Tendons** are similar structures that attach muscle to bone.

## THE GROWTH AND FORMATION OF BONE

The skeleton of a developing fetus is completely formed by the end of the third month of pregnancy. However, at this time, the skeleton is predominantly cartilage. During the subsequent months of pregnancy, ossification, the formation of bone, and growth occur. The osteoblasts invade the cartilage and convert it to bone. Longitudinal growth of bones continues until approximately 15 years of age

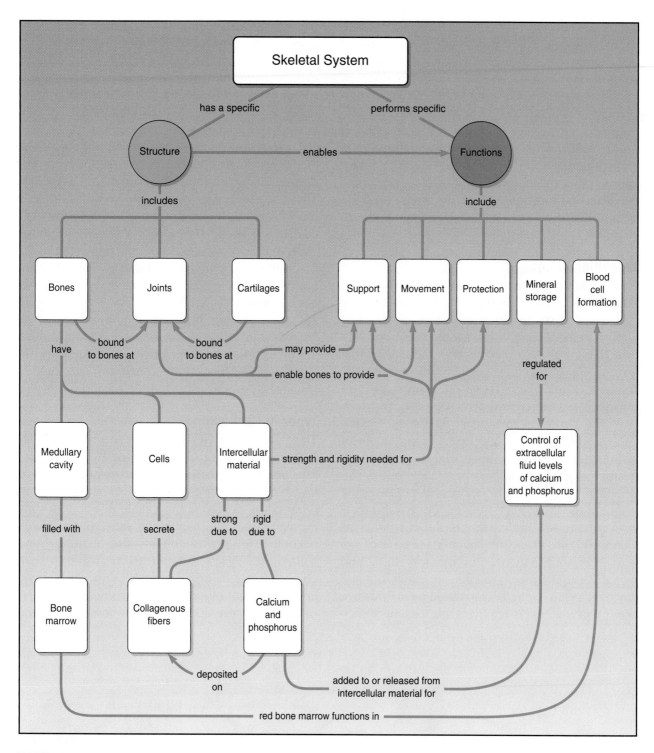

**CONCEPT MAP 7-1.** Skeletal System.

in girls and 16 years of age in boys. This takes place at the epiphyseal line or plate. Bone maturation and remodeling continue until the age of 21 in both sexes. It would be incorrect to state that cartilage actually turns into bone. Rather cartilage is the environment in which the bone develops.

The strong protein matrix is responsible for a bone's resilience or "elasticity" when tension is applied to the bone so that it gives a little under pressure. The mineral salts deposited into this protein matrix are responsible for the strength of the bone so that it does not get crushed when pressure is applied to the bone.

## Deposition of Bone

Bone develops from spindle-shaped cells called **osteoblasts** that develop from undifferentiated bone cells called **osteoprogenitor** (**oss**-tee-oh-pro-**JEN**-ih-tohr) **cells** (Figure 7-1). These osteoblasts are formed beneath the fibrovascular membrane that covers a bone called the **periosteum** (pair-ee-**AH**-stee-um) (Figure 7-2). These osteoblasts are also found in the **endosteum** (en-**DOS**-tee-um), which lines the bone marrow or medullary cavity. Deposition of bone is controlled by the amount of strain or pressure on the bone. The more strain the greater the deposition of bone. The heel bone or calcaneum is a large strong bone because it receives the weight of the body when walking. Bones (and muscles) in casts will waste away or atrophy, whereas continued and excessive strain via exercise will cause the bone and muscles to grow thick and strong. This is the reason children are told to run and play to develop strong bones during their formative years. When a cast is removed, the patient partici-

pates in physical therapy to build up the bone (and muscles) that became weak while in the cast.

A break in a bone will stimulate injured osteocytes to proliferate. They then secrete large quantities of matrix to form new bone. In addition, other types of bone cells called **osteoclasts** are present in almost all cavities of bone (see Figure 7-1). They are responsible for the reabsorption of bone. These are large cells that remove bone from the inner side during remodeling, such as when a bone is broken. These cells are also responsible for the ability of a crooked bone to become straight. If a young child is detected to be bow-legged, the physician will apply braces to the legs. Periodic tightening of the braces puts pressure on the bone so that new bone is deposited by osteocytes (mature osteoblasts), or mature bone cells, while the osteoclasts remove the old bone during this remodeling process. This process can cause a broken bone that was set improperly to heal incorrectly. To correct this, the bone must be broken again and correctly reset to straighten properly.

## Types of Ossification

There are two types of **ossification** (**oss**-sih-fih-**KAY**-shun) (the formation of bone by osteoblasts). The first type is **intramembranous ossification**, in which dense connective tissue membranes are replaced by deposits of inorganic calcium salts thus forming bone. The membrane itself will eventually become the periosteum of the mature bone. Underneath the periosteum will be compact bone with an inner core of spongy or cancellous bone. Only the bones of the cranium or skull form by this process. Because complete ossification in this way

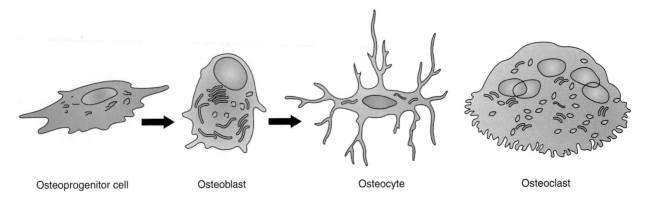

Osteoprogenitor cell          Osteoblast                    Osteocyte                     Osteoclast

**FIGURE 7-1.** The different types of bone cells.

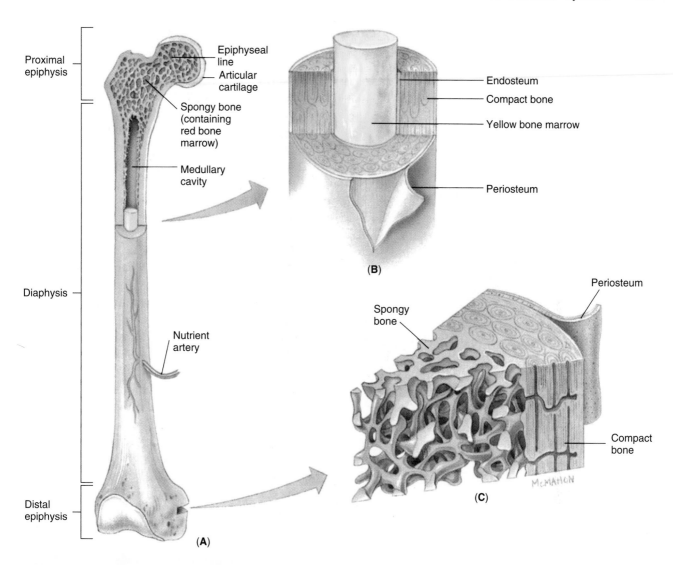

**FIGURE 7-2.** The structure of a typical long bone. (A) Diaphysis, epiphysis, and medullary cavity. (B) Compact bone surrounding yellow bone marrow in the medullary cavity. (C) Spongy bone and compact bone in the epiphysis.

does not occur until a few months after birth, one can feel these membranes on the top of a baby's skull as the *soft spot* or **fontanelle** (fon-tah-**NELL**). This allows the baby's skull to give slightly as it moves through the birth canal.

The other bones of the body are formed by the second process called **endochondral** (en-doh-**KON**-dral) **ossification** (Figure 7-3). This is the process in which cartilage is the environment in which the bone cells develop (endo = inside, chondro = cartilage). As the organic matrix becomes synthesized, the osteoblast becomes completely surrounded by the bone matrix and the osteoblast becomes a mature bone cell or osteocyte. Both types of ossification result in compact and cancellous bone.

## Maintaining Bone

In a healthy body, a balance must exist between the amount of calcium stored in the bones, the calcium in the blood, and the excess calcium excreted by the kidneys and via the digestive system. The proper calcium ion concentration in the blood and bones is controlled by the endocrine system. Two hormones, calcitonin and parathormone, control the calcium concentration in our bodies. Calcitonin causes calcium to be stored in the bones; parathormone causes it to be released into the bloodstream.

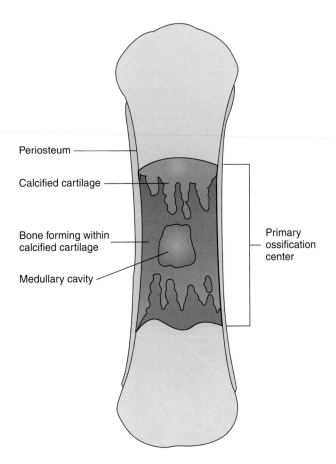

Periosteum

Calcified cartilage

Bone forming within
calcified cartilage

Medullary cavity

Primary
ossification
center

**FIGURE 7-3.** Endochondral ossification where cartilage is the environment in which bone develops.

# THE HISTOLOGY OF BONE

There are two types of bone tissue: **compact** or **dense bone**; and **cancellous** or **spongy bone** (see Figure 7-2C). In both types of tissue, the osteocytes are the same but the arrangement of how the blood supply reaches the bone cells is different. The two types of tissue have different functions. Compact bone is dense and strong, whereas cancellous bone has many open spaces giving it a spongy appearance. It is in these spaces that bone marrow can be found.

## The Haversian System of Compact Bone

The **haversian** (hah-**VER**-shan) **canal**, also called an **osteon**, was named for an English physician, Clopton Havers (1650–1702), who first described it as a prominent feature of compact bone (Figure 7-4). This system allows for the effective metabolism of bone cells surrounded by rings of mineral salts. It has several components. Running parallel to the surface of the bone are many small canals containing blood vessels (capillaries, arterioles, venules) that bring in oxygen and nutrients and remove waste products and carbon dioxide. These canals are called haversian or **central canals** and are surrounded by concentric rings of bone, each layer of which is called a **lamella** (lah-**MELL**-ah). Between two lamella or rings of bone are several tiny cavities called **lacunae** (lah-**KOO**-nee). Each lacuna

---

**Common Disease, Disorder or Condition**

## ■ RICKETS

**Rickets** is a disease caused by deficiencies in the minerals calcium and phosphorous or by deficiencies in vitamin D and sunlight. Vitamin D is necessary for calcium and phosphorous absorption. The condition causes changes in bones known as rickets in children and **osteomalacia** (**oss**-tee-oh-mah-**LAY**-she-ah) in adults. The bones fail to ossify, resulting in soft, weak bones that are easily broken. Rickets occurs in children who do not receive adequate exposure to sunlight (sunlight is necessary for vitamin D production in the body) or whose diets are deficient in vitamin D (milk is a food source of vitamin D).

## ■ FRACTURES

The breaking of bone or associated cartilage is known as a **fracture**. Because bone supports other tissues, a fracture is usually accompanied by injury to surrounding soft tissues like muscle or connective tissue. Bone fractures are classified as either open or compound if the bone protrudes through the skin, or closed or simple if this skin is not perforated. Fractures can also be categorized based on the direction of the fracture line as transverse (at right angles to a long axis), linear (parallel to a long axis), or oblique (an angle other than a right angle to a long axis).

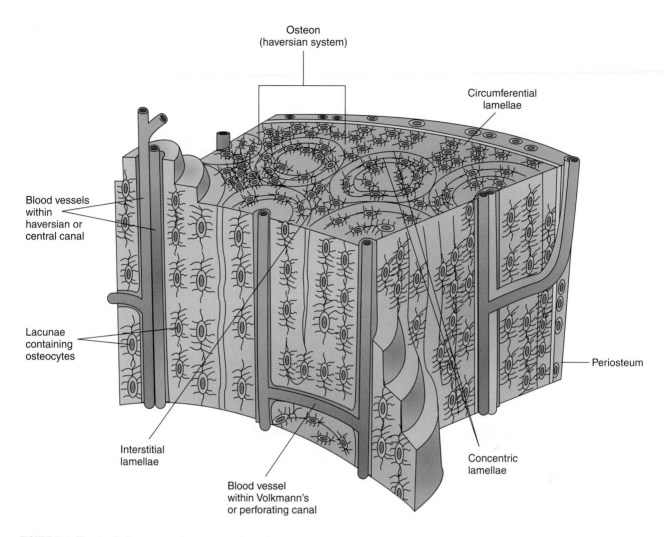

**FIGURE 7-4.** The detailed structure of compact or dense bone.

contains an osteocyte or bone cell suspended in tissue fluid. The lacunae are all connected to each other and ultimately to the larger haversian canals by much smaller canals called **canaliculi** (**kan**-ah-**LIK**-you-lye). Canals running horizontally to the haversian (central) canals, also containing blood vessels, are called **Volkmann** or **perforating canals**. It is tissue fluid that circulates through all these canals and bathes the osteocyte bringing in oxygen and food and carrying away waste products and carbon dioxide keeping the osteocytes alive and healthy.

## Cancellous Bone

Cancellous or spongy bone is located at the ends of long bones and forms the center of all other bones. It consists of a meshwork of interconnecting sec-

tions of bone called **trabeculae** (trah-**BEK**-you-lay) creating the spongelike appearance of cancellous bone. The trabeculae give strength to the bone without the added weight of being solid. Each trabecula consists of several lamellae with osteocytes between the lamellae just as in compact bone. The spaces between the trabeculae are filled with bone marrow. Nutrients exit blood vessels in the marrow and pass by diffusion through the canaliculi of the lamellae to the osteocytes in the lacunae.

## Bone Marrow

The many spaces within cancellous bone are filled with **red bone marrow**. This marrow is richly supplied with blood and consists of blood cells and their precursors. The function of red bone marrow is hematopoiesis or the formation of red and white blood cells and blood platelets. Therefore, blood cells in all stages of development will be found in red bone marrow. We shall discuss in more detail the different stages of blood cell development in Chapter 13.

In an adult, the ribs, vertebrae, sternum, and bones of the pelvis all contain red bone marrow in their cancellous tissue. These bones produce blood cells in adults. Red bone marrow within the ends of the humerus or upper arm and the femur or thigh is plentiful at birth but gradually decreases in amount as we age.

**Yellow bone marrow** is connective tissue consisting chiefly of fat cells. It is found primarily in the shafts of long bones within the medullary cavity, the central area of the bone shaft (see Figure 7-2B). Yellow bone marrow extends into the osteons or haversian systems, replacing red bone marrow when it becomes depleted.

# THE CLASSIFICATION OF BONES BASED ON SHAPE

The individual bones of the body can be divided by shape into five categories: long, short, flat, irregular, and sesamoid (Figure 7-5).

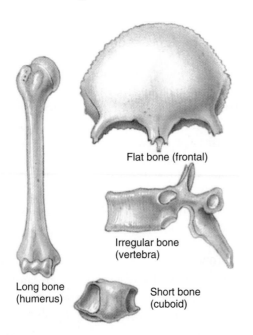

Flat bone (frontal)

Irregular bone (vertebra)

Long bone (humerus)

Short bone (cuboid)

**FIGURE 7-5.** The classification of bones based on shape.

## Long Bones

*Long bones* (see Figure 7-2) are bones whose length exceeds their width and consist of a **diaphysis** (dye-**AFF**-ih-sis) or shaft composed mainly of compact bone, a **metaphysis** (meh-**TAFF**-ih-sis) or flared portion at each end of the diaphysis consisting mainly of cancellous or spongy bone, and two extremities, each called an **epiphysis** (eh-**PIFF**-ih-sis), separated from the metaphysis by the **epiphyseal line** where longitudinal growth of the bone occurs. The shaft consists mainly of compact bone. It is thickest toward the middle of the bone because strain on the bone is greatest at that point. The strength of a long bone is also ensured by the slight curvature of the shaft, a good engineering design to distribute weight. The interior of the shaft is the **medullary cavity** filled with yellow bone marrow. The extremities or the epiphyses of the long bone have a thin covering of compact tissue overlying a majority of cancellous tissue, which usually contains red marrow. The epiphyses are usually broad and expanded for articulation with other bones and to provide a large surface for muscle attachment. Examples of obvious long bones would be the clavicle, humerus, radius, ulna, femur, tibia, and fibula. Not so obvious would be those short versions of a long bone, the metacarpals of the hand, the metatarsals of the foot, and the phalanges of the fingers and toes.

## Short Bones

*Short bones* are not merely shorter versions of long bones. They lack a long axis. They have a somewhat irregular shape. They consist of a thin layer of compact tissue over a majority of spongy or cancellous bone. Examples of short bones of the body are the carpal bones of the wrist and the tarsal bones of the foot.

## Flat Bones

*Flat bones* are thin bones found whenever there is a need for extensive muscle attachment or protection for soft or vital parts of the body. These bones, usually curved, consist of two flat plates of compact bone tissue enclosing a layer of cancellous bones. Examples of flat bones are the sternum, ribs, scapula, parts of the pelvic bones, and some of the bones of the skull.

## Irregular Bones

*Irregular bones* are bones of a very peculiar and different or irregular shape. They consist of spongy bone enclosed by thin layers of compact bone. Examples of irregular bones are the vertebrae and the ossicles of the ears.

## Sesamoid Bones

Sesamoid (**SESS**-ah-moyd) bones are small rounded bones. These bones are enclosed in a tendon and fascial tissue and are located adjacent to joints. They assist in the functioning of muscles. The kneecap or patella is the largest of the sesamoid bones. Some of the bones of the wrist and ankle could also be classified as sesamoid bones as well as short bones.

# BONE MARKINGS

The surface of any typical bone will exhibit certain projections called **processes** or certain depressions called **fossae** (**FOSS**-ee) or both. These markings are functional in that they can help join one bone to another, provide a surface for the attachments of muscles, or serve as a passageway into the bone for blood vessels and nerves. The following is a list of terms and definitions regarding bone markings.

## Processes

Processes is a general term referring to any obvious bony prominence. The following is a list of specific examples of processes.

1. *Spine*: any sharp, slender projection such as the spinous process of a vertebra (see Figure 7-20, page 156).
2. *Condyle* (**KON**-dial): a rounded or knuckle-like prominence usually found at the point of articulation with another bone such as the lateral and medial condyle of the femur (see Figure 7-21 page 157).
3. *Tubercle* (**TOO**-ber-kl): a small round process like the lesser tubercle of the humerus (see Figure 7-17, page 153).
4. *Trochlea* (**TROK**-lee-ah): a process shaped like a pulley as in the trochlea of the humerus (see Figure 7-17, page 153).
5. *Trochanter* (tro-**KAN**-ter): a very large projection like the greater and lesser trochanter of the femur (see Figure 7-21, page 157).
6. *Crest*: a narrow ridge of bone like the iliac crest of the hip bone (see Figure 7-20, page 156).
7. *Line*: a less prominent ridge of bone than a crest.
8. *Head*: a terminal enlargement like the head of the humerus and the head of the femur (see Figures 7-17 and 7-21, pages 153 and 157).
9. *Neck*: that part of a bone that connects the head or terminal enlargement to the rest of the bone, like the neck of the femur (see Figures 17-17 and 7-21, pages 153 and 157).

## Fossae

Fossae is a general term for any depression or cavity in or on a bone. The following is a list of specific examples of fossae.

1. *Suture*: a narrow junction often found between two bones like the sutures of the skull bones (see Figure 7-8, page 145).
2. *Foramen*: an opening through which blood vessels, nerves, and ligaments pass like the foramen magnum of the occipital bone of the skull or the obturator foramen of the pelvic bone (see Figure 7-20, page 156).
3. *Meatus* or *canal*: a long tube-like passage, like the auditory meatus or canal (see Figure 7-8, page 145).
4. *Sinus* or *antrum*: a cavity within a bone like the nasal sinuses or frontal sinus (see Figure 7-7A, page 144).
5. *Sulcus*: a furrow or groove like the intertubercular sulcus or groove of the humerus (see Figure 7-17, page 153).

# DIVISIONS OF THE SKELETON

The skeleton has 206 bones. The *axial* part consists of the skull (28 bones including the cranial and facial bones), the hyoid bone, the vertebrae (26 bones), the ribs (24 bones), and the sternum. The *appendicular* part of the skeleton consists of the bones of the upper extremities or arms (64 bones including the shoulder girdle bones) and the bones of the lower extremities or legs (62 bones including the bones of the pelvic girdle) (Figure 7-6).

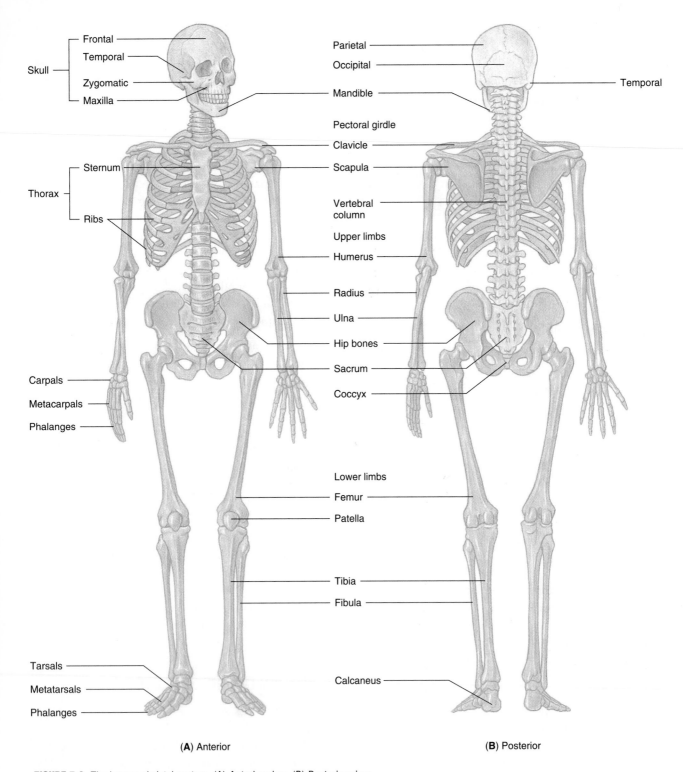

**(A)** Anterior

**(B)** Posterior

**FIGURE 7-6.** The human skeletal system. (A) Anterior view. (B) Posterior view.

# THE AXIAL SKELETON

The skull, in the correct use of the term, includes the cranial and the facial bones. We will discuss the cranial bones first.

## The Cranial Bones

The bones of the cranium have a number of important functions. They protect and enclose the brain and special sense organs like the eyes and ears. Muscles for mastication or chewing and muscles for head movement attach to certain cranial bones. At certain locations air sinuses or cavities are present that connect with the nasal cavities (Figure 7-7). All of the individual bones of the cranium are united by immovable junction lines called sutures.

The **frontal bone** is a single bone that forms the forehead, the roof of the nasal cavity, and the orbits, which are the bony sockets that contain the eyes (Figure 7-8). Important bone markings are the **orbital margin**, a definite ridge above each orbit located where eyebrows are found, and the **supraorbital ridge**, which overlies the frontal sinus and can be felt in the middle of your forehead. The **coronal suture** is found where the frontal bone joins the two parietal bones.

The two **parietal** (pah-**RYE**-eh-tal) **bones** form the upper sides and roof of the cranium. They are joined at the **sagittal suture** in the midline.

The **occipital bone** is a single bone that forms the back and base of the cranium (see Figure 7-8) and joins the parietal bones superiorly at the **lambdoid suture**. The inferior portion of this bone has a large opening called the **foramen magnum** through which the spinal cord connects with the brain. On each lower side of the occipital bone is a process called the **occipital condyle**. These processes are significant because they articulate with depressions in the first cervical vertebra (atlas), thus allowing the head to connect with and rest on the vertebrae. Other notable markings are the **external occipital crest** and the **external occipital protuberance**, which can be felt through the scalp at the base of the neck. Several ligaments and muscles attach to these regions.

The two **temporal bones** help form the lower sides and base of the cranium (see Figure 7-8). Each temporal bone encloses an ear and bears a fossa for articulation with the lower jaw or mandible. The temporal bones are irregular in shape and each consists of four parts: the squamous, petrous, mastoid, and tympanic parts. The **squamous portion** is the largest and most superior of the four parts. It is a thin flat plate of bone that forms the temple. Projecting from its lower part is the zygomatic process that forms the lateral part of the zygomatic arch or cheek bone. The **petrous part** is found deep within the base of the skull where it protects and surrounds the inner ear. The **mastoid portion** is located behind and below the auditory meatus or opening of the ear. The mastoid process is a rounded projection of the mastoid portion of the temporal bone easily felt behind the ear. Several muscles of the neck attach to this mastoid process and assist in moving your head. Finally the **tympanic plate** forms the floor and anterior wall of the external auditory meatus. A long and slender styloid process can be seen extending from the under surface of this plate. Ligaments that hold the hyoid bone in place (which supports the tongue) attach to this styloid process of the tympanic plate of the temporal bone.

The single **sphenoid bone** forms the anterior portion of the base of the cranium (Figure 7-9). When viewed from below it looks like a butterfly. It acts as an anchor binding all of the cranial bones together.

The single **ethmoid bone** is the principle supporting structure of the nasal cavities and helps form part of the orbits. It is the lightest of the cranial bones (see Figure 7-9).

The six **auditory ossicles** are the three bones found in each ear (Figure 7-7B, page 144): the **malleus** or hammer, the **stapes** (**STAY**-peez) or stirrup, and the **incus** or anvil. These tiny bones are highly specialized in both structure and function and are involved in exciting the hearing receptors.

The **wormian bones** or **sutural bones** are located within the sutures of the cranial bones. They vary in number, are small and irregular in shape, and are never included in the total number of bones in the body. They form as a result of intramembranous ossification of the cranial bones.

## The Facial Bones

Like the bones of the cranium, the facial bones are also united by immovable sutures, with one exception: the lower jawbone or mandible. This bone is

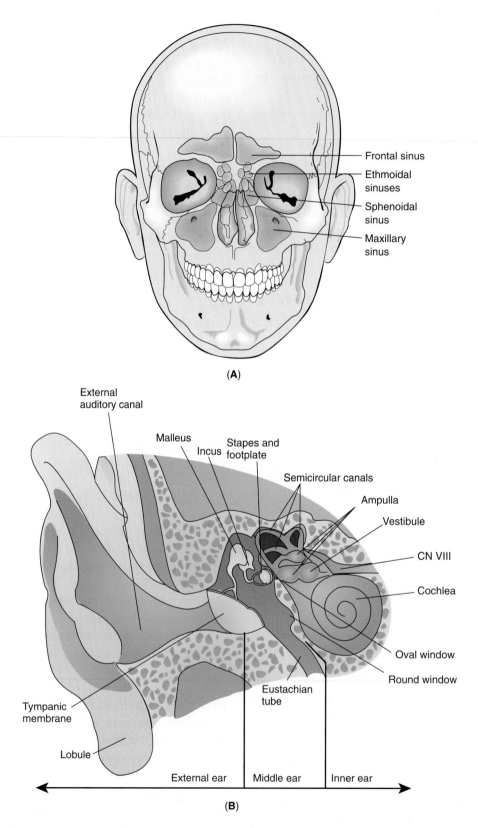

**(A)**

**(B)**

**FIGURE 7-7.** (A) The paranasal sinuses. (B) Cross section of the ear showing the ossicles.

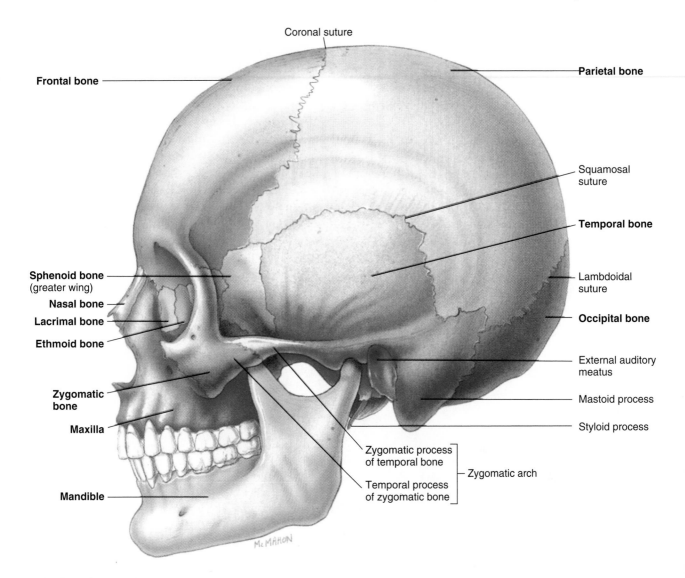

**FIGURE 7-8.** The cranial bones.

capable of movement in a number of directions. It can be elevated and depressed as in talking and it can protract and retract and move from side to side as in chewing.

The two **nasal bones** are thin and delicate bones that join in a suture to form the bridge of the nose (see Figure 7-9).

The two **palatine bones** form the posterior part of the roof of your mouth or part of the hard palate. This region is the same as the floor of the nasal cavity. Upward extensions of the palatine bones help form the outer walls of the nasal cavity.

The two **maxillary bones** make up the upper jaw (see Figure 7-9). Each maxillary bone consists

of five parts: a body, a zygomatic process, a frontal process, a palatine process, and an alveolar process. The large body of the maxilla forms part of the floor and outer wall of the nasal cavity, the greater part of the floor of the orbit, and much of the anterior face below the temple. The body is covered by a number of facial muscles and contains a large maxillary sinus located lateral to the nose. The zygomatic process extends laterally to participate in the formation of the cheek. (Processes are named according to the bone they go to, thus the zygomatic process of the maxillary bone goes toward and joins the zygomatic or cheek bone). The frontal process extends upward to the frontal

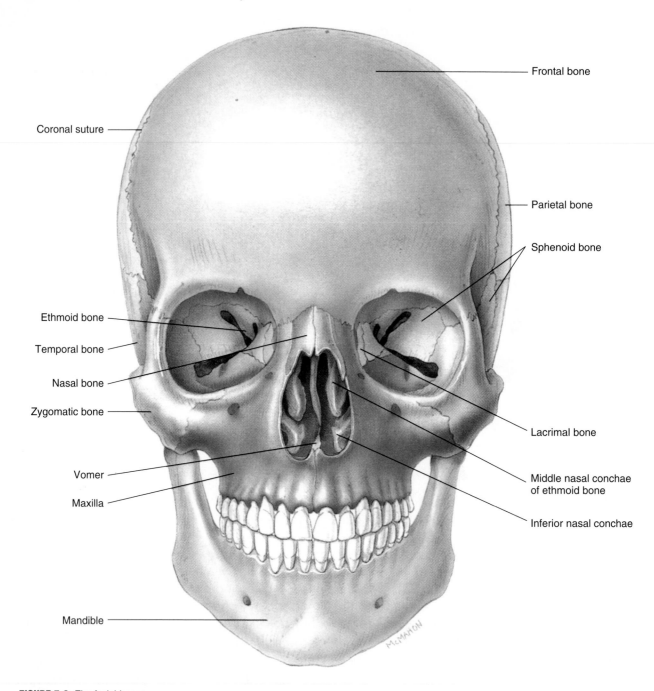

**FIGURE 7-9.** The facial bones.

bone or forehead. The palatine process extends posteriorly in a horizontal plane to join or articulate with the palatine bone and actually forms the greater anterior portion of the hard palate or roof of the mouth. The alveolar processes bear the teeth of the upper jaw, and each tooth is embedded in an **alveolus** (al-**VEE**-oh-lus) or socket. The two maxillary bones join at the intermaxillary suture. This

fusion is usually completed just before birth. If the two bones do not unite to form a continuous structure, the resulting defect is called a cleft palate and is usually associated with a cleft lip. With today's surgical techniques, the defect can be repaired early in the development of the child.

The two **zygomatic bones**, also known as the **malar bones**, form the prominence of the cheek and rest on the maxillae (see Figure 7-9). Its maxillary process joins the maxillary bone by connecting with the maxillary bone's zygomatic process. Each zygomatic bone has a frontal process extending upward to articulate with the frontal bone and a smaller temporal process that joins laterally with the temporal bone, thus forming the easily identified zygomatic arch.

The two **lacrimal** (**LAK**-rim-al) **bones** make up part of the orbit at the inner angle of the eye (see Figure 7-9). These very small and thin bones lie directly behind the frontal process of the maxilla. Their lateral surface has a depression or fossa that holds the lacrimal sac or tear sac and provides a canal for the lacrimal duct. Tears are directed from this point to the inferior meatus of the nasal cavity after they have cleansed and lubricated the eye.

The two **turbinates** or **nasal conchae bones** are very thin and fragile (see Figure 7-9). There is one in each nostril on the lateral side. They extend to but do not quite reach the bony portion of the nasal septum. They help form a series of shelves in the nasal cavity where air is moistened, warmed, and filtered.

The single **vomer bone** is a flat bone that makes up the lower posterior portion of the nasal septum (see Figure 7-9).

The single **mandible bone** develops in two parts. The intervening cartilage ossifies in early childhood and the bone becomes fused into a single continuous structure. It is the strongest and longest bone of the face (see Figure 7-9). It consists of a U-shaped body with alveolar processes to bear the teeth of the lower jaw (just like the maxillary bone's alveolar processes that bear the teeth of the upper jaw). On each side of the body are the rami that extend perpendicularly upward. Each ramus has a condyle for articulation with the mandibular fossa of the temporal bone, thus allowing for the wide range of movement of the lower jawbone.

## The Orbits

The orbits are the two deep cavities in the upper portion of the face that protect the eyes. A number of bones of the skull contribute to their formation. Refer to Figure 7-9 to view these bones. Each orbit consists of the following bones:

| Area of Orbit | Participating Bones |
| --- | --- |
| Roof | Frontal, sphenoid |
| Floor | Maxilla, zygomatic |
| Lateral wall | Zygomatic, greater wing of sphenoid |
| Medial wall | Maxilla, lacrimal, ethmoid |

## The Nasal Cavities

The framework of the nose surrounding the two nasal fossae is located in the middle of the face between the hard palate inferiorly and the frontal bone superiorly.

The nose is formed by the following bones (see Figure 7-9):

| Area of Nose | Participating Bones |
| --- | --- |
| Roof | Ethmoid |
| Floor | Maxilla, palatine |
| Lateral wall | Maxilla, palatine |
| Septum of medial wall | Ethmoid, vomer, nasal |
| Bridge | Nasal |

## The Foramina of the Skull

If one views the skull inferiorly and observes the floor of the cranial cavity, one can observe the largest foramen of the skull, the foramen magnum. One can also observe a number of much smaller foramina or openings that penetrate the individual bones of the skull. They all have names and are passageways for blood vessels and nerves entering and exiting the various organs of the skull.

## The Hyoid Bone

The single **hyoid bone** is a unique component of the axial skeleton because it has no articulations with other bones (Figure 7-10). It is rarely seen as part of an articulated skeleton in a lab. Rather, it is

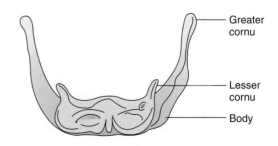

**FIGURE 7-10.** The hyoid bone (anterior view).

suspended from the styloid process of the temporal bone by two styloid ligaments. Externally you can detect its position in the neck just above the larynx or voice box a fair distance from the mandible. It is shaped like a horseshoe consisting of a central body with two lateral projections. The larger projections are the greater cornu and the smaller lateral projections are the lesser cornu. The hyoid bone acts as a support for the tongue and its associated muscles. It also helps elevate the larynx during swallowing and speech.

## How to Study the Bones of the Skull

When learning the different bones of the skull, one of the best methods is to first refer to the colored plates in your textbook where each individual bone is portrayed in a different color. Refer to Figure 7-9, the anterior view of the skull, and Figure 7-8, the lateral view of the skull. Once you get a sense of where these bones are located, use a model of a human skull (either real bone or a good plastic reproduction) and search for sutures as a guide. Remember in a real skull the older the skull the less obvious the sutures become. As we age, the sutures tend to disappear or become very faint. The colored plates will greatly assist you in learning where the bones of the skull are found.

## The Torso or Trunk

The sternum, ribs, and vertebrae make up the trunk or torso of the axial skeleton. The vertebrae are rigid and provide support for the body but the fibrocartilaginous disks between the vertebrae allow for a high degree of flexibility. The disks and vertebrae protect the delicate spinal cord contained within their articulated channels formed from successive foramina.

The spinal column is formed from a series of 26 irregular bones called vertebrae, separated and cushioned by the intervertebral disks of cartilage. A typical vertebra has the following parts or features (Figure 7-11). The *body* is a thick disk-shaped anterior portion pierced with numerous small holes for nerves and blood vessels that nurture the bone. The *neural arch* encloses a space, the *neural foramen*, for passage of the spinal cord. The arch has three processes for muscle attachment: the *spinous process*, quite large on the thoracic vertebrae, directed backward, and two *transverse processes* one on each side of the vertebra. The articular processes are used for articulating with the vertebra immediately above by the *two superior articular processes* and with the vertebra immediately below by the *two inferior articular processes*. The vertebral arch is composed of two portions on each side, the *pedicles* notched above and below for passage of nerves to

---

### Common Disease, Disorder or Condition

### ■ DISORDERS OF THE SPINE

The normal curvatures of the spine can become exaggerated as a result of injury, poor body posture, or disease. When the posterior curvature of the spine is accentuated in the upper thoracic region, the condition is called **kyphosis**. This results in the commonly referred to condition called hunchback. It is particularly common in older individuals due to osteoporosis. It can also be caused by tuberculosis of the spine, osteomalacia, or rickets. **Lordosis**, or swayback, is an abnormal accentuated lumbar curvature. It also can result from rickets or spinal tuberculosis.

Temporary lordosis is common in men with potbellies and pregnant women who throw back their shoulders to preserve their center of gravity thus accentuating the lumbar cervature. **Scoliosis** (skoh-lee-**OH**-sis), meaning twisted condition, is an abnormal lateral curvature of the spine that occurs most often in the thoracic region. It can be common in late childhood for girls but the most severe conditions result from abnormal vertebral structure, lower limbs of unequal length, or muscle paralysis on one side of the body. Severe cases can be treated with body braces or surgically before bone growth ceases.

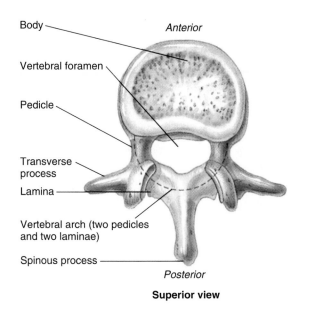

Body
Anterior
Vertebral foramen
Pedicle
Transverse
process
Lamina
Vertebral arch (two pedicles
and two laminae)
Spinous process
Posterior
**Superior view**

**FIGURE 7-11.** The characteristics of a typical vertebra.

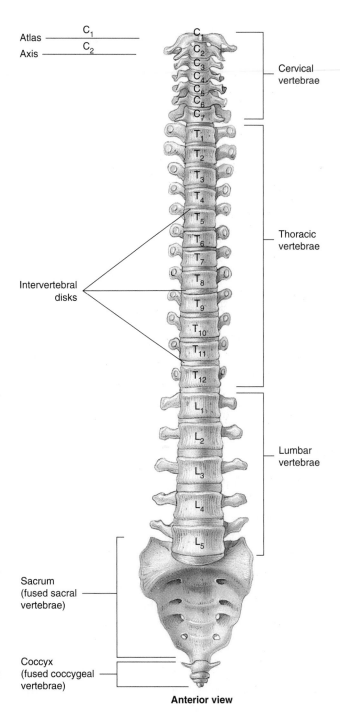

Atlas $C_1$
Axis $C_2$
Cervical
vertebrae
Thoracic
vertebrae
Intervertebral
disks
Lumbar
vertebrae
Sacrum
(fused sacral
vertebrae)
Coccyx
(fused coccygeal
vertebrae)
**Anterior view**

**FIGURE 7-12.** The vertebral column.

and from the spinal cord, and the *laminae*, which form the posterior wall of the vertebral column.

Refer to Figure 7-12 for views of the structure of the vertebral column. There are seven **cervical vertebrae**, twelve **thoracic vertebrae**, and five **lumbar vertebrae**. These all remain separate throughout life and are referred to as movable. In addition there are five **sacral vertebrae** that become fused by adult life and form the single **sacrum**. There are also four **coccygeal vertebrae** that unite firmly to form the single **coccyx** or tailbone. These last two, the sacrum and coccyx, are called fixed, hence the vertebrae are referred to in number as 26 rather than 33.

The cervical vertebrae are the smallest vertebrae. The first two have been given special names (Figure 7-13). The first is called the **atlas** (named after Atlas in Greek mythology who held up the world); it supports the head by articulation with the condyles of the occipital bone. The second vertebra is the **axis**; it acts as the pivot on which the atlas and head rotate. The thoracic vertebrae have two distinguishing characteristics: the long spinous process pointing downward and six facets, three on each side for articulation with a rib. The lumbar vertebrae are the largest and the strongest. They are modified for the attachment of the powerful back muscles. The sacrum is a triangular and slightly curved bone. The curving coccyx can move slightly to increase the size of the birth canal during delivery in the female.

In addition to providing protection for the spinal cord and support for the body, the vertebral column is also built to withstand forces of compression many times the weight of the body. The fibrocartilaginous intervertebral disks act as cushions so that landing on your feet after a jump or a fall will help prevent the vertebrae from fracturing.

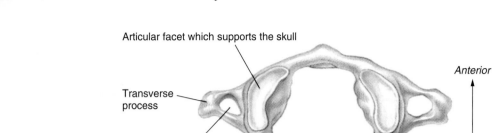

Articular facet which supports the skull

Transverse process

Transverse foramen

*Anterior*

*Posterior*

**(A) Superior view of atlas (C₁)**

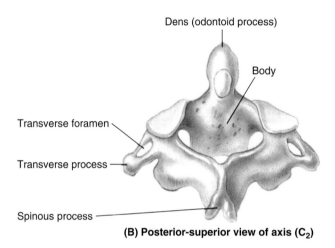

Dens (odontoid process)

Body

Transverse foramen

Transverse process

Spinous process

**(B) Posterior-superior view of axis (C₂)**

**FIGURE 7-13.** (A) Superior view of atlas (C₁) and (B) posterior-superior view of axis (C₂).

## The Thorax

The thorax or the rib cage of the body is made up of the sternum, the costal cartilages, the ribs, and the bodies of the thoracic vertebrae. This bony cage encloses and protects the heart and lungs. It also supports the bones of the shoulder girdle and the bones of the upper extremities.

## The Sternum

The **sternum** is also known as the breastbone (Figure 7-14). It develops in three parts: the **manubrium**, the **gladiolus**, and the **xiphoid** (**ZIFF**-oyd) **process**. The sternum resembles a sword, with the manubrium resembling the handle of the sword, the gladiolus or body forming the blade, and the xiphoid process forming the tip of the sword. No ribs are attached to the xiphoid but the manubrium and gladiolus have notches on each side for attachment of the first seven costal (rib) cartilages. The manubrium articulates with the clavicle

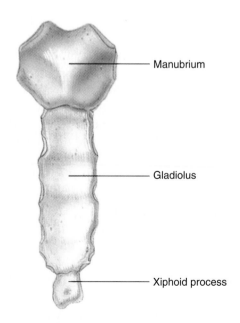

Manubrium

Gladiolus

Xiphoid process

**FIGURE 7-14.** The sternum, anterior view.

or collarbone. Between these two points of attachment is the suprasternal or jugular notch easily felt through the skin. The diaphragm and the rectus abdominis muscles attach to the xiphoid.

### The Ribs

The 12 pairs of ribs are also referred to as the **costae** (Figure 7-15). They are named according to their anterior attachments. Because the upper seven pairs articulate directly with the sternum, they are called *true ribs*. The lower five pairs are called *false ribs*. The costal cartilages of the eighth, ninth, and tenth rib pairs are attached to the cartilage of the seventh rib so they join the sternum only indirectly. Because the 11th and 12th pairs of ribs have no cartilage and do not attach at all anteriorly these "false" ribs have another name, *floating ribs*. Of course, all ribs attach posteriorly to the thoracic vertebrae.

## THE APPENDICULAR SKELETON

### The Bones of the Upper Extremities

The bones of the upper extremities include the bones of the shoulder girdle, the arm, the forearm, the wrist, the hand, and the fingers.

The bones of the shoulder girdle are the **clavicle** (**KLAV**-ih-kl) and the **scapula** (**SKAP**-you-lah). The clavicle or collarbone is a long slim bone located at the root of the neck just below the skin and anterior to the first rib. The medial end articulates with the manubrium of the sternum and the lateral end with the **acromial** (ah-**KRO**-mee-al) **process** of the scapula. The scapula or shoulder blade is a large, flat, triangular bone located on the dorsal portion of the thorax, covering the area from the second to the seventh rib (Figure 7-16). Two other prominent bony projections on the scapula are the **coracoid process**, which functions as an attachment for muscles that move the arm, and the **glenoid fossa** which receives the head of the humerus and helps form the shoulder joint.

The **humerus** (**HYOO**-mehr-us) is the largest and longest bone of the upper arm (Figure 7-17). Its head is rounded and joined to the rest of the bone by its anatomic neck. The upper part of the bone has two prominences, the greater and lesser tubercles, which function as insertions for many of the muscles of the upper extremity.

The **ulna** is the *longer*, medial bone of the forearm (Figure 7-18, page 154). Its shaft is triangular and the distal or lower end is called the head. At its

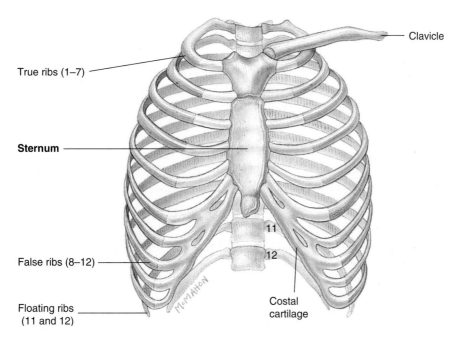

Clavicle

True ribs (1–7)

**Sternum**

11

12

False ribs (8–12)

Floating ribs
(11 and 12)

Costal
cartilage

**FIGURE 7-15.** Thoracic cage, anterior view.

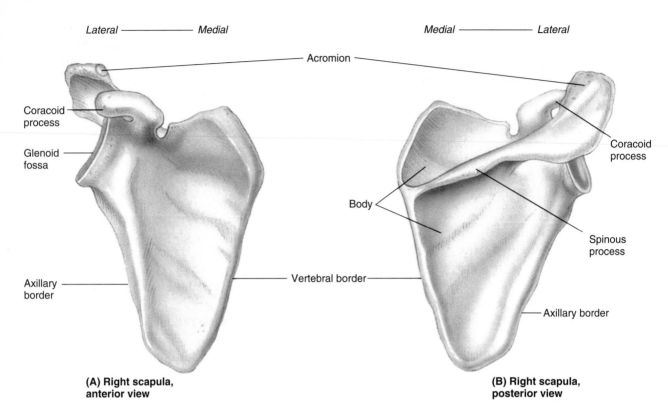

Lateral ———————— Medial          Medial ———————— Lateral

Acromion

Coracoid process

Glenoid fossa

Body

Coracoid process

Spinous process

Axillary border

Vertebral border

Axillary border

**(A) Right scapula, anterior view**

**(B) Right scapula, posterior view**

**FIGURE 7-16.** Scapula. (A) Anterior view. (B) Posterior view.

proximal end is the **olecranon** (oh-**LEK**-rah-non) **process** or elbow. When banged, nerves are pressed causing the tingling sensation, which gives it the common name of "funny bone."

The **radius** is the *shorter*, lateral bone of the forearm. It is joined to the ulna by an interosseus membrane traversing the area between the shafts of the two bones. They move as one. The styloid process of the radius articulates with some of the bones of the wrist.

The bones of the wrist are called **carpals** (Figure 7-19). They are arranged in two rows of four each. In the proximal row from medial to lateral they are the **pisiform** (**PYE**-zih-form), **trique-tral** (try-**KWEE**-tral), **lunate** (**LOO**-nate), and **scaphoid** (**SKAFF**-oyd) also known as the **navic-ular** (nah-**VIK**-you-lahr). In the distal row from medial to lateral are the **hamate**, **capitate** (**KAP**-ih-tate), **trapezoid** (**TRAP**-eh-zoyd), or lesser multiangular, and the **trapezuim** (trah-**PEE**-zee-um) or greater multiangular.

The palm of the hand is made up of the five **metacarpal bones** (see Figure 7-19). These are small, long bones, each with a base, shaft, and a head. They radiate out from the wrist bones like the spokes of a wheel rather than being parallel. They each articulate with a proximal **phalanx** (**FAY**-langks) of a finger. Each finger, except the thumb, has three **phalanges** (fah-**LAN**-jeez): a proximal, a middle, and a terminal or distal phalanx. The thumb has only a proximal and distal phalanx.

## The Bones of the Lower Extremities

The bones of the lower extremities include the pelvic girdle, which supports the trunk and provides attachment for the legs. It consists of the paired hip bones or coxal bones. Each hipbone consists of three fused parts: the **ilium** (**ILL**-ee-um), the **ischium**, (**ISS**-kee-um), and the **pubis** (**PYOO**-bis). Other bones of the lower extremity include the thigh, the kneecap, the shin, the calf, the ankle bones, the foot, and the toes.

The **pelvic girdle** is actually made up of two hip or coxal bones that articulate with one another anteriorly at the pubic symphysis. Posteriorly they articulate with the sacrum. This ring of bone is known as the pelvis.

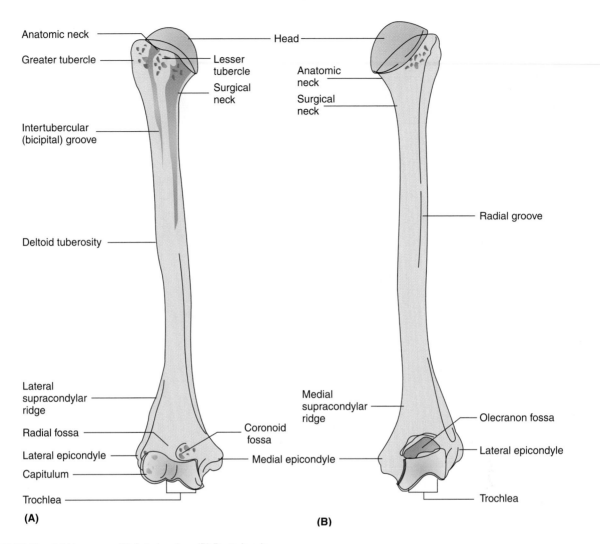

**FIGURE 7-17.** The right humerus. (A) Anterior view. (B) Posterior view.

The ilium is the uppermost and largest portion of a hipbone. It forms the expanded prominence of the upper hip or iliac crest. It is wider and broader in females and smaller and narrower in males. Its crest is projected into the anterior superior iliac spine and the anterior inferior iliac spine (Figure 7-20, page 156). The ischium is the strongest portion of a hipbone and is directed slightly posteriorly. Its curved edge is viewed from the front as the lowermost margin of the pelvis. It has the rounded and thick ischial tuberosity, which you sit on, and thus bears the weight of the body in the sitting position. The pubis is superior and slightly anterior to the ischium. Between the pubis and the ischium is the large **obturator** (OB-tuh-**ray**-tohr) **foramen**. This is the largest foramen in the body and allows for the passage of nerves, blood vessels, and tendons. On the lateral side of the hip just above the obturator foramen is the deep socket called the **acetabulum** (ass-eh-**TAB**-you-lum). All three parts of the pelvic bone meet and unite in this socket. It also receives the head of the femur to help form the hip joint.

The **femur** (**FEE**-mehr), or thigh, is the largest and heaviest bone of the body (Figure 7-21, page 157). This single large bone of the upper leg is not in a vertical line with the axis of the erect body. Rather it has a unique engineering design that allows it to bear and distribute the weight of the body. It is positioned at an angle, slanting downward and inward so that the two femurs appear as a large letter V. Its upper extremity bears a large

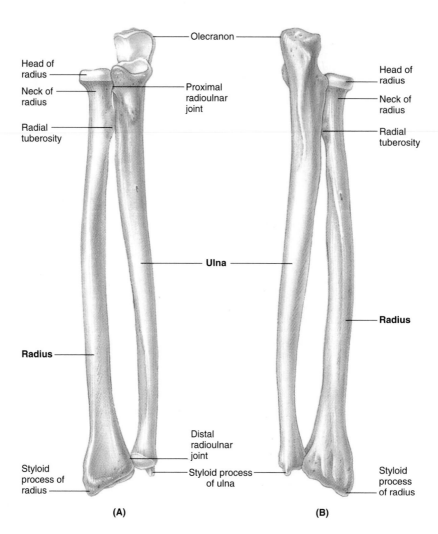

**FIGURE 7-18.** Right radius and ulna. (A) Anterior view. (B) Posterior view.

head that fits into the acetabulum of the pelvic bone with an anatomic neck. Its lower portion is widened into a large lateral condyle and an even larger medial condyle. It articulates distally with the tibia.

The **patella** (pah-**TELL**-ah) or kneecap is the largest of the sesamoid bones. It is somewhat flat and triangular lying right in front of the knee joint and is enveloped within the tendon of the quadriceps femoris muscle. Its only articulation is with the femur. It is a movable bone and it increases the leverage of the muscles that straighten out the knee.

The **tibia** (**TIB**-ee-ah) is the larger of the two bones forming the lower leg (Figure 7-22, page 158). It is also known as the shin. The rounded condyles of the femur rest on the flat condyle at the proximal end of the tibia.

The **fibula** (**FIB**-you-lah) is also known as the calf. In proportion to its length, it is the most slender bone of the body. It lies parallel with and on the lateral side of the tibia. It does not articulate with the femur but attaches to the proximal end of the tibia via its head.

The bones of the ankle are known as the **tarsal bones** (Figure 7-23, page 159). The seven short tarsal bones resemble the carpal bones of the wrist but are larger. They are arranged in the hindfoot and forefoot. The tarsal bones of the hindfoot are the **calcaneus** (kal-**KAY**-nee-us), sometimes called the calcaneum, which is the largest of the tarsal bones and forms the heel; the **talus** or ankle bone, the **navicular** (nah-**VIK**-you-lar) and the **cuboid** (**KYOO**-boyd). Because the calcaneus or heel bone receives the weight of the body when walking, it has developed

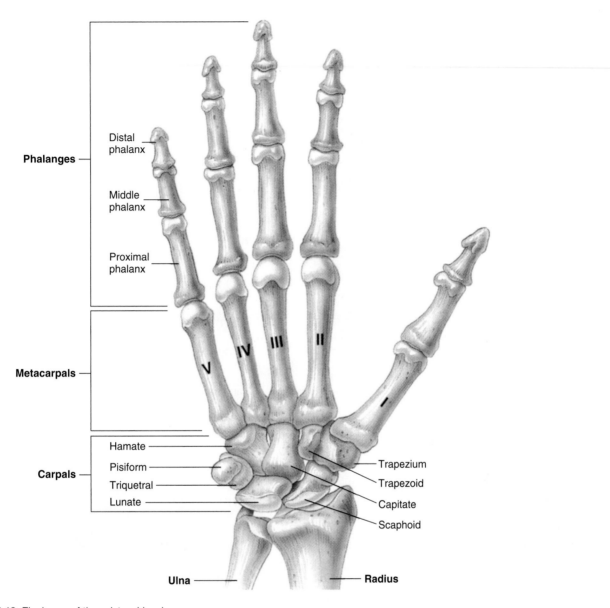

**FIGURE 7-19.** The bones of the wrist and hand.

as the largest of the tarsal bones. The tarsal bones of the forefoot are the medial (I), intermediate (II), and lateral (III) **cuneiforms** (kyoo-**NEE**-ih-formz).

The rest of the forefoot bones are the **metatarsals** and phalanges. There are five metatarsal bones in the forefoot. Each is classified as a long bone based on shape and each has a base, shaft, and a head. The heads formed at the distal ends of the metatarsals form what we call the ball of the foot. The bases of the first, second, and third metatarsals articulate with the three cuneiforms; the fourth and fifth metatarsals articulate with the cuboid. The intrinsic muscles of

the toes are attached to the shafts of the metatarsals. The first metatarsal is the largest due to its weight-bearing function during walking.

The phalanges of the toes are classified as long bones despite their short length because again they have a base, shaft, and head (see Figure 7-23B). They have the same arrangement as the phalanges of the fingers. There are two phalanges in the great toe, a proximal and distal. The proximal one is large due to its weight-bearing function when walking. The other four toes have three each, a proximal, middle, and distal phalanx.

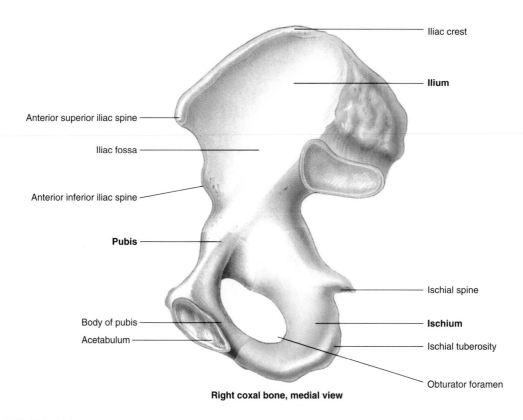

Iliac crest

Ilium

Anterior superior iliac spine

Iliac fossa

Anterior inferior iliac spine

Pubis

Ischial spine

Ischium

Body of pubis

Acetabulum

Ischial tuberosity

Obturator foramen

**Right coxal bone, medial view**

**FIGURE 7-20.** Right hipbone.

## THE ARCHES OF THE FOOT

The bones of the foot are arranged in a series of arches that enable the foot to bear weight while standing and to provide leverage while walking. There are two longitudinal arches and one transverse arch. The *medial longitudinal arch* is formed by the calcaneus, talus, navicular, the three cuneiforms, and the three medial metatarsals. This is the highest arch of the foot and can easily be noted. The *lateral longitudinal arch* is much lower and is formed by the calcaneus, the cuboid, and the two lateral metatarsals. The *transverse arch* is perpendicular to the longitudinal arches and is most pronounced at the base of the metatarsals.

The term pes planus or flatfoot indicates a decreased height of the longitudinal arches. It rarely causes any pain and can be inherited or can result from muscle weakness in the foot.

## BODY SYSTEMS WORKING TOGETHER TO MAINTAIN HOMEOSTASIS: THE SKELETAL SYSTEM

### Integumentary System
- Vitamin D is produced in the skin by UV light.
- It enhances the absorption of calcium in bones for bone and tooth formation.

### Muscular System
- Through their tendons, muscles pull on bones bringing about movement.
- Calcium from bones is necessary for muscle contraction to occur.

### Nervous System
- The cranial bones protect the brain, and the vertebrae and intervertebral disks protect the spinal cord.
- Receptors for pain monitor trauma to bones.
- Calcium from bones is necessary for nerve transmission.

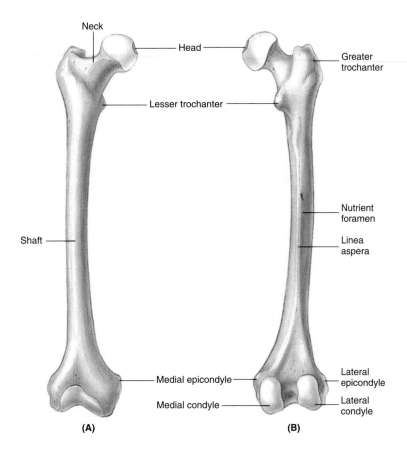

**FIGURE 7-21.** The femur. (A) anterior view. (B) Posterior view.

## Endocrine System

- The hormone calcitonin causes calcium to be stored in bones.
- The hormone parathormone causes calcium to be released from bones.
- Growth hormone from the anterior pituitary gland effects bone development.

## Cardiovascular System

- Blood cells transport oxygen and nutrients to bone cells and take away carbon dioxide and waste products.
- Calcium from bones is necessary for blood clotting and normal heart functions.

## Lymphatic System

- Red bone marrow produces lymphocytes, which function in our immune response.

## Digestive System

- Calcium, necessary for bone matrix development, is absorbed in the intestine from our daily food intake.

- Excess calcium can be eliminated via the bowels.

## Respiratory System

- Oxygen is brought into the body via the respiratory system and transported by the blood to bone cells for biochemical respiration.
- The ribs along with the intercostal muscles and diaphragm bring about breathing.

## Urinary System

- The kidneys help regulate blood calcium levels.
- Excess calcium can also be eliminated via the kidneys.

## Reproductive System

- Bones are a source of calcium during breastfeeding.
- The pelvis aids in supporting the uterus and developing fetus during pregnancy in the female.

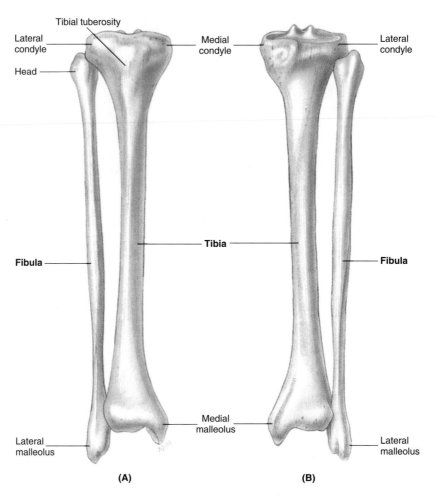

**FIGURE 7-22.** The tibia and fibula. (A) Anterior view. (B) Posterior view.

**Common Disease, Disorder or Condition**

## ■ DISORDERS OF THE SKELETAL SYSTEM

### Osteoporosis

**Osteoporosis** (oss-tee-oh-poh-**ROH**-sis) is a disorder of the skeletal system characterized by a disease in bone mass with accompanying increased susceptibility to bone fractures. This results from decreased levels of estrogens that occur after menopause in women and in both men and women in old age. Estrogens help maintain bone tissue by stimulating osteoblasts to form new bone.

Osteoporosis occurs more often in middle-aged and elderly women but it can also affect teenagers who eat too much junk food and do not eat a proper balanced diet, people allergic to dairy products, and anyone with eating disorders. The bone mass becomes depleted in such a way that the skeleton cannot withstand everyday mechanical stress. Bone fractures are common, even from normal daily activities. This disease is responsible for height loss, hunched backs, and pain in older individuals. Adequate diet and exercise can prevent osteoporosis.

(continues on page 160)

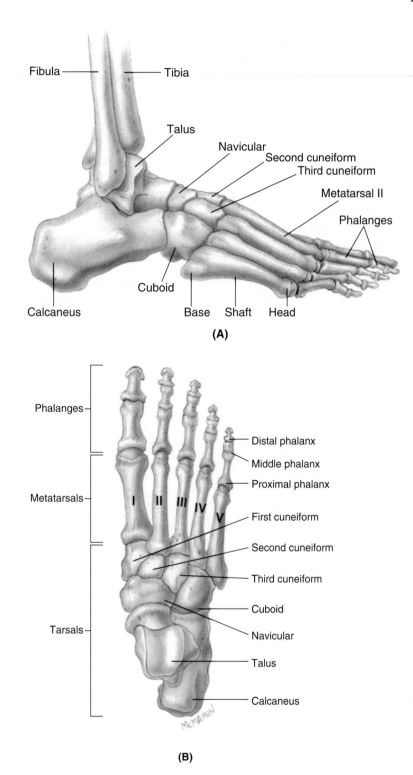

**FIGURE 7-23.** (A) Right ankle and foot lateral view. (B) Right ankle and foot superior view.

## Common Disease, Disorder or Condition *(continued)*

### Paget's disease

**Paget's disease** is a common nommeta-bolic disease of bone whose cause is unknown. It usually affects middle-aged and elderly individuals. Symptoms include an irregular thickening and softening of the bones. There is excessive bone destruction and unorganized bone repair. Areas of the body affected are the skull, pelvis, and limbs. Treatment includes a high-protein and high-calcium diet with mild but regular exercise.

### Gigantism

**Gigantism** (**JYE**-gan-tizm) is the result of abnormal endochondral ossification at the epiphyseal plates of long bones. This results in abnormally large limbs giving the affected individual the appearance of a very tall "giant."

### Dwarfism

**Dwarfism** is the opposite condition of gigantism and results from inadequate ossification occurring at the epiphyseal plates of long bones. This results in an individual being abnormally small. This condition is not to be confused with a genetic dwarf.

### Spina bifida

**Spina bifida** (**SPY**-nah **BIFF**-ih-dah) is a congenital defect in the development of the posterior vertebral arch in which the laminae do not unite at the midline. It is a relatively common disorder. It may occur with only a small deformed laminae or it may be associated with the complete absence of laminae and the contents of the spinal canal will protrude posteriorly. If the condition does not involve hernination of the meninges or the contents of the spinal canal, treatment is not required.

### Herniated disk

A **herniated disk** is a rupture of the fibro-cartilage surrounding an intervertebral disk that cushions the vertebrae above and below. This produces pressure on spinal nerve roots causing severe pain and nerve damage. The condition occurs most often in the lumbar region and is also known as a slipped disk.

## Summary Outline

### INTRODUCTION

1. The skeleton is the supporting structure of the body; it allows muscles to effect movement and breathing.
2. The solid appearance of bone is due to mineral salts that form the inorganic matrix surrounding the living bone cells.
3. Leonardo da Vinci was the first to correctly illustrate the 206 bones of the body.

### THE FUNCTIONS OF THE SKELETAL SYSTEM

The skeleton has five functions:
1. Support of surrounding tissues
2. Protect vital organs and soft tissues
3. Provide levers for muscles to pull on
4. Manufacture blood cells in red bone marrow by hematopoiesis
5. Storage area for mineral salts, especially calcium and phosphorous, and fat in yellow marrow.

### THE GROWTH AND FORMATION OF BONE

1. After 3 months, the fetal skeleton is completely formed and made primarily of cartilage. Ossification and growth then develop.
2. Longitudinal growth of bone continues until approximately 15 years of age in girls and 16 in boys.
3. Bone maturation continues until 21 years of age in both sexes.

### Deposition of the Bone

1. Bone develops from spindle-shaped embryonic bone cells called osteoblasts.
2. Osteoblasts develop into mature bone cells called osteocytes. They form under the

fibrovascular membrane covering bone, called the periosteum, and under the membrane lining of the medullary cavity, called the endosteum.

**3.** The more strain or pressure on a bone, the more the bone will develop.

**4.** Osteoclasts are large cells that are responsible for the reabsorption of injured bone. They also reabsorb bone during remodeling.

### Types of Ossification

The two types of ossification:

**1.** Intramembranous ossification is a process in which dense connective membranes are replaced by deposits of inorganic calcium salts. The bones of the cranium form in this way.

**2.** Endochondral ossification is the process whereby cartilage is the environment in which the bone cells develop. All other bones of the body develop in this way.

### Maintaining the Bone

**1.** The correct amount of calcium stored in the bones, the proper amount of calcium in the blood, and the excretion of excess calcium is controlled by the endocrine system.

**2.** The parathyroid glands secrete parathormone, which causes calcium to be released into the bloodstream. Another hormone, calcitonin, causes calcium to be stored in the bones.

### THE HISTOLOGY OF BONE

There are two types of bone tissue:

**1.** Compact or dense bone is strong and solid.

**2.** Cancellous or spongy bone has many open spaces filled with bone marrow.

### The Haversian System of Compact Bone

**1.** An English physician Clopton Havers (1650–1702) first described the histologic features of compact bone.

**2.** Haversian canals or osteons are small canals containing blood vessels running parallel to the surface of compact bone and are surrounded by concentric rings of solid bone called lamellae.

**3.** In these rings of bone are cavities called lacunae; each lacuna contains an osteocyte bathed in fluid.

**4.** Lacunae are connected to one another and eventually to the osteons by smaller canals called canaliculi.

**5.** The tissue fluid that circulates in these canals carries nutrients and oxygen to and waste away from the bone cells.

### Cancellous Bone

**1.** Cancellous bone consists of a meshwork of bone called trabeculae.

**2.** Trabeculae create the spongy appearance of cancellous bone.

**3.** The spaces between the trabeculae are filled with bone marrow.

### Bone Marrow

There are two types of bone marrow:

**1.** Red bone marrow's function is hematopoiesis, the formation of blood cells.

**2.** In an adult the ribs, vertebrae, sternum, and pelvis contain red bone marrow in their cancellous tissue.

**3.** Yellow bone marrow is found in the shafts of long bones within their cancellous tissue.

**4.** Yellow bone marrow stores fat cells.

### THE CLASSIFICATION OF BONES

The bones of the body can be classified, based on shape, into five categories.

**1.** Long bones consist of a shaft or diaphysis, a flared portion at the end of the diaphysis called a metaphysis and two extremities called epiphyses. Examples would be the clavicle, humerus, radius, ulna, femur, tibia, and fibula as well as the phalanges, metacarpals and metatarsals.

**2.** Short bones have a somewhat irregular shape. Examples would be the tarsal bones of the foot and the carpal bones of the hand.

**3.** Flat bones are flat and serve to protect or provide extensive muscle attachment. Examples would be some bones of the cranium, the ribs, scapula, and part of the hipbone.

**4.** Irregular bones have a very peculiar or irregular shape. Examples are the vertebrae and the ossicles of the ear.

**5.** Sesamoid bones are small rounded bones enclosed in tendon and fascial tissue near joints. One example is the largest sesamoid bone, the patella.

## BONE MARKINGS

1. Bones exhibit certain projections called processes. Examples of processes are spine, condyle, tubercle, trochlea, trochanter, crest, line, head, and neck.
2. Bones also exhibit certain depressions called fossae. Examples of fossae are suture, foramen, meatus or canal, sinus or antrum, and sulcus.
3. These markings are functional to help join bones to one another, to provide a surface for muscle attachment, or to serve as a passageway for blood vessels and nerves into and out of the bone.

## DIVISIONS OF THE SKELETON

1. The human skeleton has 206 bones.
2. The skeleton can be divided into the axial skeleton (skull, hyoid, vertebrae, ribs, and sternum) and the appendicular skeleton (bones of the upper and lower extremities).

## THE AXIAL SKELETON

1. The cranial bones consist of the frontal bone, the two parietal bones, the occipital bone, the two temporal bones, the sphenoid bone, the ethmoid bone, the six auditory ossicles (malleus, incus, stapes in each ear) and the varying wormian or sutural bones.
2. The facial bones consist of the two nasal bones, the two palatine bones, the two maxillary bones (upper jaw), the two zygomatic or malar bones (cheekbones), the two lacrimal bones, the two turbinates or nasal conchae, the single vomer bone, and the single lower jawbone, the mandible.

### The Orbits, Nasal Cavities, and Foramina

1. The orbits are the two deep cavities that enclose and protect the eyes. A number of bones of the skull contribute to their formation.
2. The framework of the nose surrounds the two nasal cavities made by a number of bones of the skull.
3. Foramina are passageways for blood vessels and nerves. The largest foramen of the skull is the foramen magnum for passage of the spinal cord.

### The Hyoid Bone

1. The hyoid bone does not articulate with any other bones. It is suspended by ligaments from the styloid process of the temporal bone.
2. Its function is to support the tongue.

### The Torso or Trunk

1. The sternum, ribs, and vertebrae make up the torso or trunk.
2. A typical vertebra has a number of characteristics: a disk-shaped body, an arch that encloses the spinal foramen, a spinous process and two transverse processes for muscle attachment, and two superior articular processes and two inferior articular processes for articulation with the vertebra immediately above and below.
3. There are seven cervical vertebrae: the first is called the atlas and the second the axis.
4. There are 12 thoracic vertebrae that articulate with the ribs.
5. There are five lumbar vertebrae, the strongest.
6. The single sacrum is made of five fused sacral vertebrae.
7. The single coccyx or tailbone is made up of four fused coccygeal vertebrae.
8. The sternum or breast bone develops in three parts; it looks like a sword: the manubrium or handle, the gladiolus or body that looks like the blade, and the xiphoid process that resembles the tip of the sword.
9. There are 12 pairs of ribs: the upper seven pairs articulate directly with the sternum through their costal cartilages and are called true ribs; the lower five pairs are called false ribs; because the 11th and 12th pairs have no costal cartilage to articulate indirectly with the sternum like the 8th, 9th, and 10th pairs, they are called floating ribs.

## THE APPENDICULAR SKELETON

### The Bones of the Upper Extremities

1. The bones of the shoulder girdle are the clavicle or collarbone and the scapula or shoulder blade.
2. The humerus is the bone of the upper arm.
3. The forearm bones are the ulna, the longer of the two bones, with its proximal olecranon

process or elbow, and the radius, the shorter bone that articulates with some of the wrist or carpal bones.

4. The carpal bones of the wrist are the pisiform, triquetral, lunate, and scaphoid (in the proximal row); and the hamate, capitate, trapzoid or lesser multiangular, and the trapezuim or greater multiangular (in the distal row).

5. The bones of the palm of the hand are the five metacarpals.

6. The bones of the fingers are the 14 phalanges in each hand.

### The Bones of the Lower Extremeties

1. Each hip or pelvic bone consists of three fused bones: the ischium, ilium, and pubis. They form the pelvic girdle. The female ilium is wider than in males and we all sit on our ischial tuberosity.

2. The femur or thighbone is the largest bone in the body.

3. The patella or kneecap is the largest of the sesamoid bones, it is wrapped in the tendon of the quadriceps femoris muscle.

4. The tibia or shinbone is the largest bone of the lower leg.

5. The fibula of the lower leg is the most slender bone in the body. It is also known as the calfbone.

6. The tarsal bones of the foot are the calcaneus or heel, the talus or ankle, the navicular, and the three cuneiforms.

7. The metatarsals make up the rest of the foot bones along with the 14 phalanges of the toes.

### THE ARCHES OF THE FOOT

1. The foot has three arches: the medial longitudinal arch is the highest, the lateral longitudinal arch, and the transverse arch.

2. Pes planus or flatfoot results from decreased height in the longitudinal arches.

### REVIEW QUESTIONS

1. Name five functions of the skeleton.
*2. Why should parents make sure that their young child should drink milk, exercise, and play in the sunlight on a daily basis?

3. Name the cranial bones.
4. Name the facial bones.
5. Name the carpal bones of the wrist.
6. Name the tarsal bones of the foot.

\* **Critical Thinking Question**

### Fill in the Blank
Fill in the blank with the most appropriate term.

1. The two common types of bone tissue are _____ and _____.

2. Bone develops from spindle-shaped cells called _____ found beneath the periosteum.

3. _____ are large cells, present in the cavities of bone, which function in the reabsorption of bone.

4. _____ ossification is a process in which dense connective tissue or membranes are replaced by deposits of inorganic calcium.

5. The "replacement" of cartilagenous structures with bone is called _____ ossification.

6. A disease of bone in children caused by a deficiency of vitamin D and sunlight is _____; in adults it is called _____.

7. Haversian canals are surrounded by concentric rings of bone, each layer of which is called a _____; between these are tiny cavities called _____, each containing an osteocyte.

8. _____ bone marrow's function is hematopoiesis.

9. _____ bone marrow consists chiefly of fat cells.

10. The bridge of the nose is made up of the paired _____ bones.

11. The hard palate of the roof of the mouth is made up of the two _____ bones.

12. The _____ bone, found in the axial skeleton, has no articulations with other bones, and functions as a support for the tongue.

13. The first cervical vertebra is called the _____, it supports the head; the second cervical vertebra is called the _____.

14. The sternum or breastbone develops in three parts, the _____, the body or _____, and the _____.

15. There are 12 pairs of ribs, the upper seven pairs articulate directly with the sternum and are called _____ ribs, the lower five pairs do not directly join the sternum and are called _____ ribs.

## Matching

Place the most appropriate number in the blank provided.

_____ Periosteum
_____ Osteomalacia
_____ Epiphysis
_____ Process
_____ Condyle
_____ Crest
_____ Fossa
_____ Fissure
_____ Foramen
_____ Meatus
_____ Sinus
_____ Sulcus
_____ Forehead
_____ Cheek bone
_____ Tooth socket

1. Rounded or knuckle-like prominence
2. Depression in or a bone
3. Canal, tubelike passage
4. Orifice through which vessels and nerves pass
5. Fibrovascular membrane covering bone
6. Zygomatic bone
7. Any marked, bony prominence
8. Frontal bone
9. Cavity within a bone
10. Two extremities of a long bone
11. Furrow or groove
12. Alveolus
13. Narrow ridge of bone
14. Narrow slit between two bones
15. Rickets in adults
16. Temporal bone
17. Parietal bone

## True or False

1. Cartilage actually turns into bone during ossification.                    T    F
2. The protein matrix of bone is responsible for its elasticity and the salts deposited in the matrix prevent crushing.            T    F
3. The more strain on a bone, the less the bone will develop.                       T    F
4. It is possible for crooked bones in children to become straight due to the continued process of reabsorption.             T    F
5. The proper calcium ion concentration of the blood is controlled and maintained by the parathyroid glands.                 T    F
6. The foramen magnum is the largest orifice in the skeleton and is found at the base of the parietal bone.                     T    F
7. Like the bones of the cranium, all the facial bones are united by immovable sutures.                          T    F
8. If the thoracic vertebrae become excessively curved, a condition known as kyphosis develops.                          T    F
9. The 11th and 12th ribs have another name, floating ribs, because they do not articulate at all with other parts of the skeleton.   T    F
10. The scapula is the bone whose common name is the collar bone.                   T    F

# LABORATORY EXERCISE: THE SKELETAL SYSTEM

Materials needed: An articulated human skeleton either real bone, if possible, or a good plastic reproduction; a number of skulls (one skull per 4–5 students); disarticulated examples of human bones, an articulated foot, and an articulated hand. Microscope slide of compact bone.

1. Break into groups of 4 to 5 students. Use the colored plates from your textbook and identify the cranial and facial bones with their major sutures by working with the skulls provided by your instructor.

2. Move to the articulated skeleton and identify the other bones of the body.

3. Look at an articulated hand and a foot and identify the carpal bones of the wrist and the tarsal bones of the foot.

4. Examine a hyoid bone and identify its parts.

5. Try to identify various bone markings mentioned in your text.

6. Examine a long bone that has been split open to view compact and cancellous tissue.

7. Review the histology of compact bone by viewing a microscope slide of compact bone. Identify all the parts of the haversian system.

# 8

# The Articular System

## CHAPTER OUTLINE

- **Introduction**
- **The classification of joints: structure and function:** *Synarthroses; Amphiarthroses; Diarthroses or synovial joints*
- **Movements at synovial joints**
- **The six types of diarthroses or synovial joints**
- **Bursae**

## CHAPTER OBJECTIVES

After studying this chapter, you should be able to:

1. Name and describe the three types of joints.
2. Name examples of the two types of synarthroses joints.
3. Name examples of the two types of amphiarthroses joints.
4. Describe and give examples of the six types of diarthroses or synovial joints.
5. Describe the capsular nature of a synovial joint.
6. Describe the three types of bursae.
7. Name some of the disorders of joints.

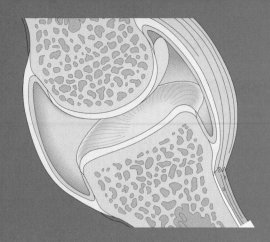

# KEY TERMS

# INTRODUCTION

An **articulation** is a place of union or junction between two or more bones, regardless of the degree of movement allowed by this union. The sutures between various bones of the skull are considered as much a part of the articular system as the knee or elbow joint. When we think of a joint, we tend to think of the freely moving joints like such as the shoulder or hip joint but other types of joints have limited or no movement at all occurring at their site.

# THE CLASSIFICATION OF JOINTS: STRUCTURE AND FUNCTION

Joints are classified into three major groups according to the degree of movement they allow (function) and the type of material that holds the bones of the joint together (structure).

## Synarthroses

**Synarthroses** (**sin**-ahr-**THRO**-seez) are joints or unions between bones that do not allow movement. Syn as a prefix means joined together. There are three examples of synarthroses or immovable joints.

The first type is a **suture** (**SOO**-chur). A suture is an articulation in which the bones are united by a thin layer of fibrous tissue. The suture joints of the skull are examples. Recall from Chapter 7 that the bones of the skull are formed by intramembranous ossification. The fibrous tissue in the suture is the remnant of that process and helps form the suture.

The second example is a **syndesmosis** (sin-dez-**MOH**-sis). Syndesmoses (plural) are joints in which the bones are connected by ligaments between the bones. Examples are where the radius articulates with the ulna and where the fibula articulates with the tibia. These bones move as one when we pronate and supinate the forearm or rotate the lower leg. Some authors consider syndesmosis as an example of an amphiarthrosis (little movement).

The third example is a **gomphosis** (gohm-**FOH**-sis). Gomphoses (plural) are joints in which a conical process fits into a socket and is held in place by ligaments. An example would be a tooth in its alveolus (socket), held in place by the periodontal ligament.

## Amphiarthroses

**Amphiarthroses** (**am**-fee-ahr-**THRO**-sis) are joints that allow only slight movement. There are two examples of amphiarthroses.

The first example of an amphiarthrosis is a **symphysis** (**SIM**-fah-sis). Symphyses (plural) are joints in which the bones are connected by a disk of fibrocartilage. An example of a symphysis would be the pubic symphysis where the two pelvic bones at the pubis are joined. During delivery this joint allows the pelvic bone slight movement to increase the size of the birth canal.

The second example of an amphiarthrosis would be a **synchondrosis** (sin-kon-**DRO**-sis). Synchondroses (plural) are joints in which two bony surfaces are connected by hyaline cartilage. The cartilage is replaced by permanent bone later in life. An example of a synchondrosis is the joint between the epiphyses (flared portions) and the diaphysis (shaft) of a long bone. Remember from Chapter 7 that this is the location of the growth plate and where long bones develop longitudinally by endochondral ossification. Some authors consider a synchondrosis as an example of a synarthrosis (no movement).

## Diarthroses or Synovial Joints

**Diarthroses** (**dye**-ahr-**THRO**-seez) or **synovial joints** are freely moving joints or articulations (Figure 8-1). They are always characterizied by the presence of a cavity enclosed by a capsule. This cavity may contain various amounts and concentrations of a number of tissues. The cavity may be enclosed by a capsule of fibrous articular cartilage. Ligaments can reinforce the capsule, and cartilage will cover the ends of the opposing bones. This capsule will be lined on the inside with synovial membrane, which produces synovial fluid. Most joints of the upper and lower limbs are diathroses.

The articular cartilage in the joint provides a smooth, gliding surface for opposing bone. This is made possible because of the lubrication caused by the synovial fluid. The opposing bones do not wear or erode over time due to the constant friction caused by movement at the joint. Articular cartilage has a limited blood supply. It receives its nourish-

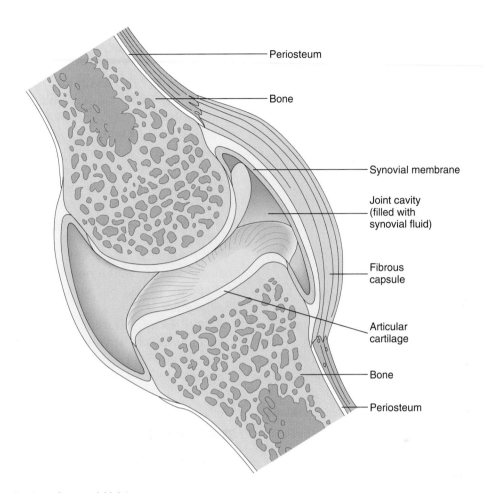

**FIGURE 8-1.** The structure of a synovial joint.

ment from the synovial fluid and from a small number of subsynovial blood vessels at the junction of the cartilage and the joint capsule. Synovial fluid has two functions: creating a smooth gliding surface for opposing bones and nourishing the articular cartilage. Cartilage also functions as a buffer between the vertebrae in the spinal column to minimize the forces of weight and shock from running, walking, or jumping.

Collagenous fibers connecting one bone to another in the synovial joint form the capsule enclosing the joint. The range of motion of the joint is related to the laxity or looseness of the joint. This is directly related to the structure of the capsule and how it is formed over the opposing bones. In the shoulder joint, which has the greatest range of movement, the capsule is loose enough to permit the head of the humerus to be drawn away from the glenoid fossa of the scapula. However, in the

hip joint the range of motion is much more restricted, because the capsule is thicker and shorter and the head of the femur sits deeply in the acetabulum of the pelvic bone. The femur is also connected to the acetabulum by a series of strong ligaments. This structure is necessary because of the need for greater strength in this joint.

In addition to the above tissues that make up the capsule, muscles and their tendons can also be found as the outermost layer of the capsule. They provide an important mechanism for maintaining the stability of a diarthrosis or synovial joint. They have advantages over ligaments because during both relaxation and contraction they maintain the joint surfaces in firm contact at every position of the joint.

In summary, synovial joints have a number of functions. First, they bear weight and allow movement; second, their construction in the form of a capsule made of ligaments, tendons, muscles, and articular cartilage provide stability; and third, synovial fluid lubricates the joint and nourishes the cartilage.

## MOVEMENTS AT SYNOVIAL JOINTS

The following movements can occur at diarthroses or synovial joints.

**Flexion** (**FLEK**-shun) is the act of bending or decreasing the angle between bones.

**Extension** (eks-**TEN**-shun) is the act of increasing the angle between bones and is the opposite of flexion. Refer to Figure 8-2A for flexion/extension and hyperextension.

**Hyperextension** increases the joint angle beyond the anatomic position.

**Abduction** (ab-**DUCK**-shun) is moving the bones or limb away from the midline of the body while the opposite is **adduction** (add-**DUCK**-shun), which is moving the bone or limb toward the midline of the body (Figure 8-2B).

**Rotation** (row-**TAY**-shun) is the act of moving the bone around a central axis; the plane of rotational motion is perpendicular to the axis, as when rotating our head.

**Circumduction** (sir-kum-**DUCK**-shun) is moving the bone in such a way that the end of the bone or limb describes a circle in the air and the sides of the bone describe a cone in the air (Figure 8-2C).

**Supination** (soo-pin-**NAY**-shun) and **pronation** (proh-**NAY**-shun) refer to the movement of the forearm and hand (Figure 8-3A). Supination is moving the bones of the forearm so that the radius and ulna are parallel. If the arm is at the side of the body, the palm is moved from a posterior to an anterior position or if the arm is extended, the palm faces up as in carrying a bowl of soup. Pronation is moving the bones of the forearm so that the radius and ulna are not parallel. If the arm is at the side of the body the palm is moved from an anterior to a posterior position, or if the arm is extended, the palm faces down.

**Eversion** (ee-**VER**-zhun) and **inversion** (in-**VER**-zhun) refer to movements of the foot (Figure 8-3B). Eversion is moving the sole of the foot outward at the ankle while inversion is moving the sole of the foot inward at the ankle.

**Protraction** (pro-**TRACK**-shun) is moving a part of the body forward on a plane parallel to the ground.

**Retraction** (rih-**TRACK**-shun) is moving a part of the body backward on a plane parallel to the ground. Refer to Figure 8-3C for protraction and retraction of the lower jaw.

**Elevation** is raising a part of the body; **depression** is lowering a part of the body. Refer to Figure 8-3D for elevation and depression of the shoulder.

**Opposition** is movement that occurs only with the thumb and is unique to primates. It occurs when the tip of the thumb and the fingers are brought together. The action allows us to use tools as when writing with a pen.

**Reposition** occurs when the digits return to their normal positions.

**Dorsiflexion** is raising the foot up at the ankle joint and **plantar flexion** is pushing the foot down at the ankle joint, actions we do when walking (Figure 8-3E).

## THE SIX TYPES OF DIARTHROSES OR SYNOVIAL JOINTS

There are six types of freely moving or synovial joints. Refer to Figure 8-4 for the geometric structure and examples of these joints that permit certain types of movements.

A **ball and socket joint** is an example of a multiaxial joint. In this type of joint a ball-shaped head fits into a concave socket. Two examples are the ball-shaped head of the femur fitting into the concave socket of the acetabulum of the pelvic bone and the head of the humerus fitting into the glenoid fossa of the scapula. This type of joint provides the widest range of motion. Movement can occur in all planes and directions. Of the two ball and socket joints, the hip and the shoulder, the shoulder has the widest range of movement.

The **hinge joint** is structured in such a way that a convex surface fits into a concave surface. In this type of a joint, motion is limited to flexion and extension in a single plane. Two examples are the elbow and knee joint. Because motion is restricted to one plane these joints are also called uniaxial hinge joints. Refer to Figure 8-5 on page 174 to see the structure of the

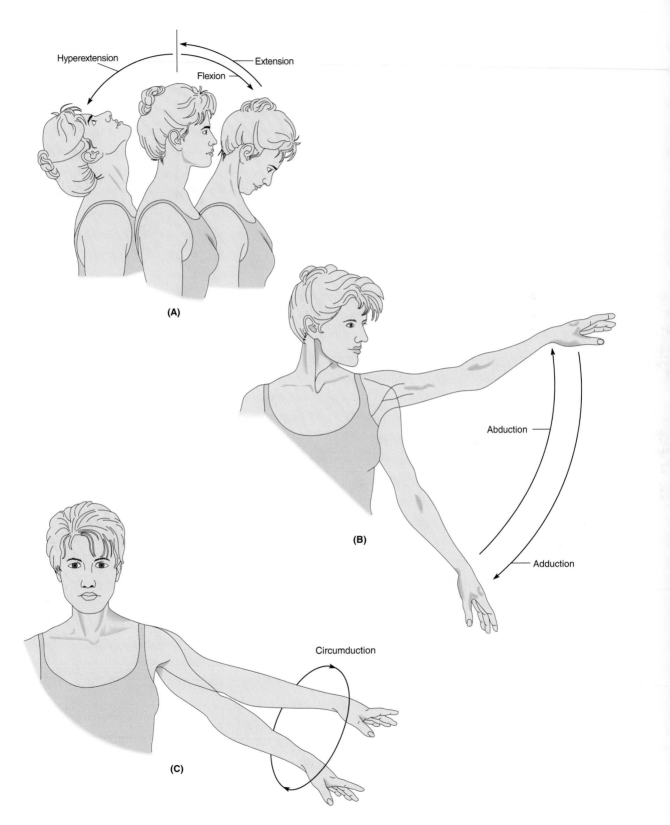

**FIGURE 8-2.** Movements at synovial joints. (A) Flexion/extension and Hyperextension. (B) Abduction/adduction. (C) Circumduction.

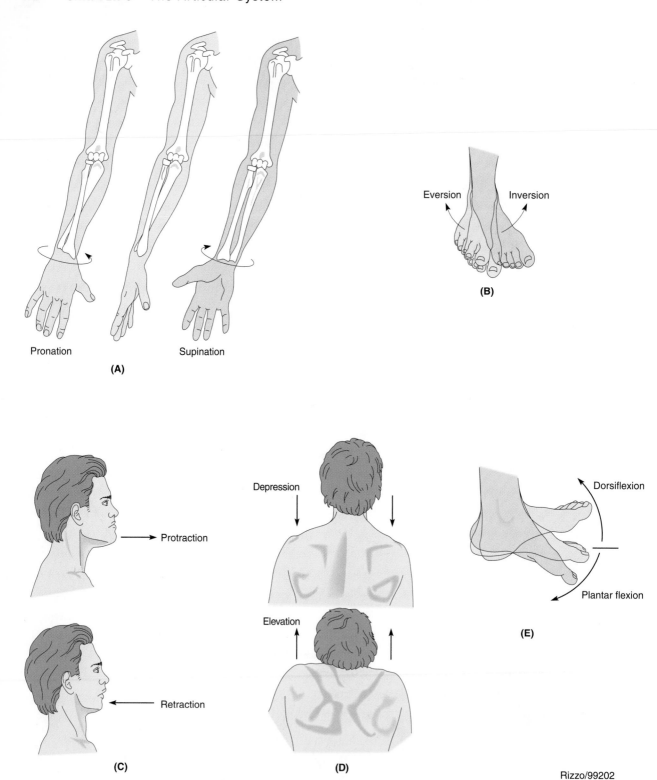

**FIGURE 8-3.** Movements at synovial joints. (A) Pronation/supination. (B) Eversion/inversion. (C) Protraction/retraction. (D) Depression/elevation. (E) Dorsiflexion/plantar flexion.

Rizzo/99202

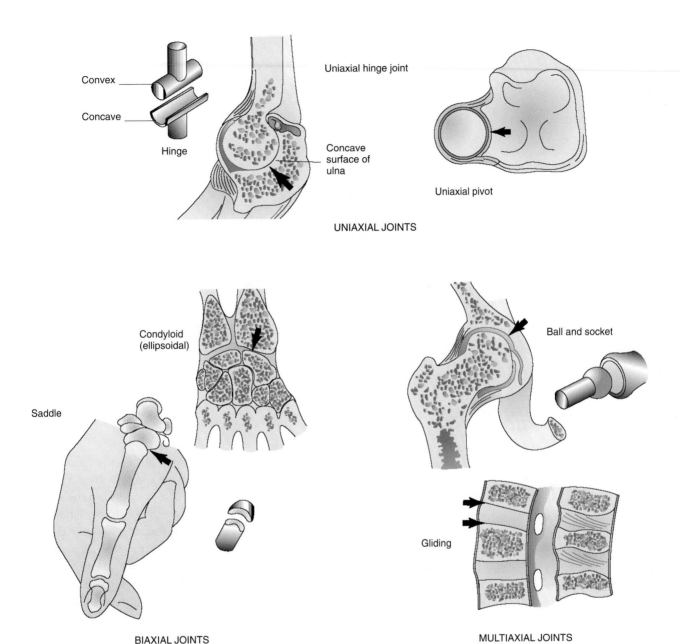

Convex

Concave

Hinge

Uniaxial hinge joint

Concave surface of ulna

Uniaxial pivot

**UNIAXIAL JOINTS**

Condyloid (ellipsoidal)

Saddle

**BIAXIAL JOINTS**

Ball and socket

Gliding

**MULTIAXIAL JOINTS**

**FIGURE 8-4.** The six types of freely moving diarthroses or synovial joints.

uniaxial knee joint. Other uniaxial hinge joints are the middle and distal phalanges of the fingers and toes.

The **pivot joint** is another uniaxial joint because motion is limited to rotation in a single plane. The joint is constructed in such a way that a pivot-like process rotates within a bony fossa around a longitudinal axis. One example is the joint between the atlas vertebra (the pivot process) that rotates within the bony fossa of the axis vertebra.

The **condyloid (KON-**dih-loyd) **joint**, sometimes called an ellipsoidal joint, is a biaxial joint that consists of an oval-shaped condyle that fits into an elliptical cavity. Motion is possible in two planes at right angles to each other. The wrist joint between the radius of the forearm and some of the carpal bones of the wrist is a condyloid joint. The hand can be flexed and extended in one plane like raising your hand in a sign to stop and returning it to

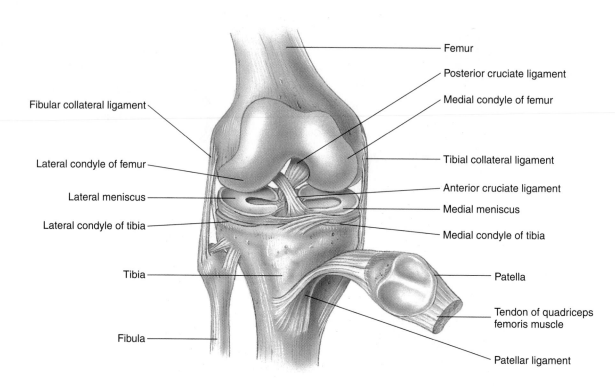

**FIGURE 8-5.** The structure of the uniaxial hinge joint of the knee.

a downward position. It can also be abducted and adducted like waving good-bye when moving the hand from side to side.

The **saddle joint**, another biaxial joint, is a bit more complex in its structure. In this type of a joint, one articular surface is concave in one direction and convex in the other (the trapezium, a carpal bone of the wrist) while the other articular surface is reciprocally convex and concave (the metacarpal bone in the thumb). Thus, the two bones fit together. Refer to Figure 8-4 to study its construction. Movement is possible in two planes at right angles to each other: flexion and extension plus abduction and adduction. This construction also permits opposition of the thumb, an evolutionary advancement allowing phenomenal dexterity of the hand to grasp and use tools.

The **gliding joint** is the last type of synovial joint and is a multiaxial joint. This type of joint is formed by either opposing planes surfaces or slightly convex and concave surfaces. This type of joint only allows gliding movement. Examples of gliding joints would be between the superior and inferior articular processes of the vertebrae in the spine.

## BURSAE

**Bursae** (burr-**SEE**) are closed sacs with a synovial membrane lining. Bursae can be found in the spaces of connective tissue between tendons, ligaments, and bones. Bursae will be found wherever friction could develop during movement. They facilitate the gliding of either muscle over muscle or tendons over bony ligamentous surfaces. Bursae are classified into three types based on where they are found.

**Subcutaneous bursae** are found under (sub) the skin (cutaneous) wherever the skin is on top of an underlying bony process (e.g., the knee joint). Between the patella or kneecap and its overlying skin is a subcutaneous bursa preventing friction between bone and skin.

**Subfascial** (sub-**FASH**-ee-al) **bursae** are located between muscles. They are found above the **fascia** (**FASH**-ee-ah) of one muscle and below the fascia of another. The fascia is the fibrous connective tissue that covers the epimysium of a muscle bundle. We will discuss fascia in Chapter 9.

**Subtendinous bursae** are found where one tendon overlies another tendon or where one tendon overlies some bony projection, as in the shoulder.

## Common Disease, Disorder or Condition

# ■ DISORDERS OF JOINTS

### Bursitis

Bursitis (burr-**SIGH**-tis) is an inflammation of the synovial bursa that can be caused from excessive stress or tension placed on the bursa. Playing tennis for long periods of time causes tennis elbow. It is an example of bursitis in the elbow joint caused by excessive stress. You may experience "canoist" elbow if you go canoeing and paddle for long hours. This is, of course, temporary. The elbow and the shoulder are common sites of bursitis. It can also be caused by a local or systemic inflammatory process. If bursitis persists, as in chronic bursitis, the muscles in the joint can eventually degenerate or atrophy and the joint can become stiff even though the joint itself is not diseased.

### Arthritis

Arthritis (ahr-**THRY**-tis) is an inflammation of the whole joint. It usually involves all the tissues of the joint: cartilage, bone, muscles, tendons, ligaments, nerves, blood supply, and so on. There are well over 100 varieties of arthritis and 10% of the population experiences this disorder, which has no cure. Pain relief is common through analgesics but these only relieve a symptom of arthritis, the pain.

### Rheumatic fever

Rheumatic fever is a disease involving a mild bacterial infection. If undetected in childhood, the bacterium can be carried by the bloodstream to the joints, resulting in a development of rheumatoid arthritis.

### Rheumatoid arthritis

Rheumatoid arthritis is a connective tissue disorder resulting in severe inflammation of small joints. It is severely debilitating and can destroy the joints of the hands and feet. The cause is unknown. A genetic factor may be involved or an autoimmune reaction in which an immune reaction develops against a person's own tissues. The synovial membranes of the joints and connective tissues grow abnormally to form a layer in the joint capsule. This layer grows into the articulating surfaces of the bones, destroying cartilage and fusing the bones of the joint.

### Primary fibrositis

Primary fibrositis is an inflammation of the fibrous connective tissue in a joint. It is commonly called rheumatism by the layman. If it is in the lower back, it is commonly called lumbago.

### Osteoarthritis

Osteoarthritis, sometimes referred to as degenerative joint disease, occurs with advancing age especially in people in their seventies. It is more common in overweight individuals and affects the weight-bearing joints. Mild exercising can prevent joint deterioration and increases the ability to maintain movement at joints.

### Gout

Gout (**GOWT**) is an accumulation of uric acid crystals in the joint at the base of the large toe and other joints of the feet and legs. It is more common in men than in women. These waste product crystals can also accumulate in the kidneys causing kidney damage.

## Summary Outline

### INTRODUCTION

An articulation or joint is a place of union between two or more bones regardless of the degree of movement allowed by the union.

### THE CLASSIFICATION OF JOINTS

1. Joints are classified into three main groups based on the degree of movement they allow and their structure: synarthroses, amphiarthroses, and diarthroses.

### Synarthroses

1. Synarthroses do not allow movement. The three examples of synarthroses are: suture, syndesmosis, and gomphosis.
2. A suture is a joint in which the bones are joined by a thin layer of fibrous connective tissue, like the sutures of the skull.
3. A syndesmosis is a joint in which the bones are connected by ligaments between the bones, like the radius and ulna articulations and the tibia and fibula articulations. Some authors classify this as an amphiarthrosis.
4. A gomphosis consists of a conical process in a socket held together by ligaments, like a tooth in its socket.

### Amphiarthroses

1. Amphiarthroses only allow slight movement. The two examples are a symphysis and a synchondrosis.
2. A symphysis is a joint in which the bones are joined by a disk of fibrocartilage, as in the pubic symphysis.
3. A synchondrosis is a joint where two bony surfaces are joined by hyaline cartilage, like the growth plate between the diaphysis and epiphysis of a long bone. Some authors classify this as a synarthrosis.

### Diarthroses or Synovial Joints

1. Diarthroses or synovial joints are freely moving joints.
2. They are characterized by having a capsular structure with an internal cavity.
3. The capsule of the joint can be made up of a number of different kinds of tissue: fibrous cartilage, ligaments, tendons, muscle, and synovial membranes.
4. The diarthroses or synovial joints have several functions. They bear weight and allow movement; the ligaments, tendons, muscles, and articular cartilage provide stability; and the synovial fluid lubricates surfaces and nourishes the cartilage.

### MOVEMENTS AT SYNOVIAL JOINTS

1. Flexion decreases the angle between bones.
2. Extension increases the angle between bones.
3. Hyperextension increases the joint angle beyond the anatomic position.
4. Dorsiflexion raises the foot upward at the ankle joint.
5. Plantar flexion pushes the foot down at the ankle joint.
6. Abduction moves a bone away from the midline.
7. Adduction moves a bone toward the midline.
8. Rotation moves a bone around a central axis, perpendicular to the axis.
9. Circumduction moves a bone so the end of it describes a circle and the sides of it describe a cone.
10. Supination moves the palm of the hand to an upright position or from a posterior to an anterior position if at the side of the body.
11. Pronation moves the palm of the hand to a downward position or from an anterior position to a posterior position if at the side of the body.
12. Eversion moves the sole of the foot outward at the ankle.
13. Inversion moves the sole of the foot inward at the ankle.
14. Protraction moves a part of the body forward on a plane parallel to the ground.
15. Retraction moves a part of the body backward on a plane parallel to the ground.
16. Elevation raises a part of the body.
17. Depression lowers a part of the body.
18. Opposition, unique to the thumb, allows the tip of the thumb and the fingers to be brought together.
19. Reposition is the opposite of opposition.

### THE SIX TYPES OF DIARTHROSES OR SYNOVIAL JOINTS

1. The ball and socket joint (multiaxial) allows the widest range of movement, as in the shoulder and hip joint.

2. The hinge joint (uniaxial) limits movement to flexion and extension, examples are the knee, elbow, and the middle and distal phalanges of the fingers and toes.

3. The pivot joint (uniaxial) limits movement to rotation in one plane, such as the atlas and axis articulation in the spine.

4. The condyloid joint or ellipsoidal (biaxial) joint allows motion in two planes at right angles to each other, as in the wrist joint between the radius and carpal bones.

5. The saddle joint (biaxial), found only in the thumb, allows movement in two planes at right angles to one another, located at the carpal-metacarpal articulation in the thumb.

6. The gliding joint (multiaxial) allows only gliding motion, as the intervertebral joints in the spine.

## BURSAE

1. There are three types of bursae. Bursae are closed sacs with a synovial membrane lining that prevents friction between overlapping tissues.

2. Subcutaneous bursae are found between skin and underlying bony processes.

3. Subfascial bursae are found where muscles overlie one another.

4. Subtendinous bursae are found where one tendon overlies another or overlies a bony projection.

## REVIEW QUESTIONS

1. Name and describe the three types of joints found in the human body.

2. Name two types of synarthroses and give an example of each.

3. Name two types of amphiarthroses and give an example of each.

*4. Why must diarthroses or synovial joints be constructed like a capsule for maximum function?

5. Name the six types of diarthroses and give an example of each.

6. Name and define the three types of bursae found in the human body.

7. How can an individual try to prevent the occurrence of osteoarthritis?

* **Critical Thinking Questions**

## LABORATORY EXERCISE: THE ARTICULAR SYSTEM

Materials needed: An articulated skeleton, anatomic models of the shoulder joint and hip joint that can be disarticulated showing muscles, tendons, bones, and cartilage.

1. Examine the ball and socket joint of the hip and shoulder. Identify the capsular nature of the joints by viewing the muscle, tendon, ligaments, and cartilage. If possible pop out the head of the femur from the acetabulum and view the structure of the joint.

2. Examine the bones of the elbow and knee joint on the skeleton, noting how the bones fit together to allow flexion and extension.

3. Study the hand: note the flexion and extension hinge joints of the fingers, and the saddle-joint of the thumb.

4. Examine the wrist joint and the ankle joint. On the wrist note the condyloid joint where the radius articulates with the carpal bones.

5. Your instructor will show you either a series of 35 mm slides or a videotape on the anatomy of human joints.

# Glossary

## A

**A bands** the dark, thick bands of the protein myosin in muscle cells

**Abdominal aorta** the part of the aorta located in the abdomen

**Abdominopelvic cavity** second subdivision of the ventral cavity that contains the kidneys, stomach, liver and gallbladder, small and large intestines, spleen, pancreas, and the ovaries and uterus (in women)

**Abducens nerve** controls movement of the eyeball

**Abduction** movement of a bone or limb away from the midline of the body

**Abductor digiti minimi** abducts little toe

**Abductor hallucis** abducts, flexes great toe

**Abductor pollicis** abducts the thumb

**ABO blood group** one of the blood groups

**Absorption** the passage of digested food from the digestive tract into the cardiovascular and lymphatic systems for distribution of the body's cells

**Accessory nerve XI** helps control swallowing and movements of the head

**Acetabulum** deep socket on the lateral side of the hipbone just above the obturator foramen

**Acetaldehyde** an intermediate product of fermentation

**Acetic acid** an intermediate product of the citric acid cycle

**Acetylcholine** neurotransmitter substance

**Acetylcholinesterase** an enzyme in the postsynaptic neuron that breaks down acetylcholine

**Acetyl-CoA** an intermediate product of the citric acid cycle

**Acid** a substance that dissociates and forms an excess of H ions when dissolved in water

**Acidosis** a condition caused by lowering of blood pH

**Acid rain** rain with a high acid concentration resulting from pollutants emitted from cars and coal-fired power planes

**Acini** exocrine glands of the pancreas

**Acromial process** bony prominence on the scapula

**Acrosome** contains enzymes that aid the sperm cell in penetrating the ovum

**Actin** thin filaments of protein in a muscle cell

**Action potential** when a muscle generates its own impulse to contract

**Active immunity** a type of immunity acquired naturally when exposed to a bacterium or virus or acquired artificially through a vaccine

**Active transport** mechanism requiring energy by which cells acquire materials against a concentration gradient

**Adam's apple** thyroid cartilage

**Addison's disease** condition in which the adrenal cortex fails to produce enough hormones

**Adduction** movement of a bone or limb toward the midline of the body

**Adductor pollicis** muscle that adducts the thumb

**Adenine** a purine nitrogen base

**Adenoids** pharyngeal tonsils

**Adenosine triphosphate (ATP)** high-enery fuel molecule the cell needs to function

**Adipose** loose connective tissue full of fat cells

**Adipose capsule** second layer of tissue that surrounds the kidney

**Adrenal cortex** outermost part of the adrenal gland

**Adrenal glands** small glands found on top of each kidney; suprarenal glands

**Adrenal medulla** inner part of the adrenal gland

**Adrenaline** a neurotransmitter also called epinephrine used by the autonomic nervous system

**Adrenocorticotropic hormone (ACTH)** stimulates the adrenal cortex to secrete the hormone cortisol

**Adventitia** the outermost layer of the wall of the alimentary canal

**Aerobic** requires oxygen

**Afferent arteriole** takes blood from the renal artery to Bowman's glomerular capsule

**Afferent lymphatic vessels** lymphatic vessels that enter the lymph nodes at various sites

**Afferent peripheral system** consists of afferent or sensory neurons that convey information from receptors in the periphery of the body to the brain and spinal cord

**Agglutination** clumping of red blood cells

**Agonists** muscles performing the actual movement

**AIDS** acquired immunodeficiency syndrome

**Albinism** the absence of skin color

**Albumin** a protein found in blood plasma that maintains osmotic pressure in blood and tissues

**Aldosterone** hormone that regulates sodium reabsorption and potassium excretion by the kidneys

**Alimentary canal** the name given to the digestive tube that runs from the mouth to the anus

**Allergies** hypersensitive reactions to common, normally harmless environmental substances

**All-or-none law** a contraction either occurs or does not occur

**Alpha cells** secrete the hormone glucagon

**Alpha-ketoglutaric acid** an intermediate product of the citric acid cycle

**Alveolar-capillary/respiratory membrane** membrane through which respiratory gases move

**Alveolar ducts** branches of respiratory bronchioles

**Alveolar sacs** two or more alveoli that share a common opening

**Alveoli** 1. milk-secreting cells; 2. cup-shaped outpouchings lined with epithelium

**Alveolus** a socket for articulation with a tooth

**Alzheimer's disease** results in severe mental deterioration

**Amine group** NH2 found in amino acids

**Ammonia** molecule that comes from the decomposition of proteins via the digestive process, and the conversion of amino acids in cellular respiration to ATP molecules

**Amnion** fluid-filled sac that surrounds the embryo

**Amphiarthroses** joints that allow only slight movement

**Ampulla of Vater** common duct of the pancreas and liver that enters the duodenum

**Amylase** the salivary enzyme that breaks down simple carbohydrates

**Anabolism** an energy-requiring process that builds larger molecules by combining smaller molecules

**Anaerobic respiration** respiration that does not require oxygen

**Anal canal** the terminal one inch of the rectum

**Anal columns** longitudinal folds of mucous membrane of the anal canal

**Anaphase** third and shortest stage of mitosis

**Anaphase I** stage of meiosis in which the centromere does not divide

**Anaphase II** stage of meiosis in which the centromeres of the chromosome divide

**Anastomosis** junction of two or more blood vessels

**Anatomy** the study of the stucture and organization of the body

**Anconeus** muscle that extends the forearm

**Androgens** male sex hormones

**Anemia** a decrease of hemoglobin in the blood

**Angina pectoris** a sensation of pain in the chest

**Antagonists** muscles that relax while the agonist contracts

**Anterior**   toward the front

**Anterior (ventral) gray horn**   part of the spinal cord

**Anterior interventricular sulcus**   separates the right and left ventricles from each other

**Anterior (ventral) root**   point of attachment of the spinal nerve to the cord, also known as the motor root

**Anterior tibial arteries**   supply blood to the leg and foot

**Anterior tibial veins**   drains the calf and foot

**Antibodies**   immunoglobulins; destroy foreign proteins

**Antidiuretic hormone (ADH)**   maintains the body's water balance; vasopressin

**Antigens**   foreign proteins that gain access to our bodies through cuts and scrapes, digestive or circulatory systems, or the urinary and reproductive systems

**Anus**   the opening of the anal canal to the exterior

**Aorta**   largest artery in the body

**Aortic arch**   the part of the aorta that arches to the left and heads down the spine through the thorax

**Aortic semilunar valve**   found in the opening where the ascending aorta leaves the left ventricle

**Apical foramen**   opening at the base of each root canal

**Aponeurosis**   wide and flat tendon

**Appendicitis**   inflammation of the vermiform appendix caused by an obstruction

**Aqueous humor**   fluid in the anterior compartment of the eye located in front of the lens

**Arachnoid mater**   the middle spinal meninx

**Arch of the aorta**   sends arteries to upper parts of the body

**Arcuate arteries**   the interlobar arteries that arch between the cortex and medulla

**Arcuate veins**   Drain filtered blood at the base of the pyramid

**Areola**   circular pigmented area of skin surrounding the nipple

**Areolar**   a type of loose connective tissue

**Arrector pili muscle**   consists of smooth muscle fibers attached to a hair follicle that causes the goose flesh appearance on the skin when we get scared or get a chill

**Arteries**   blood vessels that carry blood away from the heart

**Arterioles**   small arteries that deliver blood to capillaries

**Arthritis**   inflammation of the whole joint

**Articulation**   a place of junction between two or more bones

**Arytenoid cartilages**   move the vocal cords

**Ascending aorta**   leaves the left ventricle of the heart

**Ascending colon**   first part of the colon

**Ascending limb of Henle**   name given to the loop of Henle as it ascends toward the cortex

**Aster**   a starburst cluster of microtubules of tubulin produced by the centriole

**Astrocytes**   star-shaped cells that twine around nerve cells to form a supporting network in the brain and spinal cord

**Atherosclerosis**   disease of the arteries in which plaque accumulates on the inside of arterial walls

**Atlas**   first cervical vertebra that supports the head by articulation with the condyles of the occipital bone

**Atom**   the smallest particle of an element that maintains all the characteristics of that element

**Atomic number**   the number of protons or electrons in an atom

**Atrioventricular bundle**   bundle of His; part of the conduction system of the heart running through the top of the interventricular septum

**Atrioventricular (AV) node**   part of the conduction system of the heart located in the lower portion of the right atrium

**Atrophy**   a decrease in muscle bulk due to a lack of exercise

**Auditory tubes**   the ear canals located in the middle ear that equalize air pressure preventing hearing distortion; eustachian tubes

**Auricle**   external appendage of an atrium

**Autolysis**   the process of self-destruction in old or weakened cells

**Autonomic nervous system (ANS)**   conducts impulses from the brain and spinal cord to smooth muscle tissue, cardiac muscle tissue, and glands

**Axillary artery**   part of the subclavian artery that runs down the arm

**Axillary vein**   found in the armpit

**Axis**   the second vertebra

**Axon**   the long extension of a nerve cell body; a neuron has only one axon

**Axon endings**   the terminal portions of axons

**Axon terminals**   the endings of axons

**Azygos vein**   drains the thorax

## B

**B cells**  lymphocytes found in lymph nodes, spleen, and other lymphoid tissue where they replicate

**B lymphocytes**  cells that produce antibodies and provide humoral immunity; also known as B cells

**Ball and socket joint**  a type of synovial or diarthrosis joint, also called a multiaxial joint, like the shoulder or hip joint

**Basal cell carcinoma**  most common type of skin cancer

**Base**  a substance that combines with H ions when dissolved in water

**Basement membrane**  anchors epithelial cells to each other and to underlying tissues

**Basilic vein**  drains the medial part of the arm

**Basophils**  release heparin, histamine, and serotonin during an allergic reaction

**Beta cells**  secrete the hormone insulin

**Biceps brachii**  muscle that flexes the arm and forearm, and supinates the hand

**Biceps femoris**  flexes leg; rotates laterally after flexed

**Bicuspid valve**  mitral valve; valve between the left atrium and left ventricle

**Bile duct**  part of the liver that transports bile to the duodenum of the small intestine

**Bipolar neurons**  consist of one dendrite and one axon

**Blastula**  a hollow ball of cells produced by mitotic divisions of the zygote; blastocyst

**Blood**  specialized connective tissue

**Body**  term for the large central portion of the stomach and the pancreas

**Body of the uterus**  central tapering region of uterus

**Bonds**  formed when atoms combine chemically with one another

**Bone**  specialized connective tissue

**Bowel**  large intestine

**Bowman's glomerular capsule**  double-walled globe located in the cortex of the kidney

**Brachial artery**  extension of the axillary artery that runs down the arm

**Brachial vein**  drains the arm and empties into the axillary vein

**Brachialis**  muscle that flexes the forearm

**Brachiocephalic artery**  first branch of the aortic arch

**Brachioradialis**  muscle that flexes the forearm

**Brain stem**  one of the four major parts of the brain; it connects the brain to the spinal cord

**Breast cancer**  leading cause of death in women

**Bronchial arteries**  supply blood to the lungs

**Bronchial tree**  branching of the bronchi

**Bronchioles**  smaller branches of segmental bronchi

**Bronchitis**  inflammation of the bronchi

**Bronchomediastinal trunk**  drains lymph from the thorax, lungs, heart, diaphragm, and portions of the liver

**Bronchopulmonary segment**  segment of lung tissue that each of the tertiary bronchi supplies

**Brownian movement**  the random collision of diffusing molecules

**Brunner's glands**  secrete an alkaline mucus

**Bubonic plague**  disease of the lymphatic system

**Buccal glands**  secrete small amounts of saliva; found in the mouth

**Buccinator**  muscle that compresses the cheek

**Buffer**  a substance that acts as a reservoir for hydrogen ions

**Bulbourethral glands**  Cowper's glands; they produce an alkaline mucus

**Bursae**  closed sacs with a snyovial membrane lining

**Bursitis**  inflammation of the snyovial bursa

## C

**Calcaneus**  the heel

**Calcitonin**  hormone secreted by the thyroid that lowers the calcium and phosphate ion concentration of the blood

**Callus**  a thickened area of skin developed from an excessive amount of friction

**Calorie**  unit used to measure energy

**Canaliculi**  small canals in compact bone that connect lacunae with one another

**Cancellous bone**  forms the inner spongy tissue underneath compact bone

**Canine teeth**  teeth used to tear food

**Capillaries**  microscopic blood vessels where exchange of nutrients and oxygen and waste and carbon dioxide gas occurs between blood and tissue cells

**Capitate** one of the bones of the wrist

**Carbohydrate** made of atoms of carbon, hydrogen, and oxygen in a 1:2:1 ratio

**Carbon dioxide** chemical produced as a waste product of cellular respiration

**Carboxyl group** the COOH group found in amino acids and fatty acids

**Carcinogens** cancer-causing agents

**Carcinomas** tumors developing from epithelial tissue

**Cardia** part of the stomach that surrounds the gastroesophageal sphincter

**Cardiac muscle** muscle found only in the heart

**Cardiovascular system** body system consisting of heart and vessels that pump and distribute blood to and from all cells

**Carotene** a carotenoid pigment in plant cells that produces a red/orange color

**Carpals** bones of the wrist

**Cartilage** a type of specialized connective tissue

**Catabolism** an energy-releasing process that breaks down large molecules into smaller ones

**Catalyst** substance that increases the rate of a chemical reaction without being affected by that reaction

**Cecum** pouch-like first part of the large intestine

**Celiac trunk** the first branch of the abdominal artery

**Cell body** contains the nucleus of a neuron

**Cell cycle** process by which a cell divides in two and duplicates its genetic material

**Cell plate** first stage of a new cell wall forming at the equator of a dividing plant cell

**Cellular immunity** results of the body's lymphoid tissue

**Cellular respiration** the energy changes that occur in cells

**Cellulose** carbohydrate material that makes the cell wall of plant cells

**Cementum** substance that covers the dentin of the root of a tooth

**Central nervous system (CNS)** consists of the brain and spinal cord

**Centrioles** two centrioles make up a centrosome; they produce spindle fibers during cell division

**Centromere** portion of a duplicated chromosome that holds the two daughter chromatids together

**Centrosome** area near the nucleus made of two centrioles

**Cephalad** toward the head

**Cephalic vein** drains the lateral part of the arm and connects with the axillary vein

**Cerebellum** second largest portion of the brain concerned with coordinating skeletal muscle movements and balance

**Cerebral aqueduct** connects the third and fourth ventricles of the brain; also called aqueduct of Sylvius

**Cerebral circulation** blood circulatory route that supplies the brain with oxygen and nutrients, and disposes of waste

**Cerebral cortex** surface of the cerebrum

**Cerebral hemispheres** the right and left halves of the cerebrum

**Cerebral palsy** condition caused by brain damage during brain development or the birth process

**Cerebral peduncles** convey impulses from the cerebral cortex to the pons and spinal cord

**Cerebrovascular accident (CVA)** caused by a thrombus or embolus that blocks circulation resulting in cellular death

**Cerebrum** the bulk of the brain consisting of two cerebral hemispheres

**Cerumen** earwax

**Ceruminous glands** glands that produce earwax

**Cervical canal** interior of the cervix

**Cervical vertebrae** the seven smallest vertebrae found in the neck

**Cervix** 1. narrow, inferior portion of uterus that opens into the vagina; 2. the constricted junction between the crown and the root of a tooth, also known as the neck of a tooth

**Chancre** a sore on the penis caused by syphilis

**Chiasmata** figures of chromosomes during crossing-over

**Chief cells** secreting cells of the parathyroid glands

**Chloroplasts** organelles found only in plant cells where photosynthesis occurs; contain the pigment chlorophyll

**Chondrocytes** cells of cartilage

**Chordae tendinea** connect the pointed ends of the flaps or cusps to the papillary muscles in the ventricles

**Chorionic vesicle** a 100-cell blastocyst

**Chorionic villi** projections of the trophoblast

**Choroid** the second layer of the wall of the eye containing blood vessels and pigment cells

**Chromatids** duplicated copies of a chromosome

**Chromatin** term used to describe the genetic material inside a nucleus before duplication

**Chromoplasts** plastids in plant cells that contain the carotenoid pigments

**Chyle** lymph in the lacteals that has a high fat content and looks milky

**Chyme** the digested, viscous, semi-fluid contents of the intestine

**Cilia** small fibers found in cells that function in movement of materials across the cell's outer surface

**Ciliary body** consists of smooth muscles that hold the lens in place

**Circumduction** moving the bone in such a way so that the end of the bone or limb describes a circle in the air and the sides of the bone describe a cone in the air

**Circumvallate papillae** projections of the lamina propria that are covered with epithelium and contain taste buds; found toward the back of the tongue

**Cirrhosis** long-term degenerative disease of the liver in which the lobes are covered with fibrous connective tissue

**Cisternae** cavities of an endoplasmic reticulum that are sac- or channel-like

**Citric acid** an intermediate product of the citric acid cycle

**Clavicle** collar bone

**Cleavage furrow** pinching in of an animal cell membrane during cell division

**Clitoris** small, cylindrical mass of erectile tissue with nerves found at the anterior junction of the labia minora

**Clones** exact duplicates

**Clot** formed by fibrin at the site of a cut in a blood vessel

**CoA enzyme** converts acetic acid to acetyl-CoA

**Coccygeal vertebrae** the vertebrae of the tailbone

**Coitus** sexual intercourse

**Cold sores** small, fluid-filled blisters caused by the herpes simplex virus

**Collagen** a tough fiber found in the matrix of connective tissue

**Collecting duct** connects with the distal tubules of other nephrons

**Colon** largest part of the large intestine

**Color blindness** inability to perceive one or more colors

**Colorectal cancer** cancer of the large intestine and rectum

**Columnar epithelium** epithelial cells that are tall and rectangular; found lining the ducts of certain glands and in mucous-secreting tissues

**Common hepatic artery** supplies blood to the liver

**Compact bone** forms the outer layer of bone and is very dense

**Complement** a set of enzymes that attack foreign antigens

**Compound** formed when two or more elements combine via bonding

**Compound exocrine glands** glands made of several lobules with branching ducts

**Conduction system** generates and distributes electrical impulses over the heart to stimulate cardiac muscle fibers or cells to contract

**Condyle** rounded prominence found at the point of articulation with another bone

**Condyloid joint** a type of synovial joint, also called an ellipsoidal joint, like the wrist

**Congenital heart disease** heart disease present at birth

**Conjunctivitis** pinkeye

**Connective tissue** a type of tissue that supports or binds

**Contracture** condition in which a muscle shortens its length in the resting state

**Coracoid process** bony projection on the scapula that functions as an attachment for muscles that move the arm

**Corium** true skin; another name for the dermis

**Cornea** transparent part of the outermost layer of the eye that permits light to enter the eye

**Corniculate cartilage** cone-shaped, paired cartilages of the larynx

**Corns** caused by abrasion on bony prominences on the foot

**Coronal plane** dividing anterior and posterior portions of the body at right angles to the sagittal plane

**Coronal suture** found where the frontal bone joins the two parietal bones

**Coronary arteries** supply the walls of the heart with oxygenated blood

**Coronary circulation** supplies blood to the myocardium of the heart

**Coronary heart disease** results from reduced blood flow in the coronary arteries that supply the myocardium of the heart

**Coronary sinus** drains the blood from most of the vessels that supply the walls of the heart with blood

**Coronary sulcus** groove separating the atria from the ventricles

**Coronary thrombosis** blood clot in the vessel

**Corpus albicans** white body

**Corpus callosum** deep bridge of nerve fibers that connects the cerebral hemispheres

**Corpus hemorrhagicum** clot within a ruptured Graafian follicle

**Corpus luteum** yellow body

**Cortex** 1. smooth-textured area of the kidney extending from the renal capsule to the bases of the renal pyramids; 2. principal portion of the hair

**Cortical nodule** a dense aggregation of tissue in a lymph node

**Cortisol** hormone that stimulates the liver to synthesize glucose from circulating amino acids

**Cortisone** steroid closely related to cortisol given to reduce inflammation

**Covalent bond** a bond in which the atoms share electrons to fill their outermost shells

**Cowper's glands** bulbourethral glands

**Cramp** spastic and painful contraction of a muscle that occurs because of an irritation within the muscle

**Cranial cavity** cavity containing the brain

**Cremaster muscle** muscle in the spermatic cord that elevates the testes

**Crest** narrow ridge of bone

**Cretinism** a lack of or low level of thyroid hormones in children, resulting in mental and sexual retardation

**Cricoid cartilage** a ring of cartilage of the larynx that attaches to the first tracheal cartilage

**Cristae** the folds of the inner membrane of a mitochondrion

**Crohn's disease** chronic, inflammatory bowel disease of unknown origin

**Crossing over** the exchange of genetic material during prophase I of meiosis

**Crown** the portion of a tooth above the level of the gums

**Crypts of Lieberkuhn** pits in the mucosa of the small intestine

**Cuboid** a tarsal bone of the ankle

**Cuboidal epithelium** epithelial cells that look like small cubes; their function is secretion, protection, and absorption

**Cuneiform cartilage** rod-shaped, paired cartilages of the larynx

**Cuneiforms** the tarsal bones of the forefoot

**Cushing's syndrome** condition resulting from too much secretion from the adrenal cortex, resulting in obesity and puffiness in the skin

**Cuspids** another name for the canine teeth

**Cuticle** outermost portion of the hair

**Cyanosis** bluish discoloration of the skin caused by lack of oxygen in the blood

**Cystic fibrosis** an inherited disease of the respiratory system, usually fatal by early adulthood

**Cystitis** inflammation of the urinary bladder

**Cytochrome system** an electron carrier complex

**Cytokinesis** the phase of cell division in which division and duplication of the cytoplasm occurs

**Cytoplasm** the protoplasm outside the nucleus of a cell

**Cytosine** a pyrimidine nitrogen base

## D

**Decussation of pyramids** crossing of the tracts in the brain stem

**Deep femoral artery** supplies blood to the thigh

**Defecation** the elimination from the body of those substances that are indigestible and cannot be absorbed

**Deglutition** the process of swallowing

**Deltoid** muscle that abducts the arm

**Dendrites** receptive areas of the neuron; extensions of the nerve cell body

**Dentes** teeth

**Dentin** bone-like substance found in teeth

**Deoxyribonucleic acid (DNA)** genetic material of cells located in the nucleus of the cell that determines all the functions and characteristics of the cell

**Deoxyribose** a five-carbon sugar found in DNA

**Depolarization** reversal of electrical charge

**Depression** lowering a part of the body

**Dermis** second layer of skin; also called the corium

**Descending colon** part of the colon on the left side of the body

**Descending limb of Henle** name given to the proximal convoluted tubule as it dips into the medulla

**Descending thoracic aorta** part of the aorta located in the thorax

**Desmosomes** interlocking cellular bridges that hold skin cells together

**Detrusor muscle** three layers of smooth muscle in the bladder wall

**Diabetes mellitus** disease caused by a deficiency in insulin production

**Diaphragm** the muscle that separates the thoracic from the abdominal cavity, used in breathing

**Diaphysis** shaft composed mainly of compact bone

**Diarrhea** the passing of loose, watery stools affecting the function of the colon

**Diarthroses** freely moving joints or articulations; also called synovial joints

**Diastole** phase of relaxation of the heart

**Diencephalon** one of the four major parts of the brain consisting of the thalamus and the hypothalamus

**Diffusion** the movement of molecules through a medium from an area of high concentration of those molecules to an area of low concentration of those molecules

**Digestion** the breakdown of food by both mechanical and chemical mechanisms

**Digestive system** consists of the alimentary canal with its associated glands

**Diploid** the full complement of chromosomes

**Distal** away from the point of attachment or origin

**Distal convoluted tubule** name given to the ascending limb of Henle as it enters the cortex and becomes convoluted

**Diverticulosis** the presence of pouch-like herniations through the muscular layer of the colon

**Dopamine** a neurotransmitter

**Dorsal** toward the back

**Dorsal tectum** reflex center that controls the movement of the eyeballs and head in response to visual stimuli

**Dorsal venous arch** drains blood in the foot

**Dorsalis pedis artery** supplies blood to the dorsal part of the foot

**Dorsiflexion** raising the foot up at the ankle joint

**Duct of Wirsung** large main duct of the pancreas; also called pancreatic duct

**Ductus deferens** vas deferens

**Ductus epididymis** a single tube into which the coiled efferent ducts empty

**Duodenum** shortest and first part of the small intestine

**Dura mater** the outermost spinal meninx

**Dwarfism** the result of inadequate ossification at the epiphyseal plates of long bones that causes an individual to be abnormally small

## E

**Ectoderm** a primary germ layer that forms the skin and nervous system of a developing fetus

**Edema** swelling

**Efferent arteriole** carries blood away from the glomerular capsule

**Efferent ducts** series of coiled tubes that transfer the sperm out of the testes

**Efferent lymphatic vessels** lymphatic vessels that leave a lymph node at the hilum

**Efferent peripheral system** consists of efferent or motor neurons that convey information from the brain and spinal cord to muscles and glands

**Ejaculatory duct** duct formed from the joining of the seminal vesicle and ductus deferens that ejects spermatozoa into the urethra

**Elastic cartilage** forms the external ear, ear canals, and epiglottis

**Elastin** flexible fibers found in the matrix of connective tissue

**Electrical potential** caused by a rapid influx of sodium ions into a muscle cell

**Electron** negatively charged particle that orbits the nucleus at some distance from its center

**Electron acceptors** molecules that gain electrons during a reaction

**Electron carriers** molecules that gain electrons only to lose them to some other molecule in a very short time

**Electron donors** molecules furnishing electrons during a reaction

**Electron shells** the energy levels in which electrons are grouped

**Electron transfer/transport system** the aerobic mechanism of respiration which produces most of the ATP molecules from the breakdown of glucose

**Element** a substance whose atoms all contain the same number of protons and electrons

**Elevation** raising a part of the body

**Embolism** embolus that becomes lodged in a vessel and cuts off circulation

**Embolus** piece of blood clot that dislodges and gets transported by the bloodstream

**Emphysema** a degenerative disease with no cure that results in the destruction of the walls of the alveoli

**Enamel** protects teeth from wear and acids, found on the crown of a tooth

**Encephalitis** inflammation of brain tissue usually caused by a virus

**Endocarditis** inflammation of the endocardium

**Endocardium** innermost layer of the heart wall, including epithelial cells that line the heart

**Endochondral ossification** the formation of bone in a cartilagenous environment

**Endocrine glands** ductless glands that secrete hormones directly into the bloodstream

**Endocrine system** consists of the endocrine glands

**Endoderm** a primary germ layer that forms the lining of internal organs and glands of a developing fetus

**Endometrium** innermost layer of the uterine wall

**Endomysium** delicate connective tissue that surrounds the sarcolemma

**Endoplasmic reticulum (ER)** a complex system of membranes that form a collection of membrane-bound cavities

**Endorphins** neurotransmitters

**Endosteum** a fibrovascular membrane that lines the medullary cavity of a long bone

**Endothelial-capsular membrane** formed by the visceral layer of Bowman's capsule and the endothelial capillary network of the glomerulus

**Endothelium** epithelial cells that line the circulatory system

**Energy** the ability to do work

**Enlarged prostate** causes constriction of the urethra making urination difficult, usually occurring in elderly males

**Entamoeba histolytica** amoeba in protozoan infections caused by drinking untreated water; causes severe diarrhea

**Enzymes** protein catalysts

**Eosinophils** produce antihistamines

**Ependymal cells** line the fluid-filled ventricles of the brain; produce and move cerebrospinal fluid through the CNS.

**Epicardium/visceral pericardium** outermost layer of the heart wall

**Epidermis** top layer of skin

**Epiglottis** large, leaf-shaped piece of cartilage of the larynx that blocks food from entering the trachea when we swallow

**Epilepsy** a disorder of the brain resulting in seizures

**Epimysium** coarse, irregular connective tissue that surrounds the whole muscle

**Epiphyseal line** place where longitudinal growth of bone takes place

**Epiphysis** the extremity of a long bone

**Epithelial tissue** type of tissue that protects, absorbs, or secretes

**Erection** swelling and hardening of the penis due to retained entry blood

**Erythroblastosis fetalis** hemolytic disease of the newborn

**Erythrocytes** red blood cells (RBCs)

**Erythropoietin** hormone that stimulates red blood cell production in red bone marrow

**Escherichia coli** normal bacteria in the intestine

**Esophageal arteries** supply blood to the esophagus

**Esophageal hiatus** an opening in the diaphragm for passage of the esophagus to join the stomach

**Esophagus** collapsible, muscular tube located behind the trachea that transports food to the stomach

**Estrogen** female sex hormone

**Ethmoid bone** the principal supporting structure of the nasal cavities; forms part of the orbits

**Ethyl alcohol** a final product of fermentation

**Eukaryotic** refers to higher cells, like those of the human body, with membrane-bound organelles

**Eversion** moving the sole of the foot outward at the ankle

**Exhalation** expiration; movement of air out of the lungs

**Exocrine glands** glands that have ducts

**Exophthalmia**   bulging of the eyeballs

**Extension**   increasing the angle between bones

**Extensor carpi**   muscles that extend the wrist

**Extensor digitorum communis**   muscles involved in abducting and adducting the wrist; also extends toes and fingers

**Extensor hallucis**   extends great toe; dorsiflexes ankle

**Extensor pollicis**   muscle involved in extending the thumb

**External auditory meatus**   ear canal

**External iliac veins**   drain the pelvis

**External intercostals**   muscles that draw adjacent ribs together

**External jugular vein**   drains the muscle and skin of the head region

**External oblique**   muscle that compresses abdominal contents

**External occipital crest**   a projection of the occipital bone for muscle attachment

**External occipital protuberance**   a projection of the occipital bone for muscle attachment

**External os**   opening of the cervix into the vagina

**External respiration**   the exchange of gases between the lungs and blood

**External urinary sphincter**   surrounds the urethra as it leaves the bladder; made of skeletal muscle

## F

**Facial nerve VI**   controls the muscles of facial expression and conveys sensations related to taste

**Falciform ligament**   separates the two lobes of the liver

**Fascia**   layer of areolar tissue covering the whole muscle trunk

**Fascicle**   individual bundle of muscle cells

**Fasciculi**   skeletal muscle bundles

**Fatty acids**   along with glycerol, a building block of fats

**Fauces**   opening to the oropharynx

**Feces**   semi-solid mass of indigestible material in the large intestine

**Femoral artery**   supplies blood to the thigh

**Femoral vein**   drains blood from the thigh

**Femur**   thigh bone

**Fermentation**   process in which yeast breaks down glucose anaerobically (in the absence of oxygen)

**Fertilized egg**   zygote; organism produced by the union of two gametes

**Fetal circulation**   circulation route that exists only between the developing fetus and its mother

**Fetus**   embryo at nine weeks

**Fibrillation**   rapid, uncontrolled contraction of individual cells in the heart

**Fibrin**   long threads that form a clot

**Fibrinogen**   plasma protein

**Fibrinolysis**   dissolution of a blood clot

**Fibroblasts**   small, flattened cells with large nuclei and reduced cytoplasm that produce fibrocytes

**Fibrocartilage**   form the intervertebral disks that surround the spinal cord

**Fibrous pericardium**   outermost layer of the pericardial sac

**Fibula**   calf bone

**Filiform papillae**   found at the front of the tongue; important in licking

**Fimbriae**   finger-like projections surrounding the infundibulum

**First-degree burn**   burn involving just the epidermis and heals with no scarring

**Flagella**   long fibers that push a cell, like the sperm cell

**Flavin adenine dinucleotide (FAD)**   an electron carrier

**Flexion**   bending or decreasing the angle between bones

**Flexor carpi**   muscles that flex the wrist

**Flexor digitorum**   flexes toes and fingers

**Flexor hallucis**   flexes great toe

**Flexor pollicis**   muscles involved in flexing the thumb

**Fluid mosaic pattern**   term used to describe the arrangement of protein and phospholipid molecules in a plasma or cell membrane

**Follicle-stimulating hormone (FSH)**   stimulates development of the follicles in the ovaries of females, and the production of sperm cells in the seminiferous tubules of the testes

**Fontanelle**   soft spot on top of a baby's head

**Food bolus**   the soft mass of chewed food

**Foramen**   opening in a bone through which blood vessels, nerves, and/or ligaments pass

**Foramen magnum**   inferior portion of the occipital bone through which the spinal cord connects with the brain

**Foramen of Monroe**   connects each lateral ventricle with the third ventricle of the brain

**Foreskin**   prepuce

**Fornix**   recess in the lower portion of the birth canal

**Fossa**   any depression or cavity in or on a bone

**Fovea centralis**   a depression in the retina

**Frontal**   plane dividing anterior and posterior portions of the body at right angles to the sagittal plane

**Frontal bone**   a single bone that forms the forehead and part of the roof of the nasal cavity

**Frontal lobe**   forms the anterior portion of each cerebral hemisphere

**Frontalis**   muscle that raises the eyebrows and wrinkles the skin of the forehead

**Fructose**   a six-carbon sugar

**Full-thickness burn**   burn in which the epidermis and dermis are completely destroyed; also called third-degree burn

**Fundus**   1. the rounded portion of the stomach above and to the left of the cardia; 2. dome-shaped portion of the uterus above the uterine tubes

**Fungiform papillae**   found toward the back of the tongue; contain taste buds

## G

**Gallbladder**   pear-shaped sac located in a depression of the surface of the liver

**Gallstones**   collection of precipitated cholesterol in the gallbladder

**Gametogenesis**   the formation of the gametes

**Ganglia**   nerve cell bodies grouped together outside the central nervous system

**Gastrocnemius**   calf muscle

**Gastrointestinal tract**   the name given to the digestive tube that runs from the mouth to the anus; the alimentary canal

**Gene**   a sequence of organic nitrogen base pairs that codes for a polypeptide or a protein

**Genital herpes**   infection with simplex herpes II virus that causes lesions and blister-like eruptions on the skin of the genitals

**Genital warts**   highly contagious infection caused by a virus

**Germinal center**   part of a lymphatic node that produces lymphocytes

**Germinal epithelium**   surface of an ovary

**Gigantism**   the result of abnormal endochondral ossification at the epiphyseal plates of long bones, giving the individual the appearance of a very tall giant

**Gingivae**   the gums

**Gladiolus**   part of the sternum bone resembling the blade of a sword

**Glandular epithelium**   forms glands

**Glans**   exposed portion of the clitoris

**Glans penis**   head of the penis

**Glaucoma**   destruction of the retina or optic nerve resulting in blindness

**Glenoid fossa**   a depression in the scapula for articulation with the head of the humerus

**Glial cells**   cells that perform support and protection

**Gliding joint**   a type of synovial joint found in the spine

**Globin**   protein in hemoglobin

**Globulins**   blood plasma proteins like antibodies and complement

**Glomerulonephritis**   inflammation of the kidneys

**Glomerulus**   a capillary network surrounded by Bowman's capsule

**Glossopharyngeal nerve IX**   controls swallowing and senses taste

**Glottis**   space between the vocal cords in the larynx

**Glucagon**   a hormone produced by the pancreas that regulates blood glucose levels

**Glucose**   a six-carbon sugar

**Gluteus maximus**   muscle that extends, rotates thigh laterally

**Gluteus medius**   muscle that abducts, rotates thigh medially

**Gluteus minimus**   muscle that abducts, rotates thigh medially

**Glycerol**   - a simple molecule similar to a sugar except that it has only a three-carbon chain

**Glycogen**   animal starch

**Glycolysis**   the first step in cellular respiration in which a glucose molecule gets broken down into two molecules of pyruvic acid; does not require oxygen; occurs in the cytoplasm

**Glycosuria**   large amount of sugar in the urine

**Goblet cells**   unicellular glands that secrete mucus

**Goiter** enlargement of the thyroid gland due to an inadequate amount of iodine in the diet

**Golgi body/apparatus** consists of an assembly of flat sac-like cisternae that look like a stack of saucers or pancakes; used as a storage area in the cell

**Gomphosis** a joint in which a conical process fits into a socket and is held in place by ligaments

**Gonorrhea** venereal disease caused by a bacterial infection

**Gout** an accumulation of uric acid crystals in the joint at the base of the large toe and other joints of the feet and legs

**Graafian follicle** a mature follicle with a mature egg

**Gracilis** adducts thigh, flexes leg

**Granum** stacks of membranes found in chloroplasts

**Graves' disease** a type of hyperthyroidism caused by overproduction of thyroid hormone

**Gray matter** gray areas of the nervous system

**Great saphenous veins** longest veins in the body

**Greater vestibular glands** secrete mucus; Bartholin's gland

**Growth hormone (GH)** stimulates cell metabolism in most tissues of the body

**Guanine** a purine nitrogen base

**Gyri** folds on the surface of each hemisphere of the cerebrum

## H

**H band** slightly darker section in the middle of the dark A band; also called H zone

**Hair** one of the main characteristics of mammals

**Hair follicle** an epidermal tube surrounding an individual hair

**Hamate** one of the bones of the wrist

**Haploid** half the number of chromosomes

**Hard palate** anterior part of the roof of the mouth

**Haustrae** pouches in the colon

**Haversian canals** a feature of compact bone containing capillaries

**Head** 1. part of the pancreas closest to the duodenum; 2. terminal enlargement, like the head of the humerus

**Headache** cephalalgia; pain in the head

**Heart** major pumping organ of the cardiovascular system

**Heart failure** caused by progressive weakening of the myocardium and failure of the heart to pump adequate amounts of blood

**Helicobacter pylori** bacterium associated with the development of stomach or peptic ulcers

**Helper T cells** stimulate the production of killer T cells and more B cells to fight invading pathogens

**Hematocytoblasts** undifferentiated mesenchymal cells

**Hematopoiesis** blood cell formation

**Hematopoietic tissue** specialized connective tissue that produces blood cells

**Heme** pigment in hemoglobin

**Hemodialysis** procedure in which a dialysis machine filters blood taken from an artery and sends it back to a vein

**Hemoglobin** red pigment in erythrocytes

**Hemolytic anemia** inherited condition in which erythrocytes rupture or are destroyed at a faster rate than normal

**Hemophilia** genetically inherited clotting disorder

**Hemorrhoids** caused by inflammation and enlargement of rectal veins

**Heparin** anti-coagulant manufactured by the liver

**Hepatic portal circulation** route between the digestive tract and the liver

**Hepatic portal vein** drains the organs of the digestive tract

**Hepatitis** inflammation of the liver caused by excessive alcohol consumption or a virus infection

**Herniated disk** rupture of the fibrocartilage surrounding an intervertebral disk that cushions the vertebrae above and below

**Hilum** 1. notch in the center of the concave border of the kidney through which the ureter leaves the kidney; 2. depression on one side of a lymph node

**Hinge joint** a type of synovial joint, like the knee or elbow

**Histamine** an inflammatory substance produced in response to allergies

**Histiocytes** large, stationary phagocytic cells

**Histology** the study of tissue

**Homeostasis** maintaining the body's internal environment

**Horizontal** plane dividing the body into superior and inferior portions

**Hormones** chemical secretions, usually from an endocrine gland

**Horns** the areas of gray matter in the spinal cord

**Humerus** largest and longest bone of the upper arm

**Humoral immunity** results of the body's lymphoid tissue

**Hyaline cartilage** a type of cartilage that forms the early skeleton of the embryo

**Hydrogen bond** a type of bond that helps hold water molecules together by forming a bridge between the negative oxygen atom of one water molecule and the positive hydrogen atoms of another water molecule

**Hydroxyl group** the OH group found in sugars

**Hymen** thin fold of tissue that partially closes the distal end of the vagina

**Hyperextension** increases the joint angle beyond the anatomic position

**Hyperglycemia** chronic elevations of glucose in the blood

**Hyperopia** farsightedness

**Hyperparathyroidism** an abnormally high level of PTH secretion

**Hypertension** high blood pressure

**Hyperthyroidism** too much secretion of thyroid hormone

**Hypertonic solution** solution in which water molecules will move out of a cell and the cell will shrink, as in a 5% salt solution

**Hypertrophy** an increase in the bulk of a muscle caused by exercise

**Hypodermis** subcutaneous tissue

**Hypoglossal nerve XII** controls the muscles involved in speech and swallowing; its sensory fibers conduct impulses for muscle sense

**Hypoparathyroidism** an abnormally low level of PTH

**Hypophysis** another name for the pituitary gland

**Hypothalmus** part of the brain that controls secretions from the pituitary gland

**Hypothyroidism** a lack of or low level of thyroid hormone

**Hypotonic solution** solution in which water molecules will move into a cell and the cell will swell, as in pure distilled water

**I**

**I bands** light, thin bands of the protein actin in muscle cells

**Ileocecal valve** the opening from the ileum of the small intestine into the cecum of the large intestine

**Ileum** the third part of the small intestine measuring 12 feet in length

**Iliacus** muscle involved in flexing the thigh

**Ilium** the uppermost and largest portion of a hip bone

**Immunity** the ability of the body to resist infection from disease-causing microorganisms

**Immunoglobulin A (IgA)** type of antibody found in exocrine gland secretions, nasal fluid, tears, gastric and intestinal juice, bile, breast milk, and urine

**Immunoglobulin D (IgD)** type of antibody found on the surface of B lymphocytes

**Immunoglobulin E (IgE)** type of antibody found in exocrine gland secretions that is associated with allergic reactions

**Immunoglobulin G (IgG)** type of antibody found in tissue fluids and plasma

**Immunoglobulin M (IgM)** type of antibody that develops in blood plasma as a response to bacteria or antigens in food

**Impetigo** highly contagious skin disease of children caused by the bacterium Staphylococcus aureus

**Incisors** front teeth used to cut food

**Incus** ear bone referred to as the anvil

**Infarct** an area of damaged cardiac tissue

**Infarction** death of tissues

**Infectious mononucleosis** caused by the Epstein-Barr virus; infects lymphocytes and the salivary glands

**Inferior** lowermost or below

**Inferior meatus** one of three narrow passageways in the nasal cavity formed by the turbinate bones

**Inferior mesenteric artery** supplies blood to the large intestine

**Inferior oblique** muscle that rotates the eyeball on axis

**Inferior rectus** muscle that rolls the eyeball downward

**Inferior vena cava** brings blood from the lower parts of the body; also called posterior vena cava

**Infraspinatus** muscle that rotates the humerus outward

**Infundibulum** 1. part of the hypothalamus that connects to the pituitary gland; 2. open end of Fallopian tube

**Ingestion** the taking of food into the body

**Inhalation** inspiration; movement of air into the lungs

**Insertion** the movable attachment where the effects of contraction are seen

**Insula** lobe in the brain that separates the cerebrum into frontal, parietal, and temporal lobes

**Insulin** hormone produced by the pancreas that regulates blood glucose levels

**Integumentary system** consists of the epidermis and dermis

**Intercalated disks** structures that connect the branches of cardiac muscle cells with one another

**Intercostal arteries** supply blood to the muscles of the thorax

**Intercostal trunk** helps drain lymph from portions of the thorax

**Interlobar arteries** branches of the renal arteries in the renal columns

**Interlobar veins** run between the pyramids in the renal columns

**Internal iliac artery** supplies blood to the thigh

**Internal intercostals** muscles that draw adjacent ribs together

**Internal jugular vein** drains the dural sinus of the brain

**Internal nares** two internal openings in the nose

**Internal oblique** muscle that compresses abdominal contents

**Internal os** junction of the uterine cavity with the cervical canal

**Internal respiration** exchange of gases between the blood and body cells

**Internal urinary sphincter** located at the junction of the urinary bladder and urethra; made of smooth muscle

**Internuncial neurons** transmit the sensory impulse to the appropriate part of the brain or spinal cord for interpretation and processing; also known as association neurons

**Interossei** muscles that cause abduction of the proximal phalanges of the fingers

**Interphase** a stage of the cell cycle

**Interstitial cells of Leydig** produce male sex hormone testosterone

**Interstitial fluid** blood plasma found in the spaces between tissue cells

**Interventricular foramen** another name for the foramen of Monroe

**Interventricular septum** separates the right and left ventricles of the heart

**Intestinal glands** pits in the mucosa of the small intestine; also known as crypts of Lieberkuhn

**Intestinal trunk** drains lymph from the stomach, intestines, pancreas, spleen, and surface of the liver

**Intramembranous ossification** formation of bone by a process in which dense connective tissue membranes are replaced by deposits of inorganic calcium salts

**Inversion** moving the sole of the foot inward at the ankle

**Ion** charged atom

**Ionic bond** a bond that is formed when one atom gains electrons while the other atom loses electrons from its outermost shell

**Iris** colored part of the eye

**Iron-deficiency anemia** results from nutritional deficiencies or excessive iron loss from the body

**Ischium** the strongest portion of a hip bone

**Islets of Langerhans** pancreatic islets; form the endocrine portions of the gland

**Isometric contraction** contraction in which a muscle remains at a constant length while tension against the muscle increases

**Isotonic contraction** contraction in which tone or tension remains the same as the muscle becomes shorter and thicker

**Isotonic solution** solution in which water molecules diffuse into and out of a cell membrane at equal rates, as in normal saline solution

**Isotopes** different kinds of atoms of the same element

**Isthmus** small, constricted region between body of uterus and cervix

## J

**Jejunum** the second part of the small intestine measuring 8 feet in length

**Jugular trunk** drains lymph from the head and neck

## K

**Keratin** a protein material

**Keratinization** a process by which epidermal cells change shape, composition, and lose water as they move to the upper layers and become mainly protein and die

**Kidney stones**  stones made of precipitates of uric acid, magnesium, calcium phosphate, or calcium oxalate that can accumulate in the kidney

**Kidneys**  paired organs that regulate the composition and volume of blood and remove wastes from the blood in the form of urine

**Killer T cells**  kill virus-invaded body cells and cancerous body cells

**Kinetochore**  a disk of protein on the centromere

**Krebs' citric acid cycle**  the step after glycolysis that takes place in the mitochondria during which pyruvic acid gets broken down into carbon dioxide and water; requires oxygen

**Kupffer's cells**  eat bacteria and old white and red blood cells; found in the liver

**Kyphosis**  condition commonly referred to as hunchback

## L

**Labia majora**  two longitudinal folds of hair-covered skin

**Labia minora**  two delicate folds of skin medial to the labia majora

**Labor**  process by which the fetus is expelled from the uterus

**Lacrimal bones**  bones that make up part of the orbit at the inner angle of the eye; contain the tear sac

**Lactation**  secretion of milk from the mammary glands

**Lacteals**  lymphatic vessel that absorbs fats and transports them from the digestive tract to the blood

**Lactic acid**  the final product of anaerobic production of ATP in muscle cells

**Lactiferous ducts**  continuations of ampullae that terminate at the nipple

**Lactiferous sinuses**  expanded sinuses that store milk

**Lactogenic hormone (LTH)**  stimulates milk production in the mammary glands after delivery; also called prolactin

**Lacunae**  tiny cavities between the lamellae or rings of compact bone that contain bone cells

**Lambdoid suture**  a line where the two parietal bones connect with the occipital bone

**Lamella**  1. system of membranes that connect grana in a chloroplast; 2. layer of concentric rings surrounding the Haversian canals

**Lamina propria**  the second layer of the tunica mucosa consisting of loose connective tissue

**Large intestine**  the last part of the digestive tract measuring 5 feet in length; the bowel

**Laryngopharynx**  lowermost portion of the pharynx

**Larynx**  voice box

**Lateral**  toward the side or away from the midline of the body

**Lateral rectus**  muscle that rolls the eyeball laterally

**Latissimus dorsi**  muscle that extends, adducts, and rotates the arm medially

**Left atrium**  one of the upper chambers of the heart

**Left bundle branch**  branch of the bundle of His; part of the conduction system of the heart

**Left colic (splenic) flexure**  position where the transverse colon curves down beneath the spleen

**Left common carotid artery**  second branch of the aortic arch

**Left external carotid artery**  supplies blood to the muscles and skin of the neck and head

**Left gastric artery**  supplies blood to the stomach

**Left internal carotid artery**  supplies blood to the brain

**Left primary bronchus**  the first left division of the trachea

**Left pulmonary artery**  carries blood to the left lung

**Left renal aretery**  transports one-quarter of the total cardiac output directly to kidneys

**Left renal vein**  carries filtered blood from the interlobar veins to the hilum

**Left subclavian artery**  third branch of the aortic arch

**Left ventricle**  one of the lower chambers of the heart

**Lens**  the crystalline part of the eye

**Lesser vestibular glands**  Skene's glands; secrete mucus

**Leucoplast**  plastid in plant cells that contains no pigment but stores sugar or starch

**Leukemia**  type of cancer in which there is abnormal production of white blood cells

**Leukocytes**  white blood cells (WBCs)

**Levator labii superioris**  muscle that raises the upper lip and dilates the nostril

**Levator scapulae**  muscle that elevates the scapula

**Ligament**  connective tissue that attaches bone to bone

**Line** a less prominent ridge of bone than a crest

**Lingual frenulum** septum dividing tongue into symmetrical halves

**Lingual tonsils** located on the back surface of the tongue at its base

**Lipids** substances that are insoluble in water, like fats

**Lips** fleshy folds that surround the opening of the mouth

**Liver** largest organ of the digestive system

**Lobules** divisions of a bronchopulmonary segment

**Longitudinal fissure** fissure separating the cerebrum into right and left halves

**Loop of Henle** the U-shaped structure of the limb of Henle

**Lordosis** an abnormal accentuated lumbar curvature

**Lower esophageal sphincter** gastroesophageal sphincter; connects the esophagus with the stomach and controls the passage of food into the stomach

**Lumbar arteries** supply blood to the muscles of the abdomen and walls of the trunk of the body

**Lumbar trunk** drains lymph from the lower extremities, walls and viscera of the pelvis, kidneys and adrenal glands, and most of the abdominal wall

**Lumbar vertebrae** the five vertebrae of the lower back

**Lumen** a hollow core through which blood flows

**Lunate** a bone of the wrist

**Lung cancer** most common type of cancer

**Lunula** the white crescent at the proximal end of each nail

**Luteinizing hormone (LH)** stimulates ovulation in the ovary and production of the female sex hormone progesterone

**Lymph** the name given to interstitial fluid when it enters a lymphatic capillary

**Lymph capillaries** blind end tubes that are the origin of lymphatic vessels

**Lymph glands** lymph nodes

**Lymph nodes** lymph glands

**Lymph sinus** space between groups of lymphatic tissue

**Lymph trunks** the main draining vessels of the lymphatic system

**Lymphadenitis** inflammation of lymph nodes or glands

**Lymphangitis** inflammation of the lymphatic vessels

**Lymphatic system** consists of the lymph nodes, thymus gland, spleen, and the lymphatic vessels

**Lymphatics** lymphatic vessels that resemble veins but have more valves

**Lymphocytes** involved in the production of antibodies

**Lymphoid tissue** specialized connective tissue

**Lymphokines** chemicals released by the sensitized T lymphocytes

**Lymphoma** tumor of lymphatic tissue that is usually malignant

**Lysosomes** small bodies in the cytoplasm that contain powerful digestive enzymes that enhance the breakdown of cellular components

**Lysozyme** enzyme that destroys bacteria

## M

**Macrophages** engulf and digest antigens

**Major calyces** minor calyces joined together

**Malaria** caused by the injection of a protozoan

**Malic acid** an intermediate product of the citric acid cycle

**Malignant melanoma** skin cancer associated with a mole on the skin

**Malleus** ear bone referred to as the hammer

**Mamillary bodies** part of the diencephalon involved in memory and emotional responses to odor

**Mammary glands** produce milk in females

**Mammography** procedure in which low intensity x-rays are used to detect tumors in the soft tissues of the breast

**Mandible** the strongest and longest bone of the face; forms the lower jaw

**Manubrium** part of the sternum resembling the handle of a sword

**Masseter** muscle that closes the jaw

**Mast cells** roundish-shaped cells found close to small blood vessels that produce heparin

**Mastication** chewing

**Mastoid portion** located behind and below the auditory meatus or opening of the ear; part of the temporal bone

**Matrix** intercellular material in connective tissue

**Maxillary bones**   make up the upper jaw

**Meatus**   long tube-like passage

**Medial**   nearest the midline of the body

**Medial rectus**   muscle that rolls the eyeball medially

**Median cubital vein**   vein used to draw blood from the arm

**Mediastinum**   the space between the lungs

**Medulla**   1. middle or central portion of the hair; 2. the inner part of a kidney

**Medulla oblongata**   contains all the ascending and descending tracts that connect between the spinal cord and various parts of the brain

**Medullary cavity**   center of the shaft of long bone filled with yellow bone marrow

**Megakaryocytes**   produce thrombocytes or platelets

**Meiosis**   a reduction division that occurs in the gonads to produce egg and sperm cells

**Melanin**   pigment responsible for variations in skin color

**Melanocyte-stimulating hormone (MSH)** increases the production of melanin in melanocytes in the skin causing a darkening of the skin

**Melanocytes**   cells responsible for producing melanin

**Melatonin**   hormone produced by the pineal gland

**Membrane potential**   the ionic and electrical charge around a nerve fiber that is not transmitting an impulse; also called resting potential

**Membranous urethra**   connects the prostatic urethra to the penis

**Memory cells**   descendants of activated T and B cells

**Menarche**   first menstrual cycle

**Meninges**   a series of connective tissue membranes that surround the brain and spinal cord

**Meningitis**   inflammation of the meninges caused by bacterial or viral infection

**Menopause**   last menstrual cycle

**Menses**   cyclical shedding of the lining of the uterus

**Menstrual cycle**   cyclical shedding of the lining of the uterus

**Menstruation**   cyclical shedding of the lining of the uterus

**Mesentery**   extensions of the visceral peritoneum

**Mesocolon**   an extension of the visceral peritoneum of the colon

**Mesoderm**   a primary germ layer that forms the muscles, bone, and the rest of the body tissues in a developing fetus

**Mesothelium**   type of epithelial tissue based on function, also called serous tissue, that lines the cavities of the body that have no openings to the outside

**Messenger RNA**   a type of RNA that transcribes the genetic code of a DNA molecule

**Metabolism**   the total chemical changes that occur inside a cell

**Metacarpal bones**   bones of the palm of the hand

**Metaphase**   second stage of mitosis

**Metaphase I**   stage in meiosis in which the spindle microtubules attach to the kinetochore only on the outside of each centromere

**Metaphase II**   stage in meiosis in which the spindle fibers bind to both sides of the centromere

**Metaphysis**   flared portion at each end of long bone composed of cancellous or spongy bone

**Metastasis**   movement beyond the place of origin

**Metastasize**   defective cells spread to other parts of the body

**Metatarsals**   bones of the sole of the foot; form the arch of the foot

**Microglia**   phagocytic cell found in the central nervous system; also called neuroglia

**Microglial cells**   small cells that protect the central nervous system by engulfing and destroying microbes like bacteria and cellular debris

**Micrometer**   more common term used instead of microns

**Micron**   a cellular measurement equal to one thousandth of a millimeter

**Microtubules**   long, hollow cylinders made of tubulin

**Microvilla**   found on the free edge of villa of intestinal epithelial cells to increase the absorptive surface area of the cell

**Micturition**   urination

**Micturition reflex**   an unconscious reflex and conscious desire to urinate

**Midbrain**   mesencephalon; contains the ventral cerebral peduncles

**Middle meatus**   one of three narrow passageways in the nasal cavity formed by the turbinate bones

**Midsagittal**   plane vertically dividing the body into equal right and left portions

**Mineral salts**  composed of small ions, they are essential for the survival and functioning of the body's cells

**Minor calyx**  funnel-shaped structure that surrounds the tip of each renal pyramid

**Mitochondrion**  small oblong-shaped structure composed of two membranes; the powerhouse of the cell where ATP is made

**Mitosis**  process in which nuclear material is exactly replicated

**Molars**  teeth that grind food; also known as tricuspids

**Molecular oxygen**  necessary to convert food into chemical energy (ATP)

**Molecule**  the smallest combination or particle retaining all the properties of a compound

**Monocytes**  largest leukocytes; phagocytize bacteria and dead cells

**Monokines**  chemicals released by activated macrophages involved in the immune response

**Mons pubis**  mound of elevated adipose tissue that becomes covered with pubic hair at puberty; also called mons veneris

**Motion sickness**  caused by constant stimulation of the semicircular canals of the inner ear due to motion, resulting in nausea and weakness

**Motor neuron**  neuron that connects with muscles or glands to bring about a reaction to a stimulus; also called efferent neuron

**Motor unit**  all of the muscle cells or fibers enervated by one motor neuron

**Mucous cells**  secrete mucus

**Mucous membrane**  epithelium; lines the digestive, respiratory, urinary, and reproductive tracts; produces mucus

**Multipolar neurons**  neurons that have several dendrites and one axon

**Mumps**  disease caused by a virus that infects the salivary glands, especially in children between ages 5 and 9

**Muscle**  type of tissue that contracts and allows movement

**Muscle fibers**  muscle cells

**Muscle tissue**  tissue that can shorten and thicken or contract

**Muscle twitch**  the analysis of a muscle contraction

**Muscular dystrophy**  an inherited muscular disorder in which muscle tissue degenerates over time

**Muscular system**  consists of muscles, fasciae, tendon sheaths, and bursae

**Muscularis mucosa**  a third layer of the tunica mucosa of the small intestine

**Musculi pectinati**  muscles that give the auricles their rough appearance

**Mutation**  a mistake in the copying of genetic material

**Myalgia**  muscle pain

**Myasthenia gravis**  condition characterized by the easy tiring of muscles  or muscle weakness

**Myelin sheath**  a fatty sheath surrounding some axons

**Myeloid tissue**  red bone marrow; produce blood cells by hematopoiesis

**Myocardial infarction**  heart attack

**Myocarditis**  inflammation of the myocardium that can cause a heart attack

**Myocardium**  second layer of the wall of the heart

**Myometrium**  middle layer of wall of the uterus

**Myopia**  nearsightedness

**Myosin**  thick filaments of protein in a muscle cell

**Myositis**  inflammation of muscle tissue

**Myxedema**  accumulation of fluid in subcutaneous tissues

## N

**Nail bed**  area from which the nail grows

**Nail body**  visible part of the nail

**Nail root**  the part of the nail body attached to the nail bed

**Nasal bones**  thin, delicate bones that join to form the bridge of the nose

**Nasal cavities**  cavities of the nose

**Nasal septum**  divides the nose into right and left nasal cavities

**Nasopharynx**  uppermost portion of the pharynx located in the nose

**Navicular**  one of the bones of the wrist; also called the scaphoid bone

**Neck**  the part of a bone that connects the head or terminal enlargement to the rest of a long bone

**Negative feedback loop**  mechanism by which hormonal systems function

**Nephrons**  functional units of the kidney

**Nerve**  bundle of nerve cells or fibers

**Nervous system** consists of the brain, spinal cord, cranial nerves, peripheral nerves, and the sensory and motor structures of the body

**Nervous tissue** a type of tissue that transmits impulses

**Neuroglia** cells that perform support and protection

**Neuron** nerve cell

**Neutron** part of the central nucleus that makes up an atom; carries no charge

**Neutrophils** most common leukocytes; they secrete lysozyme

**Nicotinamide adenine dinucleotide (NAD)** an electron carrier

**Nipple** the terminal point of the mammary glands

**Nissl bodies** ribosomes attached to the rough ER in a neuron; also called chromatophilic substance

**Nodes of Ranvier** gaps in the myelin sheath; also called neurofibral nodes

**Nonpolar** compounds with unpolarized bonds

**Norepinephrine** hormone produced by the adrenal medulla

**Nostrils** openings on the undersurface of the external nose; also called external nares

**Nuclear membrane** double-layered membrane that surrounds the nucleus

**Nucleic acid** the genetic material of a cell, either DNA or RNA

**Nucleolus** a spherical particle within the nucleoplasm that does not have a covering membrane around it

**Nucleoplasm** that protoplasm inside the nucleus of a cell

**Nucleotides** complex molecules made up of a sugar, a phosphate, and a nitrogen base; the building blocks of nucleic acids

**Nucleus** a mass of nerve cell bodies and dendrites inside the central nervous system

## O

**Obturator foramen** a large opening in the hip bone for passage of nerves, blood vessels, and ligaments

**Occipital bone** a single bone that forms the back and base of the cranium

**Occipital condyle** a process for articulation with the first cervical vertebra

**Occipital lobe** functions in receiving and interpreting visual input

**Occipitalis** muscle that draws the scalp backward

**Oculomotor nerve III** controls movements of the eyeball and upper eyelid and conveys impulses related to muscle sense

**Olecranon process** a projection of the ulna known as the funny bone

**Olfactory nerve I** conveys impulses related to smell

**Olfactory sense** sense of smell

**Olfactory stimuli** odors

**Oligodendroglia** provide support by forming semi-rigid connective-like tissue rows between neurons in the brain and spinal cord

**Oocyte** immature egg

**Oogenesis** formation of the female sex cells

**Oogonia** female stem cells in a developing female fetus

**Ootid** mature egg cell

**Opponens pollicis** muscle that flexes and opposes the thumb

**Opposition** movement that occurs only with the thumb

**Optic chiasma** part of the diencephalon where optic nerves cross each other

**Optic disk** where nerve fibers leave the eye as the optic nerve

**Optic nerve II** conveys impulses related to sight

**Optic tracts** part of the diencephalon involved with the sense of sight

**Orbicularis oris** muscle that closes the lips

**Orbital margin** a definite ridge above each orbit

**Orbitals** the paths that electrons travel in an energy level

**Organelles** the building blocks of structures within the protoplasm

**Origin** the more fixed attachment of a muscle that serves as a basis for the action

**Oropharynx** second portion of the pharynx located at the back of the mouth

**Osmosis** kind of diffusion that pertains only to the movement of water molecules through a semipermeable membrane

**Ossification** formation of bone by osteoblasts

**Osteoarthritis** degenerative joint disease

**Osteoblasts** cells involved in the formation of bony tissue

**Osteoclasts** bone cells present in almost all cavities of bone responsible for reabsorbing bone during remodeling

**Osteocytes**  bone cells

**Osteomalacia**  softening of bone

**Osteon**  Haversian canal

**Osteoporosis**  disorder of the skeletal system characterized by a decrease in bone mass with accompanying susceptibility to fractures

**Osteoprogenitor cell**  undifferentiated bone cells

**Otitis media**  middle ear infection

**Ova**  female eggs

**Oval window**  one of the two openings in the middle ear

**Ovarian cycle**  the cycle beginning at puberty that produces eggs

**Ovarian follicles**  ova and their surrounding tissues in various stages of development

**Ovaries**  primary sex organs of the female reproductive system

**Ovulation**  ejection of a mature egg

**Oxaloacetic acid**  an intermediate product of the citric acid cycle

**Oxygen**  gaseous element required by all organisms that breathe air

**Oxyphil cells**  secreting cells of the parathyroid glands; also called chief cells

**Oxytocin (OT)**  stimulates contraction of smooth muscles in the wall of the uterus

**P**

**Paget's disease**  common disease of bone with symptoms that include irregular thickening and softening of the bones

**Palatine bones**  form the posterior part of the roof of the mouth or part of the hard palate

**Palatine tonsils**  tonsils commonly removed in a tonsillectomy

**Pancreas**  a large digestive gland of the alimentary canal

**Pancreatic islets**  islets of Langerhans; endocrine portion of the pancreas

**Pancreatic juice**  a mixture of digestive enzymes in the pancreas

**Papillae**  projections of the lamina propria covered with epithelium; produces the rough surface of the tongue

**Papillary ducts**  ducts that empty urine into the renal pelvis

**Papillary muscles**  small conical projections on the inner surface of the ventricles

**Papillary portion**  the layer of the dermis that is adjacent to the epidermis

**Parasympathetic division**  part of the autonomic nervous system that operates under normal non-stressful conditions

**Parathyroid hormone (PTH)**  parathormone; the hormone of the parathyroid glands

**Parenchyma**  composed of the cortex and the renal pyramids

**Parietal**  refers to the walls of a cavity

**Parietal bones**  form the upper sides and roof of the cranium

**Parietal cells**  secrete hydrochloric acid

**Parietal lobe**  control center in the brain for evaluating sensory information of touch, pain, balance, taste, and temperature

**Parietal pleura**  outer layer of the pleural membrane

**Parkinson's disease**  a nervous disorder characterized by tremors of the hand and a shuffling walk

**Parotid gland**  one of the salivary glands

**Partial pressure**  the amount of pressure that gas contributes to the total pressure

**Partial-thickness burns**  first- and second-degree burns

**Parturition**  childbirth

**Passive immunity**  occurs naturally when a fetus receives its mother's antibodies through the placenta

**Patella**  kneecap

**Pathogens**  disease-causing microorganisms

**Pathology**  the study of diseases of the body

**Pectoralis major**  muscle that flexes and adducts the arm

**Pectoralis minor**  muscle that depresses the shoulder and rotates scapula downward

**Pelvic girdle**  formed by the two hip bones

**Pelvic inflammatory disease**  bacterial infection of the uterus, uterine tubes, and/or ovaries

**Penis**  the male reproductive organ used to deliver spermatozoa into the female reproductive tract

**Pepsin**  enzyme that begins to break down proteins

**Pepsinogen**  principal gastric enzyme

**Peptide bonds**  covalent bonds that form between different amino acids to form proteins

**Pericardial cavity**  space between the epicardium of the heart and the inner layer of the pericardial sac

**Pericardial fluid**  fluid in the pericardial cavity

**Pericardial sac**   membrane covering the heart
**Pericarditis**   inflammation of the pericardium
**Pericardium**   membrane covering the heart
**Perimetrium**   outermost layer of wall of the uterus
**Perimysium**   layer of connective tissue surrounding the fascicle
**Perineum**   diamond-shaped area at the inferior end of the trunk between the buttocks and thighs of both males and females
**Periodic table**   table that arranges the elements in such a way that similar properties repeat at periodic intervals
**Periodontal ligament**   anchors the root of a tooth in its socket
**Periosteum**   fibrovascular membrane that covers a bone
**Peripheral nervous system (PNS)**   consists of all the nerves that connect the brain and spinal cord with sensory receptors, muscles, and glands
**Peristalsis**   the physical movement or pushing of food along the digestive tract
**Peritoneum**   membrane lining the abdominal cavity
**Peritubular capillaries**   surround the convoluted tubules of a nephron
**Peroneal vein**   drains the calf and foot
**Peroneus longus**   everts, plantar flexes foot
**Peroneus tertius**   dorsally flexes foot
**Petrous part**   part of the temporal bone found deep within the base of the skull where it protects and surrounds the inner ear
**Peyer's patches**   aggregated lymphatic follicles found in the wall of the small intestine
**pH**   the negative logarithm of the hydrogen ion concentration in a solution
**Phagocytic**   describing the process by which a cell eats debris and microorganisms
**Phagocytosis**   the process in which phagocytes eat cellular debris and other substances
**Phalanges**   the bones of the fingers and toes
**Phalanx**   a single bone of a finger or toe
**Pharyngeal tonsils**   adenoids
**Pharynx**   part of the digestive tract (throat) involved in swallowing
**Phimosis**   condition where the foreskin of the penis fits too tightly over the head of the penis and cannot be retracted
**Phosphocreatine**   found in muscle tissue; provides a rapid source of high-energy ATP for muscle contraction

**Phosphoglyceraldehyde (PGAL)**   an intermediate product of glycolysis
**Phosphoglyceric acid (PGA)**   an intermediate product of glycolysis
**Phosphorylation**   process by which a phosphate is added to a molecule
**Phrenic arteries**   supply blood to the diaphragm muscle
**Physiology**   the study of the functions of the body parts
**Pia mater**   the innermost spinal meninx
**Pineal gland/body**   an endocrine gland located in the epithalamus of the diencephalon that produces the hormone melatonin
**Pisiform**   a bone of the wrist
**Pituitary gland**   hypophysis; the master gland of the endocrine system
**Pivot joint**   a type of synovial joint, like the joint between the atlas and axis vertebrae
**Placenta**   a structure in the uterus through which the fetus exchanges nutrients and wastes with the mother
**Plantar flexion**   pushing the foot down at the ankle joint
**Plantaris**   plantar-flexes foot
**Plaque**   cholesterol-containing masses
**Plasma cells**   B lymphocyte cells that enter tissues and become specialized cells
**Plasma membrane**   membrane surrounding cells
**Plasmalemma**   membrane surrounding cells; also called the plasma membrane
**Pleura**   membrane that lines the thoracic cavity
**Pleural cavity**   small space between the pleural membranes
**Pleural membrane**   membrane that encloses and protects the lung
**Pleurisy**   inflammation of the pleural cavity; also called pleuritis
**Plicae**   folds in the small intestine
**Pneumonia**   pneumonitis; an infection in the lungs
**Podocytes**   epithelial cells in the innermost layer of the Bowman's glomerular capsule
**Polar**   a molecule with an unequal distribution of bonding electrons
**Polar body**   non-functional cell produced in oogenesis
**Polydipsia**   excessive thirst
**Polyphagia**   intense food cravings
**Polyurea**   increase in urine production

**Pons varolii**   bridge that connects the spinal cord with the brain and parts of the brain with each other

**Popliteal artery**   the name of the femoral artery at the knee

**Popliteal vein**   the name of the posterior tibial vein at the knee

**Popliteus**   flexes and rotates leg

**Posterior**   toward the back

**Posterior gray horn**   part of the spinal cord; also known as dorsal gray horn

**Posterior interventricular sulcus**   separates the left and right ventricles

**Posterior root**   the sensory root containing only sensory nerve fibers; also known as dorsal root

**Premenstrual syndrome (PMS)**   series of symptoms that develop in many women during the premenstrual phase of the menstrual cycle

**Premolars**   teeth with two projections or cusps; bicuspid teeth

**Prepuce**   foreskin; a section of loose skin covering the glans penis

**Presbyopia**   a decrease in the ability of the eye to accommodate for near vision

**Primary fibrositis**   inflammation of the fibrous connective tissue in a joint

**Primary oocytes**   produced by mitotic division of female stem cells or oogonia

**Primary spermatocytes**   produced by mitotic division of immature sperm cells or spermatogonia

**Primary structure**   protein structure based on amino acid sequence

**Process**   any obvious bone projection

**Progesterone**   female sex hormone

**Prokaryotic**   refers to cells that do not have membrane-bound organelles, such as bacteria

**Pronation**   moving the bones of the forearm so that the radius and ulna are not parallel

**Pronator quadratus**   muscle involved in pronating the forearm

**Pronator teres**   muscle involved in pronating the forearm

**Prophase**   the second phase of mitosis

**Prophase I**   the first stage of the first meiotic division

**Prophase II**   in each of the two daughter cells produced in the first meiotic division, the nuclear membrane disappears but no duplication of DNA occurs

**Prostate cancer**   cancer of the prostate gland that can be fatal if not detected

**Prostate gland**   secretes an alkaline fluid that is part of the semen

**Prostatic urethra**   surrounded by the prostate gland

**Protein**   covalently bonded molecule composed of carbon, hydrogen, oxygen, and nitrogen

**Protein synthesis**   process in which cells containing DNA produce proteins

**Prothrombin**   plasma protein produced by the liver that is involved in blood clotting

**Proton**   part of the central nucleus that makes up an atom; has a positive charge

**Protoplasm**   the liquid part of a cell

**Protraction**   moving a part of the body forward on a plane parallel to the ground

**Proximal**   nearest the point of attachment or origin

**Proximal convoluted tubule**   first part of the renal tubule

**Pseudostratified epithelium**   cells that have a layered appearance, but actually extend from the basement membrane to the outer free surface

**Psoas**   muscle involved in flexing the thigh

**Psoriasis**   common chronic skin disorder characterized by red patches covered with thick, dry, silvery scales

**Pterygoid**   muscles involved in raising the mandible

**Pubis**   a part of the hip bone found superior and slightly anterior to the ischium

**Pulmonary circulation**   circulatory route that goes from the heart to the lungs and back to the heart

**Pulmonary fibrosis**   black lung disease; caused by excessive exposure to asbestos, silica, or coal dust

**Pulmonary semilunar valve**   found in the opening where the pulmonary trunk exits the right ventricle

**Pulmonary trunk**   the artery that leaves the right ventricle

**Pulmonary veins**   enter the left atrium of the heart

**Pulp cavity**   a cavity in the crown of a tooth

**Pupil**   a circular opening in the iris of the eye

**Purine**   a nitrogen base consisting of a fused double ring of nine atoms of carbon and nitrogen

**Purkinje's fibers**   cause actual contractions of the ventricles; they emerge from the bundle branches

**Pyloric sphincter**   the connection between the stomach and the beginning of the duodenum

**Pylorus**   narrow inferior region of the stomach; also called the antrum

**Pyrimidine**   a nitrogen base consisting of a single ring of six atoms of carbon and nitrogen

**Pyruvic acid**   the final product of glycolysis

# Q

**Quadriceps femoris**   muscle that extends the knee

**Quaternary structure**   protein structure determined by spatial relationships between amino acids

**Quinone**   an electron carrier

# R

**Radial arteries**   supply blood to the forearm

**Radial veins**   drain blood from the forearm

**Radius**   shorter, lateral bone of the forearm

**Raphe**   external median ridge of the scrotum

**Rectum**   the last 7 to 8 inches of the gastrointestinal tract

**Rectus abdominis**   muscle that flexes the vertebral column and assists in compressing abdominal wall

**Rectus femoris**   extends leg and flexes thigh

**Red bone marrow**   found within cancellous bone; makes blood cells

**Reflex**   an involuntary reaction to an external stimulus

**Reflex arc**   the pathway which results in a reflex

**Releasing hormones**   produced by the hypothalamus, they stimulate the release of hormones from the anterior pituitary gland

**Releasing inhibitory hormones**   produced by the hypothalamus, they inhibit the release of hormones from the anterior pituitary gland

**Renal capsule**   innermost layer of tissue that surrounds the kidney

**Renal columns**   cortical substance between the renal pyramids

**Renal corpuscle**   made up of Bowman's glomerular capsule and the enclosed glomerulus

**Renal failure**   results from any condition that interferes with kidney function

**Renal fascia**   outermost layer of tissue that surrounds the kidney

**Renal papillae**   the tips of the renal pyramids

**Renal pelvis**   a large collecting funnel formed where the major calyces join

**Renal plexus**   the nerve supply to the kidneys

**Renal pyramids**   triangular structures within the medulla

**Renal sinus**   cavity in the kidney

**Renal tubule**   the general name of the tubule of a nephron

**Renin**   enzyme produced by the kidneys that helps regulate blood pressure

**Repolarization**   restoration of the original charge to the nerve cell

**Reposition**   occurs when the digits return to their normal positions

**Reproductive system**   consists of the ovaries, uterine tubes, uterus, and vagina in the female; the testes, vas deferens, seminal vesicles, prostate gland, penis, and urethra in the male

**Respiration**   the overall exchange of gases between the atmosphere, blood, and cells

**Respiratory bronchioles**   microscopic divisions of terminal bronchioles

**Respiratory distress syndrome**   condition in infants in which too little surfactant is produced, causing the lungs to collapse; also known as hyaline membrane disease

**Respiratory system**   consists of nasal cavities, pharynx, larynx, trachea, bronchi, and lungs

**Resting potential**   normal electrical distribution around a muscle cell when it is not contracting

**Rete testis**   network of ducts in the testis

**Reticular**   type of loose connective tissue that forms the framework of the liver, bone marrow, spleen, and lymph nodes

**Reticular formation**   area of dispersed gray matter in the medulla

**Reticular portion**   the layer of the dermis between the papillary portion and the subcutaneous tissue beneath

**Reticuloendothelial (RE) system**   specialized connective tissue involved in phagocytosis

**Retina**   innermost layer of the eye

**Retraction**   moving a part of the body backward on a plane parallel to the ground

**Rh blood group**   one of the blood groups

**Rheumatic fever**   disease involving a mild bacterial infection

**Rheumatic heart disease**   caused by infection with a bacterium in young children

**Rheumatoid arthritis**   connective tissue disorder resulting in severe inflammation of small joints

**Rhodopsin**   pigment found in the rod cells of the eye

**Rhomboids**   muscles involved in moving the scapula

**Ribonucleic acid (RNA)**   a type of nucleic acid

**Ribose**   a five-carbon sugar found in RNA

**Ribosomes**   tiny granules distributed throughout the cytoplasm where protein synthesis occurs

**Rickets**   disease caused by deficiencies in calcium and phosphorous or by deficiencies in vitamin D

**Right atrium**   one of the upper chambers of the heart

**Right bundle branch**   branch of the bundle of His; part of the conduction system of the heart

**Right colic (hepatic) flexure**   where the ascending colon reaches the undersurface of the liver and turns to the left

**Right common carotid artery**   transports blood to the right side of the head and neck

**Right lymphatic duct**   one of two collecting channels or ducts of the lymphatic system

**Right primary bronchus**   the first right division of the trachea

**Right pulmonary artery**   carries blood to the right lung

**Right renal artery**   transports one-quarter of the total cardiac output directly to kidneys

**Right renal vein**   carries filtered blood from the interlobar veins to the hilum

**Right subclavian artery**   transports blood to the upper right limb

**Right ventricle**   lower chamber of the heart

**Ringworm**   caused by several species of fungus; its symptoms include itchy, patchy, scale-like lesions with raised edges

**Root**   1. a projection of a tooth embedded in a socket; 2. the lowermost portion of a hair found in the hair follicle

**Root canals**   narrow extensions of the pulp cavity that project into the root

**Rotation**   moving a bone around a central axis

**Rough ER**   granular endoplamic reticulum

**Round window**   an opening on the medial side of the middle ear that connects the middle ear to the inner ear

**Rugae**   large mucosal folds of the stomach

## S

**Sacral vertebrae**   lower part of the vertebral column

**Saddle joint**   a type of synovial joint, like the carpal metacarpal joint in the thumb

**Sagittal**   any plane parallel to the midsagittal or median plane vertically dividing the body into unequal left and right portions

**Sagittal suture**   line where the two parietal bones join superiorly

**Sarcolemma**   the electrically polarized muscle cell membrane

**Sarcomas**   tumors developing from connective tissue

**Sarcomere**   the area between two adjacent Z lines

**Sarcoplasmic reticulum**   an irregular curtain around muscle fibrils

**Sarcotubular system**   membranes of vesicles and tubules that surround muscle fibrils

**Sartorius**   flexes thigh, rotates it laterally

**Saturated**   a fatty acid that contains only single covalent bonds

**Scaphoid**   one of the wrist bones; also called the navicular bone

**Scapula**   shoulder blade

**Schwann cells**   form myelin sheaths around nerve fibers in the peripheral nervous system

**Sclera**   outermost layer of the wall of the eye

**Scoliosis**   an abnormal lateral curvature of the spine

**Scrotum**   outpouching of the abdominal wall

**Sebaceous glands**   glands that secrete sebum

**Sebum**   oily substance that lubricates the skin's surface

**Second-degree burn**   a burn that involves the epidermis and dermis; may form scars

**Secondary (lobar) bronchi**   divisions of the primary bronchi

**Secondary oocyte**   produced by the first meiotic division of the primary oocyte

**Secondary spermatocyte**   produced by the first meiotic division of the primary spermatocytes

**secondary structure**   protein structure determined by hydrogen bonds between amino acids resulting in a helix or a pleated sheet

**Semen**   mixture of sperm cells and secretions of the seminal vesicles, prostate, and bulbourethral glands; also called seminal fluid

**Semimembranosus**   flexes leg, extends thigh

**Seminal plasmin**  an antibiotic in semen that can destroy certain bacteria

**Seminal vesicles**  produce an alkaline, viscous component of semen rich in fructose

**Seminiferous tubules**  tightly coiled tubules in each lobule of a testis

**Semipermeable membrane**  allows only certain materials to pass through, like water through a plasma membrane

**Semitendinosus**  flexes leg, extends thigh

**Sensory neuron**  a neuron in contact with receptors, it detects changes in the external environment; also called afferent neuron

**Septal defect**  a hole in the interatrial or interventricular septum between the left and right sides of the heart

**Septicemia**  blood poisoning

**Serosa**  the outermost layer of the wall of the alimentary canal

**Serotonin**  hormone secreted by the pineal gland that acts as a neurotransmitter and vasoconstrictor

**Serous pericardium**  innermost layer of the pericardial sac

**Serous tissue**  lines the great cavities of the body that have no opening to the outside; also called mesothelium

**Serratus anterior**  muscle that moves scapula forward

**Sertoli cells**  produce secretions that supply nutrients for the developing sperm cells

**Sesamoid**  bones enclosed in a tendon and fascial tissue, located adjacent to joints

**Shaft**  1. visible portion of the hair; 2. that part of the penis behind the head

**Shingles**  painful, vesicular skin eruptions caused by the herpes zoster or chickenpox virus

**Sickle-cell anemia**  hereditary disease found mostly in African-Americans

**Sigmoid colon**  last part of the colon

**Simple epithelium**  one cell-layer thick

**Simple exocrine glands**  glands with ducts that do not branch

**Sinoatrial (SA) node**  initiates each cardiac cycle and sets the pace for the heart rate; also called pacemaker

**Sinus**  a cavity within a bone

**Skeletal muscle**  muscle attached to bone

**Skeletal system**  composed of bones, cartilage, and the membranous structures associated with bones

**Small intestine**  place where absorption and digestion occurs

**Smooth ER**  agranular endoplasmic reticulum

**Smooth muscle**  found in hollow structures of the body like the intestines; cannot be influenced at will

**Smooth muscle tissue**  spindle-shaped cells with a single nucleus and no striations

**Soft palate**  posterior portion of the roof of the mouth

**Soleus**  plantar-flexes foot

**Solute**  substance that is dissolved in a solution

**Solvent**  a medium allowing other reactions to occur

**Somatic nervous system**  conducts impulses from the brain and spinal cord to skeletal muscle, causing us to respond or react to changes in our external environment

**Spermatic cord**  connective tissue sheath enclosing the vas deferens

**Spermatids**  secondary spermatocytes that undergo the second meiotic division

**Spermatogenesis**  production of sperm

**Spermatogonia**  immature sperm cells

**Spermatozoa**  mature sperm cells

**Sphenoid bone**  forms anterior portion of the base of the cranium

**Spina bifida**  congenital defect in the development of the posterior vertebral arch in which the laminae do not unite at the midline

**Spinal cavity**  cavity containing the spinal cord

**Spinal meninges**  a series of connective tissue membranes specifically associated with the spinal cord

**Spindle fibers**  group of microtubules formed by the centrioles to guide the daughter chromatids to opposite poles

**Spine**  any sharp, slender projection such as the spinous process of the vertebrae

**Spleen**  the largest single mass of lymphatic tissue

**Splenic artery**  supplies blood to the spleen

**Spongy (cavernous) urethra**  located within the penis; about six inches long

**Squamous cell carcinoma**  skin cancer in the epidermis

**Squamous epithelium**  epithelial cells that are flat and slightly irregular in shape and serve as a protective layer

**Squamous portion**  largest part of the temporal bone

**Stapes**  ear bone referred to as the stirrup

**Stem cells**  undifferentiated mesenchymal cells that develop into blood cells; also known as hematocytoblasts

**Stenosis**  a narrowed opening through the heart valves

**Sternocleidomastoid**  main muscle that moves the head

**Sternum**  the breast bone

**Straight tubules**  located at the tip of each lobule of a testis

**Strata (stratum)**  layers

**Stratified epithelium**  several layers of cells thick

**Stratum basale**  the lowermost or basal layer of the stratum germinativum

**Stratum corneum**  outermost layer of epidermis, consisting of dead cells

**Stratum germinativum**  regenerative layer of epidermis, lowermost layer

**Stratum granulosum**  a layer of epidermis made of flattened cells containing granules

**Stratum lucidum**  clear layer of epidermis

**Stratum spinosum**  spiny or prickly layer of epidermis

**Striated muscle**  tissue that causes movement; multi-nucleated with striations; skeletal muscle

**Subclavian trunk**  drains lymph from the upper extremities

**Subclavian vein**  drains blood from the arm

**Subcutaneous bursae**  found under the skin

**Subfascial bursae**  located between muscles

**Sublingual gland**  one of the three salivary glands

**Submandibular gland**  one of the three salivary glands

**Submaxillary gland**  one of the three salivary glands

**Submucosa**  layer of connective tissue beneath a mucous membrane

**Subtendinous bursae**  found where one tendon overlies another tendon

**Succinic acid**  an intermediate product of the citric acid cycle

**Sulcus**  a furrow or groove

**Superior**  uppermost or above

**Superior meatus**  one of three narrow passageways in the nasal cavity formed by the turbinate bones; known as the olfactory region of the nose

**Superior mesenteric artery**  supplies blood to the small intestine and colon

**Superior oblique**  muscle that rotates the eyeball on axis

**Superior rectus**  muscle that rolls the eyeball upward

**Superior vena cava**  brings blood from the upper parts of the body

**Supination**  moving the bones of the forearm so that the radius and ulna are parallel

**Supinator**  muscle that supinates the forearm

**Suppressor T cells**  slow down the activities of B and T cells once infection is controlled

**Supraorbital ridge**  overlies the frontal sinus and can be felt in the middle of the forehead

**Supraspinatus**  muscle that abducts the arm

**Surfactant**  fluid inside the respiratory membrane

**Suture**  articulation in which the bones are united by a thin layer of fibrous tissue

**Sweat glands**  simple tubular glands found in most parts of the body that secrete sweat

**Sympathetic division**  part of the autonomic nervous system that prepares the body for stressful situations that require energy expenditure

**Symphysis**  joints in which the bones are connected by a disc of fibrocartilage

**Synapses**  areas where the terminal brances of an axon are anchored close to, but not touching, the ends of the dendrites of another neuron

**Synapsis**  the lining up of homologous chromosomes in meiosis

**Synarthroses**  joints between bones that do not allow movement

**Synchondrosis**  joint in which two bony surfaces are connected by hyaline cartilage

**Syndesmosis**  joint in which bones are connected by ligaments between the bones

**Syneresis**  clot retraction

**Synergists**  muscles that assist the prime movers

**Synovial membranes**  line the cavities of freely moving joints; produce synovial fluid

**Syphilis**  a venereal disease caused by a bacterial infection

**Systemic circulation**  blood circulation to the body not including the lungs

**Systole**  phase of contraction

## T

**T lymphocytes** T cells; responsible for providing cellular immunity

**T system** tubules; part of the sarcotubular system

**Tail** terminal portion of the pancreas

**Talus** ankle bone

**Tarsal bones** bones of the ankle

**Taste buds** sensory structures that detect taste stimuli

**Taste cells** interior of the taste bud

**Telophase** final stage of mitosis

**Telophase I** stage in meiosis in which the homologous chromosome pairs have separated with a member of each pair at opposite ends of the spindle

**Telophase II** stage in meiosis that produces four haploid daughter cells, each containing one half of the genetic material of the original parent cell

**Temporal bones** form the lower sides and base of cranium

**Temporal lobe** part of the cerebral hemisphere that evaluates hearing input and smell

**Temporalis** muscle that raises the mandible and closes the mouth

**Tendinitis** inflammation of a tendon

**Tendon** dense connective tissue that attaches muscle to bone

**Tensor fascia lata** muscle that tenses fascia lata

**Teres minor** muscle that adducts and rotates the arm

**Terminal bronchioles** divisions or branches of bronchioles

**Tertiary (segmental) bronchi** divisions of secondary bronchi

**Tertiary structure** protein structure with a secondary folding

**Testes** primary sex organs of the male reproductive system that produce sperm and male sex hormones

**Testis** singular form of testes

**Testosterone** the principle male sex hormone

**Tetanus** infection caused by a bacterium that produces a neurotoxin affecting motor neurons

**Tetrad** the figure formed by the lining up of homologous chromosomes consisting of four chromatids

**Thalamus** the second part of the diencephalon

**Thalassemia** hereditary disease found in African, Mediterranean, and Asian individuals that suppresses hemoglobin production

**Third-degree burn** a burn in which the epidermis and dermis are completely destroyed; also called full-thickness burns

**Thoracic aorta** the name given to the aorta in the thorax

**Thoracic cavity** first subdivision of the ventral cavity that is surrounded by the rib cage and contains the heart

**Thoracic duct** main collecting duct of the lymphatic system

**Thoracic vertebrae** twelve vertebrae that connect with the ribs

**Thrombin** an enzyme formed from prothrombin that is necessary for the clotting mechanism

**Thrombocytes** platelets; blood cells involved in blood clotting

**Thromboplastin** a substance released from blood platelets that is involved in the clotting reaction

**Thrombosis** clotting in an unbroken blood vessel

**Thrombus** a blood clot

**Thylakoid** individual double membranes that make up a granum in a chloroplast

**Thymine** a pyrimidine nitrogen base

**Thymosin** hormone secreted by the thymus gland that causes the production of T lymphocytes

**Thymus gland** an endocrine gland located beneath the sternum that is also involved in immunity as a site for lymphocyte production and maturation

**Thyroid cartilage** Adam's apple

**Thyroid gland** an endocrine gland located along the trachea

**Thyroid-stimulating hormone (TSH)** stimulates the thyroid gland to produce its hormone

**Thyroxine** a hormone of the thyroid gland that regulates the metabolism of carbohydrates, fats, and proteins

**Tibia** larger of the two bones forming the lower leg

**Tibialis anterior** dorsally flexes foot

**Tibialis posterior** plantar flexes foot

**Tissue** groups of cells similar in size, shape, and function

**Tone** a property of muscle whereby a steady or constant state of partial contraction is maintained in a muscle

**Tongue** skeletal muscle covered with epithelium that manipulates food and forms the floor of the oral cavity

**Trabeculae** fibrous connective tissue; extension of the capsule of a lymph node

**Trabeculae carneae** irregular ridges and folds of the myocardium of the ventricles

**Trachea** windpipe

**Tract** a bundle of fibers inside the central nervous system

**Transcription** process by which messenger RNA copies the genetic code in a DNA molecule

**Transfer RNA** a type of RNA that translates the code of a DNA molecule that was copied by messenger RNA

**Transitional epithelium** several layers of closely packed, flexible, easily stretched cells; appear flat when stretched and saw-toothed when relaxed

**Translation** process by which transfer RNA reads the code on messenger RNA and gets the amino acids to make a protein

**Transverse** plane dividing the body into superior and inferior portions

**Transverse colon** the second part of the colon found under the liver

**Transversus abdominis** muscle that compresses abdominal contents

**Trapezium** a bone of the wrist, also called the greater multi-angular

**Trapezius** muscle that draws the head to one side and rotates scapula

**Triacylglycerols** types of fats found in the human body

**Triceps brachii** muscle that extends and adducts the forearm

**Trichomonas** a flagellated protozoan infection that causes inflammation of vaginal tissue with an odorous yellow-green discharge

**Tricuspid** the third layer of the wall of the alimentary canal

**Tricuspid valve** valve between the right atrium and right ventricle

**Trigeminal nerve V** largest of the cranial nerves; controls chewing movements

**Trigone** a triangular region of the bladder formed by the two openings from the ureters and the single urethral opening

**Triiodothyronine** a hormone of the thyroid gland that regulates the metabolism of carbohydrates, fats, and proteins

**Triquetral** a bone of the wrist

**Trochanter** very large projection

**Trochlea** process shaped like a pulley

**Trochlear nerve IV** controls movement of the eyeball and conveys impulses related to muscle sense

**Tropomyosin** an inhibitor substance found in muscle cells

**Troponin** an inhibitor substance found in muscle cells

**Tubercle** small round process

**Tubulin** protein fibers that make up the spindle during cell division

**Tumor** abnormal and uncontrolled growth of a cell

**Tunica adventitia** the outermost wall of an artery or vein

**Tunica albuginea** a layer of white, fibrous, connective tissue that covers each testis

**Tunica intima** the innermost layers of the wall of an artery or vein

**Tunica media** the middle layer of the wall of an artery or vein

**Tunica mucosa** innermost lining of the alimentary canal

**Tunica muscularis** the third layer of the wall of the alimentary canal

**Tunica serosa** the fourth or outermost layer of the wall of the alimentary canal

**Tunica submucosa** the second layer of the wall of the alimentary canal

**Turbinates** thin, fragile bones found on the lateral sides of the nostrils

**Tympanic membrane** eardrum

**Tympanic plate** forms the floor and anterior wall of the external auditory meatus

## U

**Ulna** longer, medial bone of the forearm

**Ulnar arteries** supply blood to the forearm

**Ulnar veins** drain blood from the forearm

**Umbilical cord** a connecting stalk of tissue that connects the developing fetus to the placenta

**Unipolar neurons** neurons that have only one process extending from the cell body; most sensory neurons are unipolar

**Unsaturated** a fatty acid that contains one or more double covalent bonds between the carbon atoms

**Ureters** transport urine from the renal pelvis into the urinary bladder

**Urethra** the tube that leads from the bladder to the outside

**Urethral orifice** the terminal opening of the urethra

**Urinary bladder** hollow muscular organ located in the pelvic cavity posterior to the pubic symphysis

**Urinary system** consists of two kidneys, two ureters, urinary bladder, and urethra

**Urine** the eliminated materials from the filtered blood

**Uterine cavity** interior of the body of the uterus

**Uterine tubes** transport ova from the ovaries to the uterus; also called fallopian tubes

**Uterus** womb

**Uvula** a conical projection hanging from the posterior border of the soft palate; functions in the swallowing process and prevents food from backing up into the nasal area

## V

**Vacuole** an area within the cytoplasm that is surrounded by a vacuolar membrane

**Vagina** the opening into the female reproductive system that leads to the uterus

**Vaginal orifice** the opening into the vagina

**Vagus nerve X** controls skeletal muscle movements in the pharynx, larynx, and palate

**Vas deferens** ductus deferens

**Vascular (venous) sinuses** veins with thin walls

**Vasectomy** an operation for birth control that severs the vas deferens preventing sperm from reaching the exterior

**Vastus intermedius** extends leg and flexes thigh

**Vastus lateralis** extends leg and flexes thigh

**Vastus medialis** extends leg and flexes thigh

**Veins** blood vessels that carry blood to the heart

**Ventilation** breathing; movement of air between the atmosphere and lungs

**Ventral** the belly side

**Ventral cerebral peduncles** convey impulses from the cerebral cortex to the pons and spinal cord

**Ventricles** cavities within the brain that connect with each other

**Venules** small vessels that connect capillaries to veins

**Vermiform appendix** twisted tube attached to the closed end of the cecum

**Vertebral artery** supplies blood to part of the brain

**Vertebral vein** drains the back of the head

**Vestibular folds** upper folds in the mucous membrane of the larynx; also called false vocal cords

**Vestibule** 1. opening between the labia minora; 2. anterior portion of the nasal cavities just inside the nostrils

**Vestibulocochlear nerve** transmits impulses related to equilibrium and hearing

**Villi** projections of the mucosal coat of the small intestine that increase absorptive surface area

**Visceral** refers to the covering of an organ

**Visceral peritoneum** another name for the tunica serosa

**Visceral pleura** covers the lungs

**Vitiligo** skin disease resulting in irregular patches of skin of various sizes completely lacking any pigmentation

**Vitreous humor** fluid that fills the posterior compartment of the eye behind the lens

**Vocal folds** lower folds in the mucous membrane of the larynx; also called true vocal cords

**Volkmann's canals** canals that run horizontally to the Haversian canals

**Vomer bone** flat bone that makes up the lower posterior portion of the nasal septum

**Vulva** external genitalia of the female; also called the pudendum

## W

**Warts** uncontrolled growth of epidermal tissue caused by human papilloma virus

**Water** the most abundant substance in living cells

**White matter** groups of myelinated axons from many neurons supported by neuroglia

**Whooping cough** respiratory disorder caused by a bacterial infection resulting in severe coughing; also called pertussis

**Wormian bones** located within the sutures of the cranial bones

## X

**Xanthophyll** a carotenoid pigment in plant cells that produces a yellow color

**Xiphoid process** the terminal portion of the sternum

## Y

**Yellow bone marrow** connective tissue consisting of fat cells

## Z

**Z line** narrow, dark-staining band found in the central region of the I band

**Zygomatic bones** form the prominence of the cheek

**Zygomaticus** muscle that draws the lip upward and outward

**Zygote** fertilized egg

**Zymogenic cells** found in the stomach, they secrete the principal gastric enzyme